"The COVID-19 pandemic and the uncertainty it generated across the world provide myriad opportunities to explore the ethical dilemmas faced and decisions made as a result of those challenges. Through multiple lenses—healthcare, education, language, technology, leadership, law—the contributors to this book provide thoughtful analysis of pandemic responses and consideration of the short and long-term effects and ethical implications of decisions made."
*Ruthanne K. Orihuela, Provost and Vice President for Academic Affairs, Community College of Denver, USA*

"For a multi-dimensional ethical assessment of the handling of the COVID-19 pandemic, these volumes will prove an essential, perhaps indispensable, but certainly highly instructive source."
*Claus Dierksmeier, Professor for Globalization Ethics at the University of Tübingen, Germany*

"The COVID-19 pandemic has left the planet now polarized in terms of how to respond to infectious diseases pandemics and with a diminishing trust in public health. The pandemic required nuance and a willingness to look at the risks and benefits of each intervention, but much of that nuance was lost. This book is the definitive resource to bring back nuance to our approach to infectious diseases, through an exploration of ethics, messaging, school closures, the impact of the pandemic on health care workers, global equity, and empathy. This book, written by a variety of experts in the field, has enormous potential to heal our divisiveness around COVID and formulate a roadmap for the next pandemic, and I provide it with my highest endorsement."
*Monica Gandhi, MD, Professor of Medicine/Infectious Diseases and Director of the UCSF Center for AIDS Research, University of California San Francisco, USA*

"All too often, in times of crisis, ethics are thrown out the window as people strive to deal quickly with the pressures of coping with the emergency. This was all too true during the global pandemic. This book highlights the myriad ethical dilemmas it caused, and suggests ways to keep focused on doing the right things for the right reasons."
*Ronald E. Riggio, Ph.D., Professor of Leadership and Organizational Psychology, Kravis Leadership Institute, Claremont McKenna College, Claremont, California, USA*

"The COVID 19 pandemic highlighted a myriad of ethical challenges in our public and professional lives, such as the tension between individual rights and collective well-being, the proper role of science and government in society, the appropriate uses of biotechnology, and the disproportionate challenges faced by different groups, among others. But the fundamental issues here are not new; the pandemic merely

## Praise for **The COVID-19 Pandemic: Ethical Challenges and Considerations** and **Ethical Implications of COVID-19 Management: Evaluating the Aftershock**

"The COVID-19 pandemic challenged more than our healthcare system, our community, our supply chains - it challenged the very foundation of the way medical research is conducted, interpreted, and presented to the public. This book highlights the key ethical challenges of the COVID era, from issues of equity in the workplace, to the dissemination of disinformation, to the challenges of vaccine distribution. If we do not learn from the COVID-19 pandemic, we are easy prey for the next virus that will emerge. Think of this book as not only a summation of lessons learned, but as preparation for the future."
*F. Perry Wilson, MD MSCE, Associate Professor of Medicine at Yale University, USA, and Author of "How Medicine Works and When it Doesn't"*

"One may say that the pandemic has been like a giant Trolley Problem for a global audience. The collection offers a unique space where several authors take up the question whether deontic, consequentialist, or utility ethics best serve action. Other authors mention Gilligan's 'ethics of care', which, for this reader at least, seems like something we could do with a lot more of. In the event, public action was largely driven by politics and the kind of moral intuition that chooses quantity of good over principle – as is illustrated in several chapters. The editors are to be congratulated and thanked for bringing together these timely and valuable essays. They would make salutary reading for the politicians who claim that the pandemic is over when it manifestly is not; that vaccines are a panacea, despite continuing excess deaths and disease; that international initiatives can be wound down because, as one UK politician says, the pandemic is a once-in-a-hundred-years event."
*Richard Temperley-Little, Professor of Sustainability Leadership IFLAS, University of Cumbria, UK*

"The COVID-19 pandemic had a devastating effect on the education of our children. While school leadership was grappling with making hard decisions to keep communities safe, parents were struggling with changing work and family dynamics. Constant bombardment from social media caused fear and confusion that disrupted the relationship between parents and school leadership. This book provides a balanced approach to understand the effects of the pandemic on our children and communities, creating a starting point for developing a plan to mitigate the social, physical, mental, and instructional effects of the pandemic."
*Lynette M. Bryan, Ph.D., Broome-Tioga Board of Cooperative Educational Services (BOCES), Binghamton, New York, USA*

forced us to confront them. This book is a much-needed exploration of these issues as we look for a 'new normal' in the post-COVID era, and it will help readers understand and negotiate these ethical dilemmas in a more thoughtful and productive way."
*Todd Weaver, Dean, College of Business & Leadership, Point University, Georgia, USA.*

"The COVID-19 pandemic of 2019-22 exposed weaknesses in our society's ability to respond to a pandemic threat. This was true not only in terms of public health interventions, but also challenges to our national and global economy, security, and social fabric. These new and important volumes address the ethical dilemmas arising with the many and complex dimensions affected by a serious virus threat."
*Peter Hotez, Dean, National School of Tropical Medicine and Professor, Departments of Pediatrics, Molecular Virology & Microbiology, Baylor College of Medicine, Houston, Texas, USA*

"These two texts provide a comprehensive and timely account of the many different ethical dilemmas posed by the COVID-19 pandemic. Ranging from a consideration of the long-term effects of on-line schooling for children to the ways in which the pandemic revealed the ugly realities of racial disparities across the globe, these texts are an invaluable resource for anyone wanting to pursue the moral questions raised by the pandemic. Additionally, they reveal the ethical choices faced by governments, businesses, health care providers as well as individual community members both during, and in the aftermath of the novel corona virus."
*Donna Ladkin, PhD, Professor of Inclusive Leadership, University of Birmingham, UK*

"These two COVID-19 volumes offer a groundbreaking look at the many ethical dilemmas associated with our current pandemic, and with important implications for those future pandemics that will inevitably follow this one. The editors of this collection, Eleftheria Egel and Cheryl Patton, have done a remarkable job, and provided a great service, by curating these diverse writings by scholars from around the world. In so doing, the collection provides a thought-provoking, deep dive into varied ethical considerations associated with this global challenge to human health and societal well-being."
*Larry C. Spears, School of Leadership Studies, Gonzaga University, Spokane, USA*

"The fallout from COVID-19 has had a wide-ranging impact on diverse social institutions and populations in developing and industrial nations. In many instances, we are still grappling with what its effects will mean for our shared future. This innovative collection provides thoughtful and useful pathways through the myriad ethical issues we face. It raises important questions and proposes valuable solutions while engaging and challenging readers with how best to move forward at this critical historical juncture. Its range is as expansive as the

problems we face. It is essential reading for those who want to navigate through the implications of the pandemic in a more ethical, deliberate, and thoughtful way."
*Valerie Palmer-Mehta, Ph.D., Professor of Communication & Communication Internship, and Director, Dept. of Communication, Journalism, & PR, Oakland University, California, USA*

"The COVID-19 pandemic has presented enormous ethical and moral challenges. In this collection the authors present their perspectives on these challenges. A very thought-provoking and timely work for our time."
*Kathryn M. Edwards M.D., Sarah H. Sell and Cornelius Vanderbilt Chair Professor of Pediatrics, Vanderbilt University Medical Center, Nashville, Tennessee, USA.*

# The COVID-19 Pandemic

*Ethical Challenges and Considerations*

Edited by

**Eleftheria Egel and Cheryl Patton**

The COVID-19 Pandemic: Ethical Challenges and Considerations

Edited by: Eleftheria Egel and Cheryl Patton

This book first published 2022

Ethics International Press Ltd, UK

British Library Cataloguing in Publication Data

A catalogue record for this book is available from the British Library



Print Book ISBN: 978-1-871891-79-9

eBook ISBN: 978-1-871891-80-5

# TABLE OF CONTENTS

## PART THREE
### LIVED EXPERIENCES



## PART FOUR
### HEALTHCARE PERSONNEL: FIGHTING IN THE FRONTLINE



## PART FIVE
### HEALTHCARE MANAGEMENT

# INTRODUCTION

On March 11, 2020, WHO declared the COVID-19 pandemic (WHO, 2020a). According to its data, the figure of people dying of or with COVID-19 rose from 171 on 30 January 2020 to 1,813,188 by 31 December 2020 (WHO, 2020b). This number very soon led to lockdowns, school closures, social distancing, travel restrictions, and mandatory masking for half of the world population with devastating consequences for the economic, physical, social, and psychological wellbeing of human beings and collectives. Since the beginning, there is a constant debate going on whether this was "the right thing" to do or if there is "one right thing" to do and how to determine it.

This book is the outcome of a year's effort. When we embarked on this project, our intention was to offer an expanded perspective of what happened by looking into the phenomenon of COVID-19 and its management through the lens of ethics. It was a fervent scientific and personal desire of both of us to understand what is really happening as we were overwhelmed by experiencing division among family members and friends' circles; by being denied access to previously non-negotiable common goods; by witnessing the exhaustion of frontline healthcare workers; by helplessly watching our elderly dying alone in long-term care facilities; by observing our children suffering as they were deprived of their friends' company; by the instrumentalization of the pandemic by all political sides to further their agenda; by witnessing how the crisis was exploited by some organizations and businesses to profit exorbitantly. Our aim with the Collection was to offer a space/ a platform where multi-disciplinary, multi-faceted, diverse, and antithetical contributions can co-exist. Along the way and while we were looking into the exceptional contributions we were receiving we reached the conclusion that much of the confusion around the topic was due to two non-resolved core ethical issues. First, the prevalence of individual rights over the common good and vice versa; and second, the nature and scope of public health and management. Part of the confusion around these ethical issues seems to stem from their definition. William James (1884) wrote in his "Essays on Pragmatism" that a definition is not only the starting point of an inquiry but also part of the entire process. This was proven true in our case. Questions like: how do we define "individual rights"? or what does "common good" mean? or how does the change in the timeline of public health management from short -term to long-term impact the definition of public health responsibility? took central position to our collective exploration aiming to understand and evaluate the phenomenon of COVID-19 and its repercussions in our lives. Reading the Collection, you will experience firsthand how setting out from a different definition has impacted the contributors' inquiry process and led them to different outcomes. One such instance is the definition of "information" and the criteria used to distinguish it from "disinformation" explored in Section A of the book. We are naturally urged to ask: how do we know which definition is the true one? Is there a way to find out?

We attempt to answer this question by looking shortly into the epistemology of knowledge. Knowledge is the relation between a conscious subject and a portion of reality (Zagzebski, 2017). This relation is mediated through a proposition the conscious subject considers to be true (propositional knowledge) or a direct experience (knowledge by acquaintance). In our case, knowledge by acquaintance is the relationship between an individual or a collective and COVID-19. An individual can have a direct experience when they are ill with COVID-19, visit an intensive care unit with COVID-19 patients, experience lockdown, wear a mask or are isolated. Our individual experiences -even when shared collectively- can vary widely as they are influenced by our perception. Our perception, in its turn, is shaped by our past experiences, values, personality, emotions, health, cultural norms, religious beliefs, locus of control, and contextual matters (Merleau-Ponty, 2004). Section C in the book describes direct experiences shared by certain groups: the health carers in New York hospitals, the citizens involved in a community network in South Africa, and the "ordinary man" in Nigeria. Section D also investigates how healthcare professionals' experience has been aggravated by the contextual factors; namely work overload, limited resources, unsafe work environment.

Knowledge by acquaintance can be used to strengthen the arguments presented in favour of a decision made or a course of action taken. However, as it is subjective, it is not adequate on its own, to determine public health policy or justify public governance. This is achieved through propositional knowledge. To reach consent, societies recur to propositional knowledge to determine what is a true -and consequently- a justified belief. Propositional knowledge uses "science" and "axiomatic ethical beliefs" to determine truth. In the case of the COVID-19 narrative we have seen a dichotomy of what is considered "true and justified belief" for the collective. Science and ethics were interpreted in a diametrically opposite way by a considerable part of the world population and experts. Sections B and E of the book look into how the interpretation of ethics and science led to social and medical polarization. In Section B the contributors explore how the utilitarian appeal to 'the greatest good of the greatest number' promoted by religious and governmental authority figures is used to promote one truth and justify consent, compliance, and obedience to a number of rules that circumvent legal and democratic decision making. This slogan (i.e., "the greatest good of the greatest number"), as it is explained in the Stanford Encyclopedia for Philosophy "is misleading… Utilitarianism commends considering what will follow (the consequences) when we make a decision and choosing maximization of the net good as the determinant of moral rightness. Accordingly, an act can increase happiness for most (the greatest number of) people but still fail to maximize the net good in the world if the smaller number of people whose happiness is not increased lose much more than the greater number gains. The principle of utility would not allow that kind of sacrifice of the smaller number to the greater number unless the net good overall is increased more than any alternative".

In Section E the contributors look into how instrumentalization of inductive truth - working mostly through analogy and generalization - has led to monopolization of "scientific truth" and led to ostracization of different scientific viewpoints. Scientific knowledge and political decision making were based on medical theories and data collected from the response to the 1918 Spanish flu (analogy); and an epidemiological modelling that forecasted a worldwide plague of COVID-19 (Ferguson et al., 2020) (generalization).

The rest is history…

We wish to thank our chapter authors, experts in various fields, for their eclectic contributions. Without them, this collection would not be possible. We also thank you, our readers. We sincerely hope that you enjoy reading this collection and, once completed, you are able to broaden your perspective on this most difficult crisis, the COVID-19 pandemic.

In order to retain our authors' authentic voice, we preserved their use of American and British English spelling and styling.

## References

Ferguson, N. M., Laydon, D., Nedjati Gilani, G., Imai, N., Ainslie, K., Baguelin, M., Bhatia, S., Boonyasiri, A., Cucunuba Perez, Z., Cuomo-Dannenburg, G., Dighe, A., Dorigatti, I., Fu, H., Gaythorpe, K. Green, W., Hamlet, A., Hinsley, W., Okell, L., Van Elsland, S, ... Ghani, A. (2020). Report 9: Impact of non-pharmaceutical interventions (NPIs) to reduce COVID-19 mortality and healthcare demand. Imperial College COVID-19 Response Team. https://doi.org/10.25561/77482

James, W. (1884). Essays on pragmatism.

Kahn, J. S., & McIntosh, K. (2005). History and recent advances in coronavirus discovery. *The Pediatric Infectious Disease Journal,* 24(11), S223-S227. doi: 10.1097/01.inf.0000188166.17324.60

Lauer, S. A., Grantz, K. H., Bi, Q., Jones, F. K., Zheng, Q., Meredith, H. R., Azman, A. S., Reich, N. G., & Lessler, J. (2020). The incubation period of Coronavirus Disease 2019 (COVID-19) from publicly reported confirmed cases: Estimation and application. *Annals of Internal Medicine, 172*(9). https://doi.org/10.7326/M20-0504

Merleau-Ponty, Maurice (2004). The World of Perception. Routledge: London

WHO (2020a). Virtual press conference on COVID-19. *World Health Organization.* https://www.who.int/docs/default-source/coronaviruse/transcripts/who-audio-emergencies-coronavirus-press-conference-full-and-final-11mar2020.pdf?sfvrsn=cb432bb3_2

WHO (2020b). The true death toll of COVID-19. *World Health Organization.* https://www.who.int/data/stories/the-true-death-toll-of-covid-19-estimating-global-excess-mortality

Zagzebski, L. (2017). What is knowledge?. *The Blackwell guide to epistemology*, 92-116.

# ABOUT THE EDITORS

**Dr Eleftheria Egel** is a scholar, business mentor for female entrepreneurs and startup founder. Her scholarly research focuses on female leadership & entrepreneurship, sustainability, and spiritual leadership. Her vision is to inspire and support positive transformative change in the way we interact by breaking down conventional barriers (assumptions); promoting new ways of thinking (holistic attributes such as compassion); and expanding the boundaries (sense-giving) of what is possible (sense-making) in our personal understanding and socio-organizational setting.

**Dr Cheryl Patton** serves as a PhD Dissertation Advisor and Adjunct Professor in the PhD in Organizational Leadership program at Eastern University, St. Davids, Pennsylvania. Her previous career was in the healthcare sector, where she spent two decades as a medical imaging technologist in a tertiary care center. Her research interests include healthcare leadership, workplace conflict, workplace ethics, and phenomenology.

# PART ONE
# Narratives:
# The (mis)information tightrope

# ALTERNATIVE NARRATIVES OF THE COVID-19 PANDEMIC: A SYMPTOM OF DISTRUST AND DIVIDE

**Ameline Vandenberghe**[1]

**Abstract:** Due to uncertain knowledge about the COVID-19 virus, mainstream discourses and containment measures disrupting people's lives have constantly varied during the pandemic. Many narratives competed to represent and interpret the events properly. This includes misleading alternative narratives, which have grown in popularity during the health crisis. Drawing mostly on narrative and communication theories, as well as other disciplinary approaches such as media studies and psychology, this chapter explores the factors and circumstances favourable to the endorsement or rejection of a certain narrative, independent of its factuality. In doing so, it shows distrust in leadership and media, prior to the health crisis, as the main element of scepticism in official information. As trust is necessary for crisis management and the proper functioning of a democratic society, this paper insists on the importance of dialogic participation, relationality, social change, and morality for reconciled narratives.

**Keywords:** COVID-19 pandemic, storytelling, alternative narratives, disinformation, crisis communication, distrust, moral power, dialogue.

## Introduction

Telling stories is our true Promethean gift to face the adversity of a chaotic and indifferent world, Algerian writer Boualem Sansal once claimed (Rencontres Internationales de Genève [RIG], 2016). Indeed, stories create meaning, define our identity and purposes, and guide our actions (Niles, 2010; RIG, 2016). Thus, naturally, countless accounts of the reality of COVID-19 have been made since its outbreak in November 2019. Partly due to its novelty and consequential unpredictability, differing political responses based on ongoing scientific research have fluctuated over time

[1] Master's Student, University of Tübingen, Germany

and from one country to another. Many crisis management strategies have been attempted and a lot of prognoses had to be revised, despite the relative confidence with which they were originally announced. In this climate of uncertainty, the accuracy of official information and adequacy of containment measures were seriously questioned by a part of the world population, who was significantly deprived of some fundamental liberties. This prompted the emergence of non-mainstream views trying to interpret the events as well, which were widely spread on social media and enabled uncooperative attitudes. The popularity of these alternative interpretations signifies the failure of decision-makers to convincingly establish their narrative to a part of the public. This rejection of the official discourse can be attributed to a lack of confidence in our knowledge but also in power-holders to act properly for the common good due to online disinformation, power disparity, and the pre-crisis situation.

Firstly, drawn upon narrative theories and progressively relying on a cross-disciplinary approach, this contribution explores the function of narratives in the meaning- and decision-making process and the difficulty to establish and recognise truthful statements. It shows the importance of persuasion and dialogical participation for the endorsement of narratives and, though not exhaustively, seeks to expose the factors accounting for the default suspicion towards organisational communication. Finally, it advocates for a moral consideration in the collaborative process of narrative sense-making.

## Human beings as *homo narrans*

Storytelling has been a fundamental part of human expression since time immemorial (Niles, 2010). As W. R. Fisher (1985) recalls, until the pre-Socratic area in Occident, there was no clear distinction between the technoscientific and the poetico-rhetorical discourse as we know it today. Both moral values and collective knowledge were embedded in *myths* performed to a community by a skilled storyteller – a practice that ensured a sense of group identity and social cohesion (Fisher, 1985; Niles, 2010). Although epistemological and normative communication systems have evolved, storytelling has not lost its legacy in the realm of public discourse. Indeed, it is still very much employed in most disciplines for its persuasive quality (Polletta et al., 2011). Ultimately, factuality imports less to people than the sense given to facts, which narrations convey. Hence, W. R. Fisher's (1984) conceptualisation of humans as essentially *narrative* instead of *rational* beings: they are *homo narrans* and therefore, their behaviours can be analysed according to a *narrative paradigm*. That is to say, by taking a look at their favoured "myths", one can attempt to comprehend their actions.

Verbal communication is inherently narrative as any transmitted account of events results from narrative methods, namely a selection of relevant information arranged in a logical, sense-making sequence; the mental construct of our environment is shaped through narration (Niles, 2010). Consequently, people live according to the narrative, i.e., the particular interpretation of objective events, they have been exposed to and have endorsed. W. R. Fisher (1984) adds that the likelihood of a person to adhere to a certain representation depends on whether the narration is coherent (*narrative probability*), and "ring[s] true" (p. 8) with their preconceptions or personal experience (*narrative fidelity*). For instance, a person is more likely to accept a rumour concerning a case of political fraud, without significant evidentiary support, if such scandals have already occurred in the past (plausible) and they believe their government to be easily corrupted (confirms pre-existing prejudices). These two factors – *narrative probability* and *narrative fidelity* – will always be more determinant than any positive factual demonstration when trying to convince a person on a certain issue (Fisher, 1984). This poses the harmful potential of fictitious narratives when deceitfully presented or wrongly interpreted as factual, as they do influence the way an audience perceives real-world events and accordingly responds to this perceived reality, ergo impacting it.

## Truthfulness and narrativity in factual and fictional accounts

Traditionally, fact and fiction are perceived as two antonymic concepts associated with what is real versus what is unreal. However, there might be narrativity in facts and factuality in fictional stories. Both categories are intersecting and there are no concrete linguistic devices capable of *consistently* asserting whether a narration is fictional or factual (Schaeffer, 2013). The reason for this is that factual information, as an account based on factual truths, is **constructed** as much as fictional realities. Indeed, facts are commonly understood as objective phenomena happening in the real world, thus as pure unbiased data; however, their grasp by human consciousness results from representational processes, and their rendition in human communication relies on narrative tools. As theorised by Schaeffer (2013), the main difference between fictional and factual communication is that fictions do not have an "ontological status" (para. 10). Hence, they are no entities of reality, whereas "factual narrative advances *claims* of referential truthfulness" (para. 1), namely, they have a pretense to reference things as they truly are or were. Still, fictional works might dispatch some truths (philosophical, sociological, moral, etc.) through imagined plots or characters. Indeed, although the terms "truth" and "fact" are often used synonymously, in reality, truth is more of a conviction based on facts (Rohra, 1998).

Rohra (1998) distinguishes three types of truths: *factual* (or scientific truths, based on physical facts grasped by the senses), *imaginative* (religious and mythic truths, which cannot be supported by positivist knowledge), and *created* (imagined truths but built upon physical facts). Created Truth is found in fictive works when the author relies on objective facts or real-world experiences to create its imaginary story (e.g., historical fiction or psychological drama); in contrast, Factual Truth is a matter of factual narrations, implying that the producer did not take any creative liberties (Rohra, 1998). However, people might easily confuse created and factual truths. A fiction, because of its verisimilitude to reality, can be mistaken for a factual narrative, even if they were produced with the explicit intent to be received as fictional (think of Orson Welles' infamous *War of the Worlds*); whereas lies, typically, are presented as facts although they are not referencing truthful events. Parents can tell their children that Santa Claus will bring them presents on Christmas Eve, they perfectly know that the colourfully wrapped gifts under the tree are not the work of an old, bearded man on a flying sleigh. Similarly, people claiming that COVID-19 is a hoax, implying that the virus does not exist altogether or is a nontransmissible exosome (Brandt, 2020), have yet to convincingly explain the waves of infections reported worldwide for their proposition to be validated as

Factual Truth, hence having an ontological status. Schaeffer (2013) suggests that only *common sense* can truly prevail for the distinction between factual and fictional representations in real-life situations, and insists that such differentiation must be made, for any confusion "can have dramatic consequences" (para. 2).

In other words, one needs to know what a true or false affirmation is. In the context of a crisis, especially, being knowledgeable enough and well-informed is crucial to decide on an adequate response that could prevent unnecessary endangerments. This response will most likely be based on scientific facts as they are considered objective, i.e., as being Factual Truth. However, as Latour's works (from 1989 to 1992) have demonstrated, "scientific facts" are not the results of unbiased findings but of a network process: collaborations within the scientific communities, work conditions, socio-political context, funding, interpretation of data, consensuses, etc. The object cannot be separated from the subject, knowledge cannot be separated from values; scientific facts are not immutable entities: they are results of *hybridisation* (Latour, as cited in Gutwirth, 1993, pp. 52-54). Also, the context surrounding scientific research, such as a health crisis and the *urgent* need for information to rapidly establish effective containment policies, will necessarily influence the resulting data (Saltelli & Giampietro, 2015). That is to say, the reliability of our factual knowledge is always limited.

## Crisis management and uncertain knowledge

Crisis management is a difficult task, particularly when knowledge is sparse and practical decisions are urgently required. Due to the unknown evolution of the crisis and the ongoing research conducted, initial truthful statements might become invalid in the light of new findings. Furthermore, there might be controversies over factual findings and the adequacy of the response to give, i.e., whether the interpretation of those facts is *right*. For instance, in the case of the COVID-19 pandemic, while the existence of SARS-CoV-2 was a recognised fact, it could not be asserted with as much confidence what measures were the most appropriate and effective. Some affirmed that a strict lockdown was necessary to save lives and not to overburden hospitals, others claimed this could have more disastrous consequences on the economy and people's mental health. Both sides stand for differing beliefs on what is best for societies and populations.

It has been advanced that the disagreements on the response to give the pandemic laid on an ideological divide making the health crisis management war of narratives (Avdaliani, 2020). Narratives are indeed always bound to their cultural and socio-political context of emergence, which explains that they necessarily bear an ideological component (Alber, 2017). One might then endorse or reject a narrative for its ideological dimension. However, the pandemic has shown the limits of dominant ideologies – especially in Occident –, such as liberalism, individualism, scientism, or social constructivism (Gregersen, 2020; McNeil-Willson, 2020). Concretely, one individual does not have *unlimited* freedom and cannot determine themselves and their reality *unconditionally*; moreover, neither our relatively secure systems nor science-based decisions are infallible. There are moral and natural limitations to what we can be or do. We are not isolated from other living beings and from nature, which is governed by the fundamental randomness of the universe (Gutwirth, 1993). Hence, our freedom of choice and interpretation is dependent upon them too. We are interconnected, part of a bigger ecological body, and subjected to the unpredictable and inevitable variations of our dynamic social and natural environment (see Gregersen, 2020).

Yet, this uncertainty about reported information and the adequacy of containment measures can arouse public scepticism towards crisis management strategies. This is why the type of crisis communication adopted by political and news media bodies – official sources of information – plays a determinant role in public cooperation. Cheng (2018) explored a wide range of studies on crisis communication strategies which all seem to highlight the importance for organisations to not only provide and adjust information but also to dialogically and empathically interact with and listen to the public (to monitor their feelings and needs) while attempting to achieve, preserve or restore a positive image (for instance by being relatable, taking responsibility, apologising, or reporting their past and present good results). Ertem Eray (2018) even posits this could be best achieved by employing storytelling strategies due to the evocative and engaging qualities of stories.

This confirms that a narrative cannot effectively impose itself based solely on its (factual) content; it also needs a convincing communicative mode. Indeed, the acceptance of a claim as truthful will rely on its persuasiveness, on its *perceived* credibility. Perceiving a proposition as veracious highly depends on the trustworthiness placed in the individual making the claim, therefore their reputation pre-crisis is an important factor (Fletcher & Park, 2017). In a situation of crisis, people's need for information, reinsurance, and guidance is traditionally met by mainstream media (Oates, 2008) and they will naturally consult news sources that they feel they can trust. Fletcher and Park (2017) identify three components of confidence in the informant: their *ability* (competence and knowledge of trustee), *integrity* (acceptable principles of trustee), and *benevolence* (good intentions of trustee towards trustor). Thus, for effective crisis management in a situation of insufficient and rapidly updated knowledge, the receptor must believe that their leaders' possible misjudgments are understandable (not due to incongruent logic) and were done in good faith. A continuous conversation between organisations (political, news, or other) and the public is supposed to be a necessary means to (re)gain their trust (Burzynski Bullard, 2013); thus, explaining its effectiveness as a (crisis) communication strategy. This dialogical contact between communicators and audiences comes about in a gathering space that the media can produce virtually. As such, leaders regularly employ mainstream media – now including social media – to reach their audience and attempt to influence their opinion in their favor (Oates, 2008), or put differently, to try and convince the public to endorse their proposed narrative.

However, with the emergence of the Internet, the creation, access, and sharing of a diversity of contents from a multitude of sources has drastically changed the public's relationship with organisational information but has not helped to foster trust – on the contrary (Romo, 2022). Some studies suggest that high exposure to user-generated online content, mostly shared on social media, might negatively impact some people's trust level resulting in them turning to non-mainstream and potentially risk-enabling narratives (Cheng, 2018; Fletcher & Park, 2017). This might be attributed to the fact that the Internet bred new narrative formats for all kinds of information that people are indistinctly confronted with, leaving them unsure of what is truthful or not.

## Online content, disinformation, and alternative narratives

Stories, like any other discourse, are actualised via a medium, be it the human voice or the Internet. Moreover, depending on the nature of the information being shared, the narrative will be constructed according to codified conventions which are medium-adapted and culturally defined (Ryan, 2014). These codes are supposed to signal to an audience what kind of narrative they are engaging with (Schaeffer, 2013). However, this implies that producing truthful seeming propositions only necessitates following the proper protocol, regardless of their (possibly lacking) ontological realism, and that ill-intentioned persons can adequately create deceitful or manipulative stories. As each technological innovation brings new improvements and expressive possibilities for the construction and transmission of narratives (Ryan, 2014), a new medium engenders further means and ways to distort or falsify information (e.g., photoshopped pictures or deep fakes). The Internet, and social media in particular, has immensely facilitated the production of and exposition to untruthful content, and thus, it has been instrumental to the increase of disinformation.

Nielsen (2021) defines "disinformation" as the general term for untrustworthy and harmful narratives, coexisting with concepts such as *misinformation* (false or misleading claims with no intent to harm), *malinformation* (factual representation manipulatively shared to harm), and *fake news* (regularly employed for content that is "neither fake nor news" (para. 2)[2]. Although their intentionality varies, all notions bear the potential to endanger the appreciator of the narrative (Nielsen, 2021). This is why tackling disinformation has become a major focus for many public organisations, especially during the COVID-19 pandemic. However, as Nielsen notes, there is no substantial agreement on what constitutes disinformation: some might regard a discourse as misleading, while others

---

[2] Nielsen bases these definitions on Wardle and Derakhshan's report to the Council of Europe (2017), arguing that the term "Fake News" can encompass many discursive entities and is thus ill-suited for framing *information disorder*. Also, in recent years, it has been exploited by politicians to discredit the information they dislike. As such, it has become a tool to target news organisations.

perceive it as legitimate counter-speech. Indeed, non-professional depictions of an event might align with and possibly complete official discourses, but they can also challenge hegemonic representations, thus facilitating the rejection of information distributed by mainstream news sources and reducing their influence over the public's opinion. We might call them *alternative narratives*.

The term "alternative narrative" can be commonly understood as a non-mainstream narrative that offers a differing interpretation of events (Imhoff & Lamberty, 2020). However, this encompasses non-hegemonic, pluralist, diversity-oriented narratives (Intercultural Cities, n.d.); *counter-narratives*, shedding light on aspects left aside and this way countering the dominant story (Bamberg, 2004); or narrative misrepresentations rejecting the official discourses and (dangerously) contributing to disinformation, e.g., conspiracy theories (Imhoff & Lamberty, 2020). Without precise delineation, indicates Nielsen (2021), an adequately scaled control of disinformation that would not censor legitimate unofficial narratives and obstruct free speech, cannot be effectively addressed. This task is all the more difficult as studies have shown people's preference for non-professional, user-generated information shared on social media (Burzynski Bullard, 2013).

## Social media for news content

Burzynski Bullard (2013) attributes the general tendency to prefer social platforms over traditional news sources to the greater liberty users have vis-à-vis the selection of received information and to the community and connective properties of social media. This appealing participatory quality is also highlighted by Fletcher and Park (2017) who remark that people are mostly interested in weighing in the interpretative stage of news reporting; that is to say, people will more likely voice online their perspective on political or social issues, probably with the intention of influencing the public discourse. They also note that people with a low trust level tend to react more to news content on social media (Fletcher & Park, 2017). This shows that people need to be *invested* in the conveyed narrative.

Considering the importance for organisations to interactively communicate with audiences and this improved dialogic space online, one might wonder why official news sources though present on social media fail to be the main source of information. Relevance and mistrust are key elements to understanding this tendency: in the context of the information overload enabled by new technologies, people might use their friends' and family's online activity as a filter to target and access content that would speak to their values and interests (Romo, 2022). Moreover, people are aware that a great number of false or manipulative narratives circulate online and that organisations can use media to share their own. International surveys have shown that the majority of participants were concerned about the trustworthiness of online content, and saw social media as the main platform of disinformation with politicians as the principal actors of misleading information (Edelman, 2022; Newman et al., 2021). Also, journalistic news production depends upon "a country's political environment, the media norms, media regulation, ownership of media outlets" (Oates, 2007, p. 4); media biases and political control influences news coverage, which can politicise events that should not be such as pandemics (Abbas, 2020). Hence, any suspicion towards the neutrality, "censoredness" or propagandistic potential of news media might bring people to favor content their close social circle judges trust- and shareworthy, which would also fulfill their need to belong by valuing the same narratives as their peers (D'Ardenne, 2020). As such, social media is said to enhance tribalism, forming communities of like-minded people but much less receptive to ideas divergent from their in-group perception (Javanbakht, 2020). Consequently, debates on controversial topics or with no objective truths lead to competitive conversations aiming at winning the argument rather than exchanges towards consensuses (Fisher et al., 2018).

Unsurprisingly, news consumption surrounding the COVID-19 health crisis has largely taken place on social networks where alternative narratives proliferated as well. In the attempt to combat unreliable information, social network companies have expanded their content moderation rules (Nielsen, 2021). Similarly, many governments have been attentive to the media coverage as they are worried that some reports might lead people to the wrong conclusion (Newman et al., 2021). However, greater control of online and news content, even for dismantling disinformation, could be perceived as censorship confirming people's mistrust of organisations (The Royal Society, 2022). It would seem that people are suspicious of official narratives when they feel (or fear being) manipulated or controlled. This would invite them to reject official reports, tune to alternative stories and endorse those that resonate with their perception of reality. As the pandemic has distinguished itself by the rise in the appreciation of non-mainstream narratives, the circumstances that make them accord more with people's experiences should now be further explored.

## Control deprivation and narrative control retrieval

The outbreak of the COVID-19 pandemic has significantly disrupted citizens' daily life. Restrictions regulating people's spatial movements, social contacts, and actions have continuously been introduced, updated, retracted, and reinstated according to varying narratives reflecting the persistent attempt to frame and manage the crisis properly. This, however, with no concrete guarantee of the expected results. Furthermore, the constant discussions surrounding the regulations have taken place between health experts and the rulers, who were solely in charge of the decision-making process – thus, excluding the layman's participation or approval. This left many people with a feeling of helplessness and disempowerment, but also doubt about the capacities and good intentions of their decision-makers. For these persons, alternative narratives were the expression of their discontentment with the crisis management and their disagreement with the official representation of the crisis. Arguably, as the issues of misrepresentations had to be addressed, this created a dialogue that had failed to take place. As such, alternative narratives were a means for control retrieval.

In situations of limited influence over one's environment, narratives serve as a strategy to compensate for the control privation by enhancing a sense of agency and power. This lies in the very fact that stories guide human conduct and actions affect one's reality which will reciprocally react, possibly causing the desired outcome (Chen et al., 2017). Additionally, as knowledge is power (Imhoff & Lamberty, 2020), stories help define the unknown and this way, provide answers. As Ertem Eray (2018) stated: "If people don't know what is going on, they tell stories" (p. 135) and if organisations fail to offer satisfactory narrations, the public will. For instance, the scientific discourse attributed the source of the COVID-19 outbreak to a natural mutation of the SARS-CoV-2 virus, but unconvinced people speculated on a bioweapon or laboratory leak, mostly fuelled by misleading information accessible online but also by recent scientific scandals in China and some U.S. or Chinese officials' accusations (Knight, 2021). This last narrative is revelatory of a general mistrust in institutional manoeuvres. According to the adopted view on the health situation, people could position themselves in the form of a personal narrative, i.e., the way they wished to be perceived (Bamberg, 2004). Thus, those believing in alternative narratives of mismanagement from organisations assumed the persona of a non-conformist critical thinker and even resistant figure concerned with preventing power abuses. Such responses to crisis management and communication, as any other, contribute to the always unpredictable outcome of the pandemic.

## Science trust crisis and rejection of science-based policies

For any unplanned change or disturbance in our social systems must come a response. The ability to decide on the appropriate reaction is a form of power that is almost exclusively entrusted to governments in case of crises, where executive power is necessarily (and normally, temporarily) expanded (Ng, 2020). Expectedly, political leaders responded to the COVID-19 health crisis according to a science-based narrative provided by appointed health experts.

The fact that governments have relied on scientists' consulting for the health crisis management seems logical on the principle, for political leaders need to be reliably informed and advised to take the right actions. This aligns with the persistent modernist idea that searchers can render "pure scientific facts" on which legislation can then be justly built (Saltelli & Giampietro, 2015). Yet, the beginning of the pandemic, especially, was marked with scientific uncertainty. Also, the appointment of some experts over others poses the uneasy politicised dimension of scientific reliance. A few commentators have raised concerns that the collaboration between politicians and scientists for decision-making might negatively impact the exercise of science. For example, Prasad and Flier (2020) regretted that respected scientists expressing disagreements with the official views on COVID-19 were personally attacked without considering their alternative opinions for an enrichment of the debate around the best containment measures. More controversially, Esfeld (2021) goes as far as claiming that this relation might settle scientism, which could lead politicians to use the authority of science for then indisputable coercive purposes. Not to forget that the privileged status accorded to scientific truths and the in-network conditions of scientific findings have already been responsible for past malpractices, sometimes motivated by conflicts of interests (Saltelli & Giampietro, 2015).

This is at the heart of the increasing trust crisis in science that we have more clearly witnessed throughout the coronavirus pandemic. But the distrust in scientific institutions and science-based policies seems to have reached a paroxysmal point during the vaccination campaign which achieved to polarise populations worldwide between two main narratives: some considered that the politicians were dutifully taking the necessary actions to protect their citizens given the information they disposed of, but many worried that the pandemic has given governments and pharmaceutical companies the legitimacy to exert an abusive power (Ng, 2020) or make immoral profits under the guise of stemming the virus[3]. In both cases, it refers to the amount of power confided in political leaders or other groups of high stature which is asymmetrical to the level of citizens' control over social norms (Imhoff & Lamberty, 2020). This asymmetry has also been observed in the minimal (economic) impact of COVID-19 restrictions on elites, especially for those working in fields that could contribute to the management of the crisis; perceived as unfair, this drove a part of the more affected population to anti-science narratives (Pazzanese, 2020).

## Power asymmetry and decredibilising stories

According to Imhoff and Lamberty (2020), the disproportional power distribution is prone to enhancing conspiracy mentality, especially

---

[3] For further information on this question, see: ActionAid International. (2021, September 15). *Pharmaceutical companies reaping immoral profits from Covid vaccines yet paying low tax rates.*

among people of particularly low power resources (low income, low education, etc.). Hence, the rejection by some people of official science-based narratives and endorsement of alternative stories to discredit major institutions (Hotez, 2021). By criticising them, crisis management is made more difficult and has to be adapted. This can be seen as a form of participation. Inversely, to describe the persons disregarding health recommendations, the term "covidiot" has been coined; they have been characterised, among other qualifiers, as "selfish," more concerned about their self-interests than the common good, and others' safety (Miller, 2020, para. 12). But whether this criticism is founded and people are more upset about the dispossession of their comfortable pre-crisis lifestyle than public health, or not, this does not change the fact that in their chosen narrative, their actions are motivated by democratic values (i.e., people's sovereignty, liberty, equality, rule of law, transparency, etc.) that they perceived are threatened. Therefore, it is critical to understand that they do not intend to disregard moral considerations towards their more vulnerable Others.

In the case of reasonable beliefs in an abusive attempt of coercion by politicians, it is indeed necessary that people take action (Imhoff & Lamberty, 2020). Also, historical instances have shown that some expanded executive power granted to governments has never returned to their prior state post-crisis (Ng, 2020). Considering this, citizens' vigilance on the matter is not unreasonable. Problematic, however, is the practically *automatic* assumption that governments or other powerful organisations make ill-usage of their power and the default defiance towards authority, when sustained by narratives with no concrete factual grounding but plausibility at best.

## Trust crisis in power structures, social divide, and democratic challenges

This default suspicion against power-holders is central to most misleading alternative narratives, particularly conspiracy theories. Conspiracy theories can generically be described as the belief that a small group of people detain formal or informal power plots *secretly* to achieve (world) domination and control over the population(s). It is mostly grounded on the negative perception of power as a potential threat and source of abuse (Imhoff & Lamberty, 2020). Therefore, the increase of such alternative narratives during the pandemic cannot only be accredited to the exceptional circumstances of the crisis; they also reflected and arguably exacerbated a distrust that roots deeper and pre-existed COVID-19 in some countries. Indeed, depending on the historical, economic, socio-politico, and cultural context, the tropic belief in corrupted political leaders working for their interests might be a population's *dominant* narrative (Imhoff & Lamberty, 2020; Lammers et al., 2015). That is, they have failed to be perceived as benevolent and having integrity, as such, they could not gain or maintain people's trust.

Damico et al. (2000) hypothesised that political trust depended on socialisation and the implication in community associations: should a person grow in an unstable and socially poor environment (limited interactions with people or a certain social group) or live distanced from institutional intern structures, then their capability for trust would be negatively affected. Typically, individuals who are financially insecure, low-educated, and feel unrepresented by politicians (*distanciation*) will tend to mistrust institutions (Imhoff & Lamberty, 2020). More generally, social and economic disparity is the mark of a government's ineffectiveness which, in turn, is likely to engender a lack of confidence in the political apparatus (lack of *ability*; Edelman, 2022). However, Damico et al. (2000) found out that the main contributor to such mistrust is (past or present) scandals and conflicts linked to power-holders. Looking at the current world situation and some contextual factors at play in the endorsement of alternative narratives, we could cite three major issues pre-pandemic: the gap between the wealthiest and the poorest is widening, climate change has become a pressing matter despite world leaders failing to propose sufficient regulating policies, and racial tensions are rising, especially in the United States. These instances and many others account for the erosion of social ties, a reduced sense of connectedness with members of other groups (e.g., the leading class and the population), the lack of adequate reactions to urgent issues, and the disagreements on the right solutions to provide. That is to say, COVID-19 was born in already very divisive times.

Because distrust and divide are a huge obstacle to the exercise of democracy and cooperative attitudes, fixing the problem of alternative narratives rooted in this climate of insecurity requires "repairing" changes. Representatives must prove with concrete actions and reforms that they effectively work for the common good and the public's interest rather than their own or that of a small elite (Duncan, 2018). In other words, power-holders must lead deontologically. The key concept towards this goal should thus be, besides transparency and accountability, *morality*.

## Towards social change: the concept of moral power

Equaling power-holders with untrustworthiness infers a lack of morality particularly attributed to politicians. This reason is that power has a disinhibiting effect and induces a focus on the Self; namely, powerful people tend to indulge more in immoral behaviours oriented towards their own needs as they are more independent from others and might feel less obligated to follow social and moral norms (Lammers et al., 2015). However, in a conceptual essay, Mehta and Winship (2010) insist on tempering this conception of political leaders destitute of any moral consideration, arguing that morality is an inherent dimension of leadership. As they state, a trustworthy leader is a person disposing of solid moral power to respond effectively to world events. Concretely, – and similarly to the three components of trust – a leader should be *morally well-intentioned, morally capable,* and have *moral standing,* i.e., be perceived as morally good. For this last aspect to succeed, a leader has to perform well, which involves acting consistently with what they preach, entertaining *relational connections* to the community, and appearing authentic. Doing so, implementing their narrative would be a non-coercive, collaborative, and less hierarchical act (Mehta & Winship, 2010).

Yet, the current distrustful environment proves that leaders failed to meet these criteria or some of them. Moreover, it could be argued that the performative dimension of leadership still poses the potential of strategically feigning good morality and using this decisive power resource for self-serving purposes. This is the reason why Lammers et al. (2015) suggest that the power-induced disinhibition should be redirected towards realising moral actions, which would require undermining self-centeredness with better perspectives (for decisions that would benefit others) and with accountability. Thus, honestly observing the moral dimension of power might be the solution to the trust crisis in our democratic societies. This involves achieving a collective consensus on what is good for society so that people can obey authority not because they must, but because they are convinced that they are working on this common project and that it is right (Mehta & Winship, 2010).

## Conclusion

In situations of health crises involving drastic changes in people's daily life, convincing communication strategies that would ignite everyone's cooperation and sense of responsibility are necessary (Ertem Eray, 2018). For this enterprise to succeed, dialogic participation is key. However, when objective truth is lacking to determine the *rightness* of practical decisions, conversations might become ideological, politicised, or confrontational; oriented towards affirming one's truth rather than finding an agreement on what is truly best (Following Fisher et al., 2018). In such battles of narratives, the participants' motives might be questioned, especially given the amount of power they might possess. Also, new technologies and social media have given further possibilities to weigh in the dispute or to weaponise narratives, possibly misleading or manipulating the public's opinion. As a relinquishment of agency was required of people during the COVID-19 pandemic, they had to believe that it was for a good cause. This chapter has thus shown that trust in those in charge of the meaning- and decision-making process is an essential part of crisis communication, but that power holders failed to gain it during and prior to the crisis. The reason is that leaders have not responded properly to their population's needs, nor engaged sufficiently with them to be perceived as morally well-intentioned and provide a narrative they could endorse and would guide their actions. This failure is at the heart of alternative stories resisting the idea that decision-makers acted dutifully in the public's interest, but with the intention to possibly make it happen.

Presumably, the majority of misleading narratives will lose their persuasiveness once we will return to a new normality, sinking into the deep waters of the "overinformation" flow. But for this stability to happen, social changes must be made, for we cannot write the future on unresolved issues of distrust and divide. The COVID-19 health crisis has been a reminder of the need for reconciled narratives to face challenging times together. Throughout the pandemic, it has been repeatedly suggested that these exceptional times should be the opportunity to reimagine the post-pandemic world, to change the course of the (hi)story. Hence, overcoming distrust narratives implies taking actions based on morality, that is to say, the will to do the right thing for the common good, which future narratives of human experience could account for, and people could identify with. Finally, as narratives conduct actions impacting the world, there should be a re-exploration of the ethical dimension in the creation of informative content. For the liberty to tell anything does not exempt anyone from the responsibility towards the truth and others. The starting question we should then ask collectively is: *what do we want this story to be?*

## References

Abbas, A. H. (2020). Politicizing the pandemic: A schemata analysis of COVID-19 news in two selected newspapers. *International Journal for the Semiotics of Law - Revue Internationale de Sémiotique Juridique*, 1–20. https://doi.org/10.1007/s11196-020-09745-2

ActionAid International. (2021, September 15). *Pharmaceutical companies reaping immoral profits from Covid vaccines yet paying low tax rates*. https://actionaid.org/news/2021/pharmaceutical-companies-reaping-immoral-profits-covid-vaccines-yet-paying-low-tax-rates

Alber, J. (2017). Introduction: The ideological ramifications of narrative strategies. *Storyworlds: A Journal of Narrative Studies, 9*(1), 3–25. https://doi.org/10.5250/storyworlds.9.1-2.0003

Avdaliani, E. (2020, May 13). *The battle of the coronavirus narratives*. Begin-Sadat Center for Strategic Studies. https://besacenter.org/coronavirus-narratives/

Bamberg, M. (2004). Considering counter narratives. In M. Bamberg & M. Andrews (Eds.), *Considering counter-narratives: Narrating, resisting, making sense* (pp. 351–371). John Benjamins. https://doi.org/10.1075/sin.4.43bam

Brandt, J. (2020, July 03). COVID-19 is a hoax. *Cook County News Herald.* https://www.cookcountynews-herald.com/articles/covid-19-coronavirus-is-a-hoax/

Burzynski Bullard, S. (2013). Social media and journalism: What works best and why it matters. *Faculty Publications, College of Journalism & Mass Communications,* 75. https://digitalcommons.unl.edu/journalismfacpub/75/

Chen, C. Y., Lee, L., & Yap, A. J. (2017). Control deprivation motivates acquisition of utilitarian products. *Journal of Consumer Research, 43*(6), 1031-1047. https://doi.org/10.1093/jcr/ucw068

Cheng, Y. (2018). How social media is changing crisis communication strategies: Evidence from the updated literature. *Journal of Contingencies and Crisis Management, 26*(1), 58–68. https://doi.org/10.1111/1468-5973.12130

Damico, A. J., Conway, M. M., & Damico, S. B. (2000). Patterns of political trust and mistrust: Three moments in the lives of democratic citizens. *Polity, 32*(3), 377–400. https://doi.org/10.2307/3235357

D'Ardenne, K. (2020, October 29). *Anti-science thinking: Why it happens and what to do about it.* ASU News. https://news.asu.edu/20201029-anti-science-thinking-why-it-happens-and-what-do-about-it

Duncan, G. (2018, November 9). *How to restore trust in governments and institutions.* The Conversation. http://theconversation.com/how-to-restore-trust-in-governments-and-institutions-106547

Edelman. (2022). *Edelman trust barometer 2022.* https://www.edelman.com/sites/g/files/aatuss191/files/2022-01/2022%20Edelman%20Trust%20Barometer%20FINAL_Jan25.pdf

Ertem Eray, T. (2018). Storytelling in crisis communication. *Online Journal of Communication and Media Technologies, 8*(2), 131–144. https://doi.org/10.12973/ojcmt/2358

Esfeld, M. (2021, January 11). *The abuse of science in the corona crisis.* American Institute of Economic Research. https://www.aier.org/article/the-abuse-of-science-in-the-corona-crisis/

Fisher, M., Knobe, J., Strickland, B., & Keil, F. C. (2018). The tribalism of truth: As political polarization grows, the arguments we have with one another may be shifting our understanding of truth itself. *Scientific American, 318*(2), 50–53.

https://www.scientificamerican.com/article/are-toxic-political-conversations-changing-how-we-feel-about-objective-truth/

Fisher, W. R. (1984). Narration as a human communication paradigm: The case of public moral argument. *Communication Monographs, 51*(1), 1–22. https://doi.org/10.1080/03637758409390180

Fisher, W. R. (1985). The narrative paradigm: In the beginning. *Journal of Communication, 35*(4), 74–89. https://doi.org/10.1111/j.1460-2466.1985.tb02974.x

Fletcher, R., & Park, S. (2017). The impact of trust in the news media on online news consumption and participation. *Digital Journalism, 5*(10), 1281–1299. https://doi.org/10.1080/21670811.2017.1279979

Gregersen, N. H. (2020). The corona crisis unmasks prevailing social ideologies. *Dialog, 59*(2), 68–70. https://doi.org/10.1111/dial.12558

Gutwirth, S. (1993). Autour du contrat naturel. In Ph. Gérard, F. Ost, & M. van de Kerchove (Eds.), *Images et usages de la nature en droit* (pp. 75–131). Publications des FUSL. https://works.bepress.com/serge_gutwirth/33/

Hotez, P. J. (2021, March 29). *The antiscience movement is escalating, going global and killing thousands*. Scientific American. https://www.scientificamerican.com/article/the-antiscience-movement-is-escalating-going-global-and-killing-thousands/

Imhoff, R., & Lamberty, P. (2020). Conspiracy beliefs as psycho-political reactions to perceived power. In M. Butter & P. Knight (Eds.), *Routledge Handbook of Conspiracy Theories* (pp. 192–205). Routledge.

Intercultural Cities. (n.d.). *Alternative narratives and inclusive communication.* Council of Europe. https://www.coe.int/en/web/interculturalcities/alternative-narratives-and-inclusive-communication

Javanbakht, A. (2020, November 14). Social media, the matrix, and digital tribalism. *Psychology Today*. https://www.psychologytoday.com/us/blog/the-many-faces-anxiety-and-trauma/202011/social-media-the-matrix-and-digital-tribalism

Knight, D. (2021). COVID-19 Pandemic origins: Bioweapons and the history of laboratory leaks. *Southern Medical Journal, 114*(8), 465–467. https://doi.org/10.14423/SMJ.0000000000001283

Lammers, J., Galinsky, A. D., Dubois, D., & Rucker, D. D. (2015). Power and morality. *Current Opinion in Psychology, 6,* 15–19. https://doi.org/10.1016/j.copsyc.2015.03.018

McNeil-Willson, R. (2020). *Framing in times of crisis: Responses to COVID-19 amongst Far-Right movements and organisations*. International Centre for Counter-Terrorism. https://doi.org/10.19165/2020.1.04

Mehta, J., & Winship, C. (2010). Moral power. In S. Hitlin and S. Vaisey (Eds.), *Handbook of the sociology of morality* (pp. 425-438). Springer. https://doi.org/10.1007/978-1-4419-6896-8_22

Miller, K. (2020, July 15). *What does 'Covidiot' mean?* Health. https://www.health.com/condition/infectious-diseases/coronavirus/what-does-covidiot-mean

Newman, N., Fletcher, R., Schulz, A., Andi, S., Robertson, C. T., & Nielsen, R. (2021). *The Reuters Institute Digital News Report 2021*. Reuters Institute for the Study of Journalism. https://reutersinstitute.politics.ox.ac.uk/sites/default/files/2021-06/Digital_News_Report_2021_FINAL.pdf

Ng, Y.-F. (2020, September 29). *Have our governments become too powerful during COVID-19?* The Conversation. http://theconversation.com/have-our-governments-become-too-powerful-during-covid-19-147028

Nielsen, R. K. (2021, February 19). *How to respond to disinformation while protecting free speech*. Reuters Institute for the Study of Journalism. https://reutersinstitute.politics.ox.ac.uk/news/how-respond-disinformation-while-protecting-free-speech

Niles, J. D. (2010). *Homo narrans: The poetics and anthropology of oral literature*. University of Pennsylvania Press. https://doi.org/10.9783/9780812202953

Oates, S. (2008). *Introduction to media and politics*. SAGE.

Pazzanese, C. (2020, October 30). What caused the U.S.' anti-science trend? *Harvard Gazette*. https://news.harvard.edu/gazette/story/2020/10/what-caused-the-u-s-anti-science-trend/

Polletta, F., Chen, P. C. B., Gardner, B. G., & Motes, A. (2011). The sociology of storytelling. *Annual Review of Sociology, 37*(1), 109–130. https://doi.org/10.1146/annurev-soc-081309-150106

Prasad, V., & Flier, J. S. (2020, April 27). *Scientists who express different views on Covid-19 should be heard, not demonized*. STAT. https://www.statnews.com/2020/04/27/hear-scientists-different-views-covid-19-dont-attack-them/

Rencontres Internationales de Genève. (2016, November 1). *Boualem Sansal – "Écrire dans la violence du monde"* [Video]. YouTube. https://www.youtube.com/watch?v=sjmBOGi6VxQ

Rohra, S. (1998). Factual truth and created truth. *Indian Literature, 42*(5 (187)), 167–171.

Romo, J. (2022, January 26). *The impact of social media on trust*. The Twofourseven Blog. https://www.twofourseven.co.uk/blog/26/1/2022/the-impact-of-social-media-on-trust

Ryan, M.-L. (2012/2014). Narration in various media. In P. Hühn, J. C. Meister, J. Pier, & W. Schmid (Eds.), *The living handbook of narratology*. Hamburg University. https://www.lhn.uni-hamburg.de/node/53.html

Saltelli, A., & Giampietro, M. (2015). *The fallacy of evidence-based policy*. [Draft for special issue on FUTURES]. Cornell University. https://arxiv.org/pdf/1607.07398.pdf

Schaeffer, J.-M. (2013). Fictional vs. factual Narration. In P. Hühn, J. C. Meister, J. Pier, & W. Schmid (Eds.), *The living handbook of narratology*. https://www.lhn.uni-hamburg.de/node/56.html

The Royal Society. (2022). *The online information environment: Understanding how the internet shapes people's engagement with scientific information*. https://royalsociety.org/-/media/policy/projects/online-information-environment/the-online-information-environment.pdf?la=en-GB&hash=691F34A269075C0001A0E647C503DB8F

Wardle, C., & Derakhshan, H. (2017). *Information disorder. Toward an interdisciplinary framework for research and policymaking*. Council of Europe Report. https://rm.coe.int/information-disorder-report-november-2017/1680764666?ct=t()

## Author Note

Acknowledgements: I would like to thank Dr. Eleftheria Egel, Cheryl M. Patton Ph.D., and the Research and Writing Center of the University of Tübingen for their helpful support and suggestions. I have no conflict of interests to disclose.

# ETHICS AND INTERTEMPORAL CHOICE: AN ANALYSIS OF LINGUISTIC VARIATION AND PANDEMIC POLICY

**Jayme Neiman Renfro**[1]

**Abstract:** Can the way a group of people speaks affect the way they perceive time, and thus impact their politics and policies? There are differences between languages in terms of how they encode time. Previous research suggests that languages that grammatically associate the future and the present foster future-oriented behavior such as saving toward retirement, and practicing healthier lifestyle behaviors. This research posits that this is related to intertemporal choice—when language separates the future from the present, it is easier for an individual to "put off" the future, and when the future and the present are more closely linked in language, speakers feel the future more immediately and act accordingly. Intertemporal decision making is key in the creation of policy and relies heavily on the ethical choices involved in weighing relative utility. This project examines the relationship between future-oriented language and pandemic policy. It explores whether the same mechanism that connects language and economic choice is at play when it comes to governments preparing for future healthcare costs and crises, and finds that the results vary by specific healthcare policy.

Intertemporal choices are decisions that involve making a choice between current and future benefits--decisions that have consequences in more than one time-period. These decisions require the decision-maker to assign a relative value to two or more payoffs in the present and in the future, and require them to trade off those costs and benefits at different points in time. These decisions may be at the individual level, about saving, health, exercise, education and the like, or alternatively, they may be made at the group level such as with business investing or committee project planning, or about policy as I will discuss in this chapter.

[1] Associate Professor, University of Northern Iowa, USA

Since the early twentieth century, economists have primarily used the discounted utility model to analyze intertemporal decisions (Samuelson, 1937). The discounted utility model makes it possible to compare costs and benefits in different time periods by expressing their values in present terms. This is done by creating a formula estimating how much people discount their future preferences, or in other words, how much people prefer benefitting today than benefitting (or potentially benefitting) in the future (EPA.gov, 2010). Discounted utility has been used to illustrate how people actually make intertemporal choices and because of this it is commonly used in the development of public policy.

It has long been established that these sorts of intertemporal decisions are, at their heart, ethical decisions. When people place different values on things that happen at different times, and particularly when they discount the future (and potentially future generations), they are not acting morally temperate in the Aristotelian sense. In this chapter I am concerned with healthcare policy, particularly as related to potential pandemic outbreaks as could affect either the future self or could skip generations completely and solely affect future generations.

Prior to the winter of late 2019 and early 2020, when none of us had heard of COVID-19, the threat of a pandemic was not even among the top answers when the Pew Research Center's poll asked Americans about the major problems facing the country. Thus, when spending on pandemic preparedness in the U.S. fell steadily over the 15 years leading up to 2020, many Americans took no notice (Greenburg, 2020).

Of course, spending on healthcare and policies regarding topics like pandemic planning vary widely around the world. Unsurprisingly, countries with higher per capita GDPs tend to exhibit substantially higher expenditure on healthcare as a share of their income (Ortiz-Ospina & Roser, 2017). There are cultural factors that drive policy variation as well. For example, a 2011 study found that a difference between entitlement versus accountability culture contributes to variation in per capita healthcare spending (Kaufman, 2011). A 2014 study analyzed the relationship between consumer culture and the provision of healthcare (Sturgeon, 2014). And another 2014 paper looked at differences in a culture's tolerance of error and how that drove medical excess (Hoffman & Kanzaria, 2014).

The cultural difference that I will focus on in this chapter is language. There is evidence from previous research that suggests that differences between languages in terms of how they encode time is related to intertemporal decision-making, specifically future-discounting (Chen 2013). Studies indicate that languages that grammatically associate the future and the present foster future-oriented behavior, and others force a separation (i.e., Hechavarria et al., 2020; Kim et al., 2021; Tang et al., 2021). Previous research posits that when language separates the future from the present, it is easier for an individual to "put off," or discount the future, and when the future and present are more closely linked in language, speakers feel the future more immediately and act accordingly.

For this project I investigate this relationship as it relates to variation in pandemic policy around the world. Countries vary in their healthcare policies and the decisions they make have consequences. Consider a country that decided to lock down during a COVID-19 wave. They made a decision that would have a short-term effect on their economy, hoping that the longer-term benefits for the health of their citizenry would outweigh those effects. Other countries found that not to be an acceptable tradeoff, considering we didn't really know what the long-term situation was going to be. Or, a country can spend significant money and energy creating a national stockpile of PPE and keep a highly paid team of scientists and doctors on staff just in case someday there is an epidemic. Or that country can spend that money on something else-something more immediate, even if that thing is less serious, it is more likely. If, as I hypothesize, countries whose languages separate the future from the present, have less or a slower response and worse outcomes, we must consider that the moral philosophers discussed above are correct and discounting is ethically problematic.

## Intertemporal Choice

There have traditionally been two main approaches to studying intertemporal choice: economic and psychological. Economists study how individuals allocate resources to maximize utility and meet goals—in other words decision makers are seen as solving problems of constrained optimization (Hardisty et al., 2012; Pindyck & Rubinfeld, 2008). People try to satisfy their desires and meet their goals using consistent criteria while strategically navigating constraints and boundaries, such as monetary and time limitations.

In this way, economists treat intertemporal choices like any other kind of choice--the decision comes down to a trade-off between costs and benefits, only in these cases the costs and benefits may occur at different times. For example, if a government is deciding whether to build a new sports arena, they must look at the trade-off between the costs of building and maintaining the stadium, and the benefit of the tourism and sales tax dollars that will come later. The merit of the project is evaluated by comparing the costs and benefits predicted to come from building the plant.

In general though, we know that it is largely considered desirable to acquire benefits as quickly as possible and push off costs as far into the future as possible. For example, getting $100 today is better than getting $100 in ten years because the immediate $100 could be put in the bank to earn interest in the meantime. Furthermore, $100 today is relatively more useful today than it will be in the future because most people (and nations) grow richer over time (Ackerman & Heinzerling, 2002). Thus, according to economic analysis it is perfectly rational, even advisable, to discount future costs and benefits. The net present value of a project or choice is a single number meant to indicate its worth, after adjusting for a time delay. It is calculated by subtracting the discounted costs from the discounted benefits.

Psychologists and behavioral economists, on the other hand, have focused on describing the cognitive, emotional, motivational, and contextual factors that the anomalies in human behavior, where the actual choices made are not explained by economic models. Things like bounded rationality (Simon, 1955) and motivational factors, like a desire to fit in with a group, to live up to the expectations of others, and to be evaluated positively when compared to others also affect intertemporal choice (Shultz et al., 2007). Variations in these factors lead to variations in how people make intertemporal choices. For example, if a tasty treat is not right in front of you, it is easier to resist (Liberman & Trope 2008; Metcalfe & Mischel 1999; Mischel & Baker, 1975). Thus, one's time preference for dessert now versus health and waistlines in the future can vary substantially (Appelt et al., 2011; Dinner et al., 2011).

Philosophers too have wrestled with the morality aspect of future discounting for millennia and largely agree that *not* discounting the future can be considered a moral virtue related to prudence and impartiality (i.e., Smith, 1790). For example, Aristotle considered "phronesis," or prudence, as a central intellectual virtue. He also highlighted the virtue of temperance, "For moral excellence is concerned with pleasures and pains; it is on account of the pleasure that we do bad things and it is on account of the pain that we abstain from noble ones." (Aristotle, 2000) For Aristotle, an imprudent and intemperate person has an appetite for life's pleasures and chooses them at the cost of other, higher goods. More recently Brink (2010) also considered the temporal aspects of prudence but in terms of distributive justice and argued that temporal neutrality is required of temperance. Discounting the future may not be ethical.

Some economists have even jumped into the philosophical side of this discussion. In 1928, F.P. Ramsey was considering the optimal savings rate of a country. In his discussion he calls discounting later benefits as "ethically indefensible" and "aris[ing] merely from the weakness of the imagination" (Ramsey, 1928, p. 543). In 1948, R.F. Harrod agreed and called discounting a product of a "lack of telepathic faculty" and "conquest of passion over reason" (pp. 38, 40). An ethical debate, indeed.

## Language

Intertemporal choice has many factors and thus varies widely among people and groups. One factor that is not as widely studied is language. According to the Sapir-Whorf hypothesis, otherwise known as the principle of linguistic relativity, language may influence thought through perception, or to put it differently, "speakers of different languages think and perceive reality in different ways and...each language has its own world view" (Hussein, 2012, p. 642). As Lakoff (1993) argued, language is often used metaphorically and languages use different cultural metaphors that reveal something about how speakers of that language think.

The "go-to" illustration of this is that the Inuit have many words for snow because it is so salient to their daily lives and they needed to be more specific (chat with some American skiers for a similar experience). This example isn't quite right though as an example of linguistic relativity, as it is more about how language rules and patterns force the speaker to make inferences and categorizations themselves, which they then internalize (Korskrity, 2000). A better example would be how gendered language (doing things like calling the boys' team the Blue Jays and the girls' team the Lady Jays) perpetuates misogyny in college sports (Messner et al., 1993).

Current research suggests that while certainly not deterministic, language may indeed affect thought, and there is evidence that language influences worldviews and perceptions (Boroditsky, 2001; Deutscher, 2010; Levinson, 1996; Lucy, 1992). For instance, in the Proceedings of the Annual Meeting of the Berkeley Linguistics Society, Slobin (2011) describes a process that he deemed "thinking for speaking" in which pre-linguistic perceptional data get translated into linguistic terms for the purpose of communication. He uses a series of pictures with no words and shows them to children who speak four different languages to show that the variation in the languages themselves influence how the children perceive the pictures and thus tell a story about what is happening in them.

Slobin (2011) was using variation in how languages encode motion for his study. Keith Chen (2013) points to future-time reference as another area in which variation may impact worldview. Languages differ widely in both how and when they require the speaker to signal that they are talking about the future. For example, English primarily marks the future with either "will" or forms of "be going to." In contrast, some languages mark future events using a much larger and more diverse set of constructions. For example, Bittner (2005) documents that Kalaallisut (West Greenlandic) has at least 28 distinct constructions which mark future time. And some languages don't require the distinction at all. For instance, if someone wanted to explain in English what they are doing over winter break, they are obligated to say something along the lines of "I (am going, will go, have to go) to Puerto Rico" If I were having the same conversation in Mandarin Chinese, I might instead say something like, "I go to Puerto Rico" since the timing of the trip in the future would be handled by the context of the conversation (I was asked what I was going to do over winter break). Thus, English obligates its speakers to distinguish between the present and future in a way that Mandarin does not. This distinction, a central characteristic of the weak versus strong future time reference classification (Thieroff, 2000), is the one that Chen (2013) uses in his work, and is the difference between languages used in this study as well.

Future-time reference differences between languages are surprisingly widespread and occur not only between neighboring countries in the same region, but sometimes occur within countries with multiple languages. In Europe, languages range from Finnish, which only rarely marks a difference between present and future time to French, which has very specific future forms of verbs. Switzerland and Belgium both have both languages with obligatory future-tense references and languages without as official languages in their countries.

In his 2013 work, Chen found that speakers of languages that do not force a distinction between present-time and future-time are more likely to save more money, smoke less, have safer sex and have more money for retirement. These are issues of intertemporal choice—making some sort of sacrifice in the present to benefit oneself in the future. As Chen (2013) puts it:

> Being required to speak in a distinct way about future events leads speakers to take fewer future-oriented actions. This hypothesis arises naturally if grammatically separating the future and the present leads speakers to disassociate the future from the present. This would make the future feel more distant, and since saving involves current costs for future rewards, would make saving harder. On the other hand, some languages grammatically equate the present and the future. Those speakers would be more willing to save for a future which appears closer. Put another way, I ask whether a habit of speech which disassociates the future from the present, can cause people to devalue future rewards. (p. 1)

Chen is hypothesizing that there is variation in the amount of discounting that the speakers are doing about the future utility of costs and rewards.

He figures that when people are forced, by virtue of the very words that they speak regularly, to consider the future over and over again, that they will act as if that future is soon and important. They will make the ethical evaluation, temperance, to take actions like save money, use condoms, and not smoke cigarettes so that their older selves and future generations will be happier and healthier. On the flip side of this, when speakers are able to disassociate from the future by linguistically separating it and making it feel "other," they are able to act more in the present, perhaps even selfishly so.

## COVID-19

Coronavirus disease 2019, or COVID-19 is a contagious respiratory and vascular disease caused by severe acute respiratory syndrome coronavirus 2 (EBioMedicine, 2020). Common symptoms include fever, cough, fatigue, shortness of breath, and loss of taste and smell and generally begin between one and fourteen days after exposure. Most people who are infected experience only mild symptoms, however some develop acute respiratory distress syndrome, cytokine storms, multi-organ failure, septic shock and blood clots. Organ damage has been observed in some patients, as well as other long-term symptoms such as fatigue, memory loss, muscle weakness, and cognitive issues (Chen et al., 2020).

The first known human COVID-19 infections were in Wuhan, Hubei, China in December of 2019, and the first related death in China was officially recorded on January 11, 2020. The first human-to-human transmission of the virus was confirmed by the World Health Organization (WHO) on January 20, 2020 and linked to a seafood market in Wuhan. Within one month of the first death, China had recorded over one thousand deaths—worse than the entire death toll from the 2002-2003 SARS outbreak in Asia. On January 23, 2020 Wuhan was placed under lockdown (Feng, 2021).

The modern world is extremely globalized though, and the lockdown came too late. There were 654 recorded cases and 18 deaths on the day Wuhan went into lockdown, but only a week later, when the UK announced its first confirmed case, there were 9,927 cases confirmed worldwide and 213 deaths (Clarke et al., 2020). And Europe was about to be hit hard. Italy recorded its first local case in late February, though it is clear that the virus had been lurking for at least a month prior, if not longer (Saplakoglu, 2020). Spain and France both began to see spikes in cases, leading to a variety in national and local measures to try to slow the spread. Belgium in particular struggled, as their three regions disagreed over the proper policies to enact to balance economic losses with disease control (Amaro, 2020). As of late November, there had been almost 15 million cases reported in Europe (Clarke et al. 2020).

By March 2020 the WHO had declared COVID-19 a pandemic. The Middle East, and Iran in particular, were badly affected. The United States passed a $2 Trillion emergency package. In April the world hit 1 million recorded cases. The world hit 1.5 million only 6 days later (Clarke et al., 2020). Worldwide, from the beginning of January 2020 until the end of March, 2022, there have been around 467 million cases of COVID-19 reported, including approximately 6.1 million deaths (Clarke et al., 2020).

## Methods and Hypotheses

Those millions of cases exist in countries where there is a large amount of variation, and I am interested in whether decisions about pandemic planning can be linked to future time reference in language. Basically, do countries who, because of the structure of the language they speak, make policy decisions that had different outcomes in the beginning of the COVID-19 pandemic? And what are the moral implications of this? For the purpose of this study I used the beginning of the pandemic, the time period including the first few months that we knew about COVID-19 and countries began implementing policy to deal with it to look at the policy stringency measures. I chose to look at the beginning of the pandemic as a more rigorous test of the effects of the country's pre-planning for crises such as these, rather than their ability to pivot after a crisis is already occurring. Additionally, there are three ways that I looked at how hard the pandemic has hit each country—cumulative cases per million, cumulative deaths per million, and fatality rate, and for each of these measures there are countries that have fared relatively well and countries that have suffered worse (see Table 1). For these measures I examined data a little further into the pandemic (November 2020) in order to be able to include more countries in the data and more variability. In terms of cumulative cases per million, the range varied from only 3 cases in Laos and Vanuatu all the way to 49,958 in Bahrain. Likewise, cumulative deaths per million hovered at or near zero in several countries (Tanzania, Vietnam, Taiwan, Burundi, Thailand, and Papua New Guinea), but reached as high as 1,265 in Belgium. The fatality rate was essentially zero in Cambodia, Eritrea, Mongolia, Bhutan, the Seychelles, Fiji, and Singapore, however in Yemen, where the pandemic and a preexisting humanitarian crisis collided, there was a fatality rate of 29.2% (Roser et al., 2020).

**Table 1:** *Descriptive Statistics of Pandemic Severity Measures (The range of how bad things were in each included country as of November 2020)*

| | Number of Countries Included | Minimum | Maximum | Mean | Std. Deviation |
|---|---|---|---|---|---|
| **Cumulative Cases Per Million** | 173 | 3 | 49,958 | 9908.84 | 12,016.72 |
| **Cumulative Deaths Per Million** | 162 | 0 | 1,265 | 194.04 | 255.96 |
| **Fatality Rate** | 168 | 0 | 29.2 | 2.2 | 2.58 |

Another way to compare countries' pandemic results is through their policy responses. Researchers at Oxford University's Blavatnik School of Government have a COVID-19 Government Response Tracker project in which they systematically collect information on policy indicators from countries around the world (Hale et al., 2020). These policies are common policy measures, such as stay-at-home orders, mask mandates, and restrictions on gatherings (see Appendix A for full list). The researchers have then indexed the results of the responses to each category, resulting in an additive score for each country. They note that these scores should only be used in a comparative manner and not interpreted as a rating of how well any given country is handling the pandemic (Hale et al., 2020).

The severity of the COVID-19 pandemic in any given country could also be related to other factors, such as geographic location, state wealth, or the availability of healthcare to the general population in that country. To account for these, I used both per capita gross domestic product (World Bank, 2020), a categorical continent variable, and a dummy variable for universal healthcare. For our purposes, countries with universal healthcare are those that offer healthcare to "more than 90% of their citizens" and "regulate the healthcare system to ensure that the care given is sufficient and that taking advantage of this care does not provide a financial hardship to citizens" (World Population Review, 2020).

The independent variable of interest for this study is what Chen (2013) refers to as Strong FTR (strong future-time reference), as opposed to what Dahl (2000) describes as "futureless" (and what I refer to as Weak FTR): those languages that do not require a future-time reference in a prediction-based context. This criterion was adopted from the European Science Foundation's Typology of Languages in Europe (EUROTYP) project (Dahl, 2000) and has been used as a proxy for how future time is treated by a language (Chen, 2013). The working group that developed the EUROTYP project created an exhaustive program to categorize languages, however Chen (2013) performed additional validation using coding of online weather forecasts finding strong evidence in favor of the EUROPYP classifications. See Appendix B for a list of countries, languages, and their FTR classification.

In 2013 work, Chen found that weak FTR language speakers are more likely to implement practices with long-term benefits. These are issues of intertemporal choice—making some sort of sacrifice in the present for the sake of future benefits. Healthcare policy generally, but pandemic planning specifically by its very nature, is a matter of intertemporal choice. By investing time and resources into planning for a pandemic that may or may not one day happen, a nation will necessarily forgo other things to which that time and money could have gone. If Chen is correct, and speakers of languages in which the future "feels more distant" have a harder time planning for the future when there is a cost involved in the present, countries whose official language does not require a future-time reference should have stronger healthcare policies and be better prepared to handle a pandemic. My hypotheses are thus:

H1: Countries with weak FTR will have better health outcomes with regard to the COVID-19 pandemic (a lower cumulative cases per million, cumulative deaths per million and fatality rate)

H2: Countries with weak FTR will have had stronger initial policy responses to the virus (higher levels of stringency in February 2020)

## Results and Discussion

In order to test the first hypothesis, I estimated a linear regression model that included variables for 2019 GDP, the continent where each country is located, and the dummy variable for universal healthcare along with the variable for Strong or Weak FTR, first with cumulative cases per million as the dependent variable (Table 2). A significant regression equation was found ($F(4,153)=19.802$, $p<.001$), with an $R^2$ of .341. All of the non-constant variables included contributed significantly to the model.

The next model looked at cumulative deaths per million as the dependent variable (Table 3), and again, a significant regression equation was found ($F(5, 138)=12.479$, $p<.001$), however in this model only universal healthcare and continent independently contribute. So, while the model does predict COVID-19 deaths per million, there is no indication that FTR contributes in this particular model.

The parallel model (Table 4) does not significantly predict the COVID-19 fatality rate at all ($F(4,150)=1.436$, $p=.225$). Surprisingly, even if FTR is removed from the model, GDP, universal healthcare and continent don't predict fatality rate either.

**Table 2:** *Regression Analysis FTR and Cumulative Cases Per Million*

| | B | Standard Error | Significance | R2 | Significance |
|---|---|---|---|---|---|
| Constant | -.5222.492 | 2886.34 | .072 | | |
| Strong FTR | 5832.132 | 2490.454 | .020 | | |
| GDP Per Cap | .265 | .048 | .000 | | |
| Univ Health | 4551.275 | 1847.64 | .015 | | |
| Continent | 1844.021 | 738.615 | .014 | | |
| | | | | | |
| Model | | | | .341 | .000 |

**Table 3:** *Regression Analysis FTR and Cumulative Deaths Per Million*

| | B | Standard Error | Significance | R2 | Significance |
|---|---|---|---|---|---|
| Constant | -126.729 | 62.766 | .045 | | |
| Strong FTR | 57.468 | 54.041 | .289 | | |
| GDP Per Cap | .002 | .001 | .152 | | |
| Univ Health | 77.664 | 41.552 | .046 | | |
| Continent | 92.864 | 16.454 | .000 | | |
| | | | | | |
| Model | | | | .306 | .000 |

**Table 4:** *Regression Analysis FTR and Fatality Rate*

| | B | Standard Error | Significance | R2 | Significance |
|---|---|---|---|---|---|
| Constant | 2.651 | .755 | .001 | | |
| Strong FTR | -.151 | .652 | .817 | | |
| GDP Per Cap | -1.673E-5 | .000 | .188 | | |
| Univ Health | -.705 | .495 | .156 | | |
| Continent | .186 | .197 | .347 | | |
| | | | | | |
| Model | | | | .037 | .225 |

The second hypothesis was regarding policy stringency in February 2020, back in the early days of the pandemic. To test this, I estimated a regression model similar to the above, however I used the policy stringency variable taken from the Oxford Coronavirus Government Response Tracker project as the dependent variable. A significant regression equation was found ($F(4,149)=2.693$, $p<.05$), and both FTR and universal healthcare contribute significantly at the .05 threshold, providing support for the hypothesis.

**Table 5:** *Regression Analysis FTR and Policy Stringency February 2020*

| | B | Standard Error | Significance | R2 | Significance |
|---|---|---|---|---|---|
| Constant | 13.651 | 3.107 | .000 | | |
| Strong FTR | -6.321 | 2.681 | .020 | | |
| GDP Per Cap | -1.994E-5 | .000 | .696 | | |
| Univ Health | 3.944 | 1.981 | .048 | | |
| Continent | -.873 | .794 | .273 | | |
| | | | | | |
| Model | | | | .069 | .033 |

## Discussion and Conclusion

Countries are all working with limited budgets and are only able to allocate money to so many things. There are things that demand immediate attention, such as employee salaries and military equipment purchases and things where the payoff isn't quite so immediate. Money spent on climate change initiatives, for example, would fall into this category. Any expenditures that we make on the prevention of global warming isn't meant to benefit us today, but in the indeterminate future. Sacrificing programs and items that we could have now for things that could potentially be good for us someday isn't easy or even desirable for everyone, and there is variation across people and across cultures in how we approach this balance.

When it comes to pandemic planning, we find a good example of this very question. The administration of healthcare policy can be expensive. For example, in the United States the budget for the Center for Disease Control and Prevention is currently around $15.5 Billion per year and the National Institutes of Health's is over $43 Billion. You could buy textbooks for every schoolkid in the country for that, with money left over to pave some bumpy highways. But is it the *right* thing to do, to only buy the things that we can use now, or to make policy decisions that are beneficial to the people that are around now? As discussed above, many philosophers would say no.

A surface-level understanding of "temperance" would perhaps limit one's understanding to situations like, not indulging in rich foods today in order to preserve one's health later in life. This is not incorrect; however, we can expand this idea into a broader understanding of the ethical implications. Societies could, perhaps, have an ethical obligation to temper their behavior and spending on items and programs that are only beneficial immediately in order to invest in the future. Not replace everyone's school books every year and stockpile some personal protection equipment instead.

In this study I had hypothesized that there would be a relationship between futured language, and the outcomes related to pandemic planning. I find only mixed support for the hypothesized connection, however. While future time reference did contribute to a model estimating cumulative deaths and stringent pandemic policy, it did not contribute to the model estimating cumulative deaths per million, and the model estimated for fatality fate didn't work at all. The sporadic nature of these results leads me to believe that this very cursory first look at the data may be missing variables that are necessary for accurately modeling public health outcomes such as these. I continue to have confidence in my hypotheses, however future studies should add variables to account for potentialities such as the age and health of the populations, preexisting conditions in the populations, the quality of the medical facilities and healthcare in the country, and the population's general attitude toward the severity of the virus. Any of these things could be an intervening factor in the outcomes that I looked at in this study.

More importantly, this study adds a new element to the discussion of how policies are formulated to prepare for things that may or may not happen in the future. Yes, factors such as state wealth and politics have clear impacts on how countries prepare (or don't prepare) for events like pandemics, however there are likely more cultural factors at play as well. There is evidence that there is an element of shortsightedness that is endemic to some cultures and may be related to the very foundational structures of their society, such as those sociolinguistic and existential ones discussed in this chapter. This being the case, any successful measures for social or environmental responsibility and sustainability will consider these kinds of cultural variables at their very core.

## References

Ackerman, F., & Heinzerling, L. (2002). Pricing the priceless: Cost-benefit analysis of environmental protection. *University of Pennsylvania Law Review, 150*(5), 1553-1584.

Amaro, S. (2020*). Belgium has become a Covid hotspot, and there are four reasons why*. CNBC. https://www.cnbc.com/2020/11/06/belgium-has-become-a-covid-hotspot-and-there-are-four-reasons-why.html/.

Appelt, K. C., Hardisty, D. J., & Weber, E. U. (2011). Asymmetric discounting of gains and losses: A query theory account. *Journal of Risk and Uncertainty, 43*, 107-126.

Aristotle. (2000). *Nicomachean ethics*. (R. Crisp, Trans.). Cambridge University Press.

Bittner, M. (2005). Future discourse in a tenseless language. *Journal of Semantics, 22*, 339-387.

Bhatt, V. (2014). No discounting as a moral virtue in intertemporal choice models. *Keio-IES Discussion Paper Series*, Institute for Economics Studies, Keio University. https://ideas.repec.org/p/keo/dpaper/2014-003.html.

Boroditsky, L. (2001). Does language shape thought?: Mandarin and English speakers' conceptions of time. *Cognitive Psychology, 43*, 1-22.

Brink, D. O. (2011). Prospects for temporal neutrality. *Oxford Handbooks Online*.

Broome, J. (1994). Discounting the future. *Philosophy and Public Affairs, 23*, 128–156.

Chen, M. K. (2013). The effect of language on economic behavior: Evidence from savings rates, health behaviors, and retirement assets. *American Economic Review, 103*(2), 690-731.

Chen, N., Zhou, M., Dong, X., Qu, J., Gong, F., Han, Y., Qiu, Y., Wang, J., Liu, Y., Wei, Y., Xia, J., Yu, T., Zhang, X., & Zhang, L. (2020). Epidemiological and clinical characteristics of 99 cases of 2019 novel coronavirus pneumonia in Wuhan, China: A descriptive study. *Lancet, 395*(10223), 507–513.

Clarke, S., Voce, A., Gutierrrez, P., & Hulley-Jones, F. (2020). How coronavirus spread across the globe-visualized. *The Guardian*. https://www.theguardian.com/world/ng-interactive/2020/apr/09/how-coronavirus-spread-across-the-globe-visualised.

Dahl, O. (2000). The grammar of future time reference in European languages. In Ö Dahl (Ed.), *Tense and aspect in the languages of Europe* (pp. 309-328). Mouton de Gruyter.

Deutscher, G. (2010). *Through the language glass: Why the world looks different in other languages*. Metropolitan Books.

Dinner, I. M., Johnson, E. J., Goldstein, D. G., & Liu, K. (2011). Partitioning defaults: Why people choose not to choose. *Journal of Experimental Psychology: Applied, 17*(4), 332-341. https://doi.org/10.1037/a0024354

EBioMedicine. (2020). COVID-19 and vascular disease. *EBioMedicine, 58*, 102966.

EPA. (2010). *Guidelines for preparing economic analyses: Discounting future benefits and costs.* https://19january2021snapshot.epa.gov/sites/static/files/2017-09/documents/ee-0568-06.pdf.

Esty, D., Levy, M., Srebotnjak, T., de Sherbinin, A., Kim, C., & Anderson, B. (2006). *Pilot 2006 Environmental Performance Index.* Yale Center for Environmental Law & Policy, and Palisades NY: Center for International Earth Science Information Network (CIESIN), Columbia University.

Feng, E. (2021). Wuhan's lockdown memories 1 year later: Pride, anger, deep pain. *NPR.* https://www.npr.org/sections/goatsandsoda/2021/01/23/959618838/wuhans-lockdown-memories-one-year-later-pride-anger-deep-pain

Greenberg, J. (2020). Federal pandemic money fell for years. Trump's budgets didn't help. *PolitiFact.* https://www.politifact.com/article/2020/mar/30/federal-pandemic-money-fell-years-trumps-budgets-d/.

Hale, T., Webster, S., Petherick, A., Phillips, T., & Kira, B. (2020). *Government Stringency Index.* Oxford COVID-19 Government Response Tracker, Blavatnik School of Government.

Hardisty, D. J., Orlove, B., Krantz, D. J., Small, A. A., Milch, K. F., & Osgood, D. E. (2012). About time: An integrative approach to effective environmental policy. *Global Environmental Change, 22*, 684-694.

Harrod, R. (1948). *Towards a dynamic economics*. Macmillan.

Hechavarria, D., Brieger, S., & Terjesen, S. (2020). Cross-cultural implications of linguistic future time reference and institutional voids on social entrepreneurship. *SSRN.* https://papers.ssrn.com/sol3/papers.cfm?abstract_id =3634263.

Hoffman, J. R., & Kanzaria, H. K. (2014). Intolerance of error and culture of blame drive medical excess. *BMJ, 49*. doi: 10.1136/bmj.g5702

Hsu, A., Emerson, J., Levy, M., de Sherbinin, A., Johnson, L., Malik, O., Schwartz, J., & Jaiteh, M. (2014). *The 2014 Environmental Performance Index*. Yale Center for Environmental Law and Policy. http://www.epi.yale.edu.

Hume, D. (1739) *A treatise on human nature*. Clarendon Press.

Hussein, B. A. S. (2012). The sapir-whorf hypothesis today. *Theory and Practice in Language Studies,* 2(3), 642-646.

Kaufman, N. S. (2011). A practical roadmap for the perilous journey from a culture of entitlement to a culture of accountability. *Journal of Healthcare Management, 56*(5), 299–304.

Kim, J., Jeong, E., & Jun, J. (2021). The effect of future time reference on consumers' travel and dining-out spending across countries. *Current Issues in Tourism, 25*(8), 1325-1340.

Lakoff, F. (1993). The contemporary theory of metaphor. In A. Ortony (Ed.), *Metaphor and Thought* (2nd ed.; pp. 202-251). Cambridge University Press.

Levinson, S. (1996). Frames of reference and Molyneux's question: Cross linguistic evidence. In P. Bloom & M. Peterson (Eds.), *Language and Space* (pp. 109-169) MIT Press.

Liberman, N., & Trope, Y. (2008). The psychology of transcending the here and now. *Science, 322*(5905), 1201-1205.

Lucy, J. (1992). *Grammatical categories and cognition: A case study of the linguistic relativity hypothesis.* Cambridge University Press.

Messner, M. A., Duncan, M. C., & Jensen, K. (1993). Separating the men from the girls: The gendered language of televised sports. *Gender & Society, 7*(1), 121–137.

Metcalf, J., & Mischel W. (1999). A hot/cool analysis of delay of gratification: Dynamics of willpower. *Psychological Review, 195,* 254-261.

Mischel, W., & Baker N. (1975). Cognitive appraisals and transformations in delay behavior. *Journal of Personality and Social Psychology, 31,* 254-261.

Ortiz-Ospina, E., & Roser, M. (2017). Financing healthcare. *Our World in Data.* https://ourworldindata.org/financing-healthcare.

Pindyck, R., & Rubinfeld, D. (2008). *Microeconomics.* Pearson Education Inc.

Ramsey, F. P. (1928). A mathematical theory of saving. *The Economic Journal, 38*(152), 543–589.

Roser, M., Ritchie, H., Ortiz-Ospina, E., & Hasell, J. (2020). Coronavirus pandemic (COVID-19). *Our World in Data.* https://ourworldindata.org/coronavirus

Samuelson, P. A. (1937). A note on measurement of utility. *The Review of Economic Studies, 4*(2), 155–161.

Saplakoglu, Y. (2020). *How early was the coronavirus really circulating in Italy?* Live Science. https://www.livescience.com/coronavirus-circulating-italy-earlier-thought.html.

Shultz, P. W., Nolan, J. M., Cialdini, R. B., Goldstein, N. J., & Griskevicius, V. (2008). The constructive, destructive, and reconstructive power of social norms. *Psychological Science, 18*, 429-434.

Simon, H. A. (1955). A behavioral model of rational choice. *Quarterly Journal of Economics, 69*(1), 99-118. https://doi.org/10.2307/1884852

Slobin, D. (2011). Thinking for speaking. *Annual Meeting of the Berkeley Linguistics Society, 13*. https://doi.org/10.3765/bls.v13i0.1826

Smith, A. (2017). *The theory of moral sentiments ... to which is added a dissertation on the origin of languages*. Hard Press.

Sturgeon, D. (2014). The business of the NHS: The rise and rise of consumer culture and commodification in the provision of healthcare services. *Critical Social Policy, 34*(3), 405–416.

Tang, J., Yang, J., Ye, W., & Khan, S. A. (2021). Now is the time: The effects of linguistic time reference and national time orientation on innovative new ventures. *Journal of Business Venturing, 36*(5). doi: 10.1016/j.jbusvent.2021.106142

Thieroff, R. (2000). On the areal distribution of tense-aspect categories in Europe. *Empirical Approaches to Language Typology, 6*, 265-308.

Pew Research Center. (2020). *Views of the major problems facing the country views of major problems facing the U.S.* https://www.pewresearch.org/politics/2019/12/17/views-of-the-major-problems-facing-the-country/.

World Population Review. (2020). *Countries with universal healthcare 2020.* https://worldpopulationreview.com/country-rankings/countries-with-universal-healthcare.

## Appendix A

Stringency Index: Oxford COVID-19 Government Response Tracker

The specific policy and response categories are coded as follows:

School closures:

0 - No measures
1 - recommend closing
2 - Require closing (only some levels or categories, e.g., just high school, or just public schools)
3 - Require closing all levels
No data – blank

Workplace closures:

0 - No measures
1 - recommend closing (or work from home)
2 - require closing (or work from home) for some sectors or categories of workers
3 - require closing (or work from home) all but essential workplaces (e.g., grocery stores, doctors)
No data – blank

Cancel public events:

0- No measures
1 - Recommend cancelling
2 - Require cancelling
No data – blank

Restrictions on gatherings:

0 - No restrictions
1 - Restrictions on very large gatherings (the limit is above 1000 people)
2 - Restrictions on gatherings between 100-1000 people
3 - Restrictions on gatherings between 10-100 people
4 - Restrictions on gatherings of less than 10 people
No data – blank

Close public transport:

0 - No measures

1 - Recommend closing (or significantly reduce volume/route/means of transport available)

2 - Require closing (or prohibit most citizens from using it)

Public information campaigns:

0 -No COVID-19 public information campaign

1 - public officials urging caution about COVID-19

2 - coordinated public information campaign (e.g., across traditional and social media)

No data – blank

Stay at home:

0 - No measures

1 - recommend not leaving house

2 - require not leaving house with exceptions for daily exercise, grocery shopping, and 'essential' trips

3 - Require not leaving house with minimal exceptions (e.g., allowed to leave only once every few days, or only one person can leave at a time, etc.)

No data – blank

Restrictions on internal movement:

0 - No measures

1 - Recommend movement restriction

2 - Restrict movement

International travel controls:

0 - No measures

1 - Screening

2 - Quarantine arrivals from high-risk regions

3 - Ban on high-risk regions

4 - Total border closure

No data – blank

Testing policy

0 – No testing policy

1 – Only those who both (a) have symptoms AND (b) meet specific criteria (e.g., key workers, admitted to hospital, came into contact with a known case, returned from overseas)

2 – testing of anyone showing COVID-19 symptoms

3 – open public testing (e.g., "drive through" testing available to asymptomatic people)

No data

Contract tracing

0 - No contact tracing

1 - Limited contact tracing - not done for all cases

2 - Comprehensive contact tracing - done for all cases

No data

Face coverings

0- No policy

1- Recommended

2- Required in some specified shared/public spaces outside the home with other people present, or some situations when social distancing not possible

3- Required in all shared/public spaces outside the home with other people present or all situations when social distancing not possible

4- Required outside the home at all times regardless of location or presence of other people

# Appendix B

| Country | Language | Strong\ FTR=1 |
|---|---|---|
| Afghanis | Persian | .00 |
| Albania | Albanian | 1.00 |
| Algeria | Arabic | 1.00 |
| Angola | Portuguese | 1.00 |
| Antigua | English | 1.00 |
| Argentina | Spanish | 1.00 |
| Armenia | Armenian | 1.00 |
| Australia | English | 1.00 |
| Austria | German | .00 |
| Azerbaijan | Azerbai | 1.00 |
| Bahamas | English | 1.00 |
| Bahrain | Arabic | 1.00 |
| Bangladesh | Bengali | 1.00 |
| Barbados | English | 1.00 |
| Belarus | Belarusian | 1.00 |
| Belgium | Dut/Fr/G | .00 |
| Belize | Spanish | 1.00 |
| Benin | French | 1.00 |
| Bolivia | Spanish | 1.00 |
| Bosnia | Serbo-Cr | 1.00 |
| Botswana | English | 1.00 |
| Brazil | Portuguese | 1.00 |
| Brunei | Malay | .00 |
| Bulgaria | Bulgaria | 1.00 |
| BurkinaF | French | 1.00 |
| Burundi | En/Fr/Ki | 1.00 |
| Cameroon | En/Fr | 1.00 |
| Canada | English | 1.00 |
| Cape Verde | Portuguese | 1.00 |
| CenAfRep | Sango/Fr | 1.00 |
| Chad | Arabic/F | 1.00 |
| Chile | Spanish | 1.00 |
| China | Man/Cant | .00 |
| Colombia | Spanish | 1.00 |
| Comoros | Ar/Fr/Co | 1.00 |
| Congo | French | 1.00 |
| Costa Ri | Spanish | 1.00 |
| Cote d'Ivoire | French | 1.00 |
| Croatia | Serbo-Cr | 1.00 |
| Cuba | Spanish | 1.00 |
| Cyprus | Gr/Turk | 1.00 |
| Czech | Czech | 1.00 |
| Denmark | Danish | .00 |
| Djibouti | Fr/Arabi | 1.00 |
| Dominica | English | 1.00 |
| DomRep | Spanish | 1.00 |
| DRCongo | French | 1.00 |
| Ecuador | Spanish | 1.00 |
| Egypt | Arabic | 1.00 |
| El Salvador | Spanish | 1.00 |
| EqGuinea | Sp/Fr/Po | 1.00 |
| Eritrea | Tig/Ar/E | 1.00 |
| Estonia | Estonian | .00 |
| Ethiopia | Amharic | .00 |
| Fiji | En/Hindi | 1.00 |
| Finland | Finnish | .00 |
| France | French | 1.00 |
| Gabon | French | 1.00 |
| Gambia | English | 1.00 |
| Georgia | Georgina | 1.00 |
| Germany | German | .00 |
| Greece | Greek | 1.00 |
| Grenada | English | 1.00 |
| Guatemala | Spanish | 1.00 |
| Guinea | French | 1.00 |
| GuineaBi | Portuguese | 1.00 |
| Guyana | English | 1.00 |
| Haiti | French | 1.00 |
| Honduras | Spanish | 1.00 |
| Hungary | Hungarian | 1.00 |
| Iceland | Icelandic | .00 |
| India | Hindi | 1.00 |

| | | | | | |
|---|---|---|---|---|---|
| Indonesia | Indonesian | .00 | Pakistan | Urdu | 1.00 |
| Iran | Persian | .00 | Palau | English | 1.00 |
| Iraq | Ar/Kurdi | 1.00 | Panama | Spanish | 1.00 |
| Ireland | English | 1.00 | Paraguay | Spanish | 1.00 |
| Israel | Hebrew | 1.00 | Peru | Spanish | 1.00 |
| Italy | Italian | 1.00 | Phillipi | Tagalog | 1.00 |
| Japan | Japanese | .00 | Poland | Polish | 1.00 |
| Jordan | Arabic | 1.00 | Portugal | Portuguese | 1.00 |
| Kazakhstan | Kaz/Rus | 1.00 | Qatar | Arabic | 1.00 |
| Kenya | Eng/Swa | 1.00 | Rwanda | Fre/Eng | 1.00 |
| Kiribati | English | 1.00 | Romania | Romanian | 1.00 |
| Kuwait | Arabic | 1.00 | Russia | Russian | 1.00 |
| Kyrgyzstan | Kyr/Russ | 1.00 | SaudiAr | Arabic | 1.00 |
| Latvia | Latvian | 1.00 | Senegal | French | 1.00 |
| Lebanon | Arabic | 1.00 | Serbia | Serbo-Cr | 1.00 |
| Lesotho | Sotho/En | 1.00 | Seychelles | Fr/Eng | 1.00 |
| Liberia | English | 1.00 | SierraLe | English | 1.00 |
| Libya | Arabic | 1.00 | Singapore | Tamil | 1.00 |
| Lithuania | Lithuanian | 1.00 | Slovak | Slovak | 1.00 |
| Luxembourg | Lu/Ger/F | .00 | Slovenia | Slovene | 1.00 |
| Macedonia | Macedonian | 1.00 | Solomon | English | 1.00 |
| Madagasc | Mal/Fr | 1.00 | Somalia | Ar/Som | 1.00 |
| Malawi | English | 1.00 | South Africa | English | 1.00 |
| Malaysia | Malay | .00 | South Korea | Korean | 1.00 |
| Mali | French | 1.00 | Spain | Spanish | 1.00 |
| Malta | Maltese | .00 | Sri Lanka | Tamil | 1.00 |
| Mauritania | Arabic | 1.00 | Sudan | Ar/Eng/S | 1.00 |
| Mauritius | Eng/Fr | 1.00 | Suriname | Dutch | .00 |
| Mexico | Spanish | 1.00 | Swaziland | Swazi/En | 1.00 |
| Moldova | Moldovan | 1.00 | Sweden | Swedish | .00 |
| Montenegro | Monteneg | 1.00 | Switzerland | Ger/Fr/R | .00 |
| Morocco | Arabic | 1.00 | Syria | Arabic | 1.00 |
| Mozamb | Portuguese | 1.00 | Taiwan | Mandarin | .00 |
| Namibia | English | 1.00 | Tajikistan | Persian | .00 |
| Netherlands | Dutch | .00 | Tanzania | Swah/Eng | 1.00 |
| NewZea | English | 1.00 | Thailand | Thai | 1.00 |
| Nicaragua | Spanish | 1.00 | Timor | Tet/Port | 1.00 |
| Niger | French | 1.00 | Togo | French | 1.00 |
| Nigeria | English | 1.00 | Tonga | Ton/Eng | 1.00 |
| Norway | Norwegian | .00 | TrinTob | English | 1.00 |
| Oman | Arabic | 1.00 | Tunisia | Arabic | 1.00 |

| | | | | | |
|---|---|---|---|---|---|
| Turkey | Turkish | 1.00 | Uzbek | Uzbek | 1.00 |
| UAE | Arabic | 1.00 | Vanuatu | Bis/Fr/E | 1.00 |
| Uganda | Eng/Swah | 1.00 | Venezuela | Spanish | 1.00 |
| UK | English | 1.00 | Vietnam | Vietnamese | .00 |
| Ukraine | Ukrainian | 1.00 | Yemen | Arabic | 1.00 |
| Uruguay | Spanish | 1.00 | Zambia | English | 1.00 |
| US | English | 1.00 | Zimbabwe | Sotho/En | 1.00 |

# COVID-19 MISINFORMATION ON SOCIAL MEDIA: ETHICAL QUESTIONS OF RESEARCH AND REGULATION IN THE CANADIAN CONTEXT

**Karmvir Padda[1], Sarah-May Strange[1], Barry Cartwright[1], and Richard Frank[2]**

**Abstract:** This chapter reports on Canadian research into online misinformation pertaining to the COVID-19 pandemic. The qualitative research reported on herein forms part of our longer-term goal, i.e., the development of an artificial intelligence (machine-learning) tool to assist social media platforms, online service providers and government agencies in identifying and responding to misinformation on social media. In this chapter, we consider the ethical and legal issues pertaining to qualitative analysis of social media posts and the pages and hashtags on which they appear, and the degree to which COVID-19 misinformation on social media could and should be regulated by governments and/or by the social media platforms themselves. We argue in favour of a balanced, harm-based approach, wherein rights to freedom of speech and privacy should only be abrogated when the potential harm exceeds the importance of those rights.

## Introduction

This chapter discusses the context, process and unique ethical and legal issues relating to a qualitative analysis carried out for the purpose of furthering the detection and potential regulation of COVID-19 misinformation on social media, which we carried out at the request of a Canadian governmental body. The chapter is written with a focus on the Canadian context. Such a perspective is informative, as many researchers worldwide will be navigating their nation's own legislative and

[1] International CyberCrime Research Centre, Simon Fraser University, Burnaby, B.C.

[2] School of Criminology, Simon Fraser University, Burnaby, B.C.

sociopolitical milieus; however, it is also salient given that Canada is the birthplace of the COVID-inspired "freedom convoy" protest (described below), and the origin of many COVID-19 misinformation narratives (Meyers et al., 2022; U.S. Department of State Global Engagement Center, 2020). We discuss the ethical and legal issues of social media misinformation and freedom of expression as they apply to narratives found in our analysis of social media posts: namely, amongst extreme conspiratorial themes, we found narratives decrying potential censorship and asserting fear about losing freedom of speech. Further, we review legal and ethical considerations in order to shed light on the complexities and pitfalls that legislators, social media platforms, and researchers may encounter when seeking to remediate the threat posed by COVID-19 misinformation, while balancing the need to protect citizens' rights and freedoms (Radu, 2020).

For our research purposes, we have defined disinformation as the type of propaganda that is spread intentionally through campaigns that are funded and orchestrated by hostile foreign actors (or possibly but less likely by well-heeled domestic actors) with specific political objectives in mind (e.g., influencing elections, stirring up political dissent, or undermining confidence in the targeted country and its leaders). The much-investigated and well-documented efforts by the Russian Internet Research Agency (IRA) to interfere in the 2016 Brexit referendum in the UK and the 2016 and 2020 U.S. Presidential elections would be prime examples of disinformation campaigns that were designed and carried out by a hostile foreign actor in order to disrupt normal democratic processes (Intelligence and Security Committee, 2020; Mueller, 2019; National Intelligence Council; 2021). Misinformation, on the other hand, is typically less organized and less sinister in intent, and is often spread more by grass-roots movements, sometimes (but not necessarily) based on genuine misunderstandings. The purveyors of misinformation could believe what they were saying and trying to persuade others of the legitimacy of their viewpoint. Examples of misinformation might include messages insisting that the earth is flat or that the moon landing never took place.

To express it differently, misinformation lacks the degree of orchestration, sophistication, malicious intent and/or defined set of objectives associated with disinformation campaigns, and may actually be believed by the individuals or groups that are spreading it amongst themselves. The type of COVID-19 messaging found on small Facebook groups that we examined, such as Hugs Over Masks, Illuminati Exposed, and No More Lockdowns Canada – e.g., that COVID-19 is a hoax, that COVID-19 vaccines are being used to microchip people, or that COVID-19 is part of an "elite conspiracy to de-populate the planet" – would be other prime examples of misinformation (Pennycook et al., 2020; Suarez-Lledo & Alvarez-Garcia, 2021).

## Harm

The harms associated with COVID-19 should not be underestimated. According to the World Health Organization, as of July 2022, there had been over half a billion confirmed cases of COVID-19 around the world and close to 6.5 million COVID-related deaths (WHO, 2022). According to the Centers for Disease Control and Prevention (CDC, 2022), as of July 2022, there had been over 90 million cases in the United States, and well over a million COVID-related deaths. In Canada, there had been close to four million cases and over 40,000 COVID-related deaths as of July 2022 (Government of Canada, 2022). Beyond the harm created by the virus itself, COVID-19 (and sequelae of measures intended to address it and lessen its spread) has had a massive negative impact on the economy at the local levels and national levels, while decreasing social cohesion and wellbeing (Prasad, 2020).

Over the past 20 years, people have come to rely increasingly on social media for their personal health and medical information (Suarez-Lledo & Alvarez-Garcia, 2021). COVID-19 misinformation has been likened to an "infodemic" – fast-spreading and effective false information disseminated primarily on social media, which (if left unchecked) can cause real harm by persuading people to act contrary to scientific guidance, public health policies and regulations (Yang et al., 2021). COVID-19 misinformation is especially harmful when linked to spread of the virus and to the spread of far-right ideology and violence, as seen in the so-called "freedom convoys" in Canada (Gilmore, 2022; Yang et al., 2021), which included members from the far right along with an explosion of conspiratorial, far-right media (Caddell, 2022; Gisondi et al., 2022; Gosselin-Malo, 2022). The type of far-right ideology expressed by these "freedom convoys" included ethnic nationalism (e.g., White Supremacy), xenophobia (e.g., prejudice toward ethnic minorities) and hatred of anything strange or "other" (e.g., fear or hatred of the LGBTQ+ community) (Donahue, 2021; Mieriņa & Koroļeva, 2015).

These freedom convoys were comprised of truck drivers and COVID-denial activists who came *en masse* to the Canadian capital city of Ottawa, where they blockaded (occupied) the city center with their tractor-trailers, parked on the Cenotaph, danced on the Tomb of the Unknown Soldier, urinated on the National War Memorial, stole food from the charity group Shepherds of Good Hope, and blew their air-horns night and day to ensure that the residents got no sleep (Caddell, 2022). It has been reported that White nationalists and QAnon conspiracy theorists were involved in organizational aspects of the convoy (Gosselin-Malo, 2022), and that a number of the occupiers were seen to be wielding Nazi, Confederate and pro-Trump flags (Drake, 2022; McLaren, 2022). Although ostensibly about masking requirements, lockdowns, and vaccinations, this went far beyond a simple protest against COVID-19 mandates extending to threatening people who wore masks and targeting local members of the LGBTQ+ community (Drake, 2022). Demonstrating their ignorance of the Canadian political system, the "organizers" or self-appointed "spokespersons" demanded that Canadian Prime Minister Justin Trudeau be charged with treason, and further demanded the resignation of Canadian Senators (political appointees with limited powers) and the Governor General (another political appointee who is primarily a "figurehead" representing The Queen) if they failed to get on board with the demands (Caddell, 2022). The "freedom convoys," which also involved the blockading of two of the busiest border crossings between Canada and the U.S. (Gosselin-Malo, 2022; McLaren, 2022) cost taxpayers tens of millions of dollars in security expenses, several billions in estimated business losses and disruption of international trade, while creating new political platforms for the far right (O'Connell, 2022).

We conducted our research in the earlier stages of the pandemic, prior to – or in the beginning of – the extreme politicization of COVID-19. When our data was gathered, many Canadians still went onto their balconies to cheer and bang pots and pans every evening at 7 p.m. to thank healthcare workers; now, healthcare workers face violence and anger (Johnson, 2021).

At the time of our research, one out of three people reported encountering false or misleading information about COVID-19 on social media (OECD, 2020). In the same period, 30% of people believed this misinformation, also sharing that misinformation with others (Pennycook et al., 2020).

Early COVID-19 misinformation promoted claims that the virus was a hoax, a biological weapon, or curable by home remedies, while denigrating social distancing and/or wearing masks as ineffective, and insisting that only the elderly were at risk of death (Pennycook et al., 2020). While much of this misinformation was spread on social media by misinformed individuals and groups, not to mention the usual conspiracy theorists, some of it was spread by medical professionals themselves (Rubin, 2022), whose messaging was often picked up on and amplified by the denizens of the Internet. One of the key phrases that we were on the lookout for during our research was the much re-circulated "Great Barrington Declaration," in which a group of doctors argued that government-mandated preventative measures were causing more harm than COVID-19. This declaration ran contrary to accepted medical science (Alwan et al. 2020; Archer, 2020; Rubin, 2022), yet was widely cited by people with no medical knowledge whatsoever as proof that COVID-19 was a hoax. During our research, we encountered many such COVID-19-related conspiracies, misinformation narratives, and anti-government movements in their nascent forms (Velásquez et al., 2021).

COVID-19 misinformation on social media creates undeniable harm: nevertheless, the question remains – how can Western-style democracies legally and ethically justify regulating the expression of personal opinion on social media, while proclaiming that they are in favour of free speech and user rights? Beyond this, how can researchers ethically address their participation in these efforts?

## Methodological Approach

The qualitative team followed a pre-established, well-defined set of research guidelines. That said, these guidelines evolved several times during the research process, to accommodate new discoveries and/or to refine the classification process. For example, we added "not applicable" to the other categories of "real information," "misinformation," "uninformed opinion" and "unclassified" to the drop-down menu for the classification column of our highly-articulated and rigorously-developed Excel spreadsheet. We also issued new coding guidelines, indicating that the posts should only be categorized as "not applicable" if the message was on a topic totally unrelated to COVID-19. The team commenced by manually classifying the first 100 messages in the 800 message dataset that had been manually harvested from Twitter, Facebook, Reddit, and Instagram and that had been formatted in the pre-configured Excel spreadsheet. After that, we met to review the classifications for each message on a case-by-case basis, discuss any discrepancies in coding and take into consideration any new key words, key phrases or narratives that had emerged. Thereafter, we broke into smaller teams, each team member classifying 200 messages on their own, and then meeting with the other members to again review the classifications, discuss discrepancies in coding and reconcile any differences.

After the manual coding, the data was input to NVivo (Elg & Ghauri, 2019; Wiltshier, 2011), where the team sought to extract language or discourse used in the "real information" and "misinformation" narratives and to identify the codes and sub-codes within each of those narratives that appeared in the dataset of 2,500 messages.

## Qualitative Analysis

Overall, of the 2,500 messages that were manually classified by the qualitative research team, 1,096 (43.8%) were classified as real information, 810 (32.4%) were classified as misinformation, while 594 were classified as not applicable.

For the purpose of this chapter, we will focus on misinformation – messages that contained inaccurate or misleading information, or were patently false, wildly exaggerated, or clearly designed to provoke unwarranted anger or instil unnecessary fear. Some forms of online misinformation were easy to spot – for example, the medical doctor who filmed himself wearing a surgical mask whilst vaping to demonstrate that smoke could escape from the mask (Kertscher, 2021), side-stepping the fact that surgical masks do have a proven degree of efficacy (otherwise, doctors, dentists and other medical practitioners wouldn't bother wearing them when performing medical procedures) and that nobody claimed that surgical masks were 100% airtight or impenetrable (if they were, the wearer would not be able to breathe) (Howard et al., 2021). Another example would be the "empty hospitals" campaign that consisted of COVID-deniers posting videos of empty hospital reception areas and emergency rooms as proof that the COVID-19 pandemic was a hoax (Ahmed et al., 2020), ignoring the fact that people were being told to avoid hospitals altogether unless they were extremely ill, and that hospital staff were fully occupied in other areas of the hospitals, treating extremely ill COVID patients. Other types of blatant misinformation that we have mentioned above – and that we came across with regularity in the data we analysed – include the fanciful notion that COVID-19 vaccines were being used to microchip people, or that COVID-19 was part of an elite conspiracy to de-populate the planet.

In many cases, the pages and hashtags from which we extracted and analysed this misinformation – #Chinavirus, #covidhoax2020, Covid Unmasked, #FilmYourHospital, Illuminati Exposed, #NoVaccineForMe, #plandemic and #scamdemic – spoke for themselves. That said, each post was read carefully, several times by several different researchers, and if there was uncertainty, we would check out the information on reputable sites that were presumed to offer reasonably reliable information, such as the World Health Organization, the U.S. Centre for Disease Control, or the Government of British Columbia's Centre for Disease Control, to name a few.

In our qualitative analysis, four narratives accounted for 759 (98.7%) of the 810 messages that were coded as misinformation. The most prevalent narrative (n = 228, 28.1%) concerned what we referred to as "The Instrumental Use of COVID-19 to Push Hidden or Secret Agendas." The second most prevalent narrative, "Vaccines/Treatments/Preventative Measures Aren't Safe/Don't Work," accounted for 185 (22.8%) of the messages. The third most prevalent narrative, "COVID-19 is a Hoax/Doesn't Exist/is Vastly Over-Exaggerated" appeared in 22.2% (180 messages). The "Rights/Freedoms/The Economy More Important than People's Lives" referred to issues regarding how the COVID-19 pandemic did not justify the associated harms such as lockdowns, mandatory mask-wearing, enforced social isolation, or keeping children out of school, and that people had the right to work, travel, and socialize as they saw fit.

People who posted these messages seemed proud of their resistance to efforts to restrict their movements and/or their leisure activities, with one person saying that: "I wasn't scared of getting fines or arrest on May 2nd 2020 at my first #EndLockdown Protest at Queens Park - not about to start now." Another said: "Happy to report I did four ferries this weekend without owning or wearing a face diaper. #NoCompliance #TakeOffYourMask #BreatheOxygen #ShowYourSmile #NoMasks."

Another message from #HugsOverMasks lamented the closure of gyms and other fitness facilities:

*In case people forgot how healthy & fit people workout - these are some of the best of the best within fitness industry !! unfortunately this industry like most others - the leaders are being too careful... About shining bright light on the whole assault on healthy active lifestyle & humanity, between mandating masks for all during exercise, forcing all fitness / wellness facilities shutting down... WAKE UP NOW BEFORE THE TIME IS UP...*

There was a lot of messaging about large protests, where people were evidently coming together without wearing masks, practicing social distancing or complying with lockdown mandates:

*October 17th, Toronto. Look at all these beautiful people standing up for their rights and freedoms. What a magical energy when we all come together! Post a photo of your latest activist moment and tag us @100millionmoms and #100millionmoms. We can't wait to see all the action you're taking to demand better for our kids and their future #activist #activistlife #freedomrally #idonotconsent #toronto #protest #hugsovermasks #riseupcanada #thelinecanada #standup*

One lengthy message, posted on Reddit by an individual who had immigrated to Toronto described measures such as lockdowns, curfews, and other controls as "draconian" and "ideological brainwashing":

*As an immigrant who relishes in the west's individuality and freedom, seeing it all fleet away is heartbreaking. So just for some background, I'm an immigrant living in Toronto with a middle eastern background. I moved here a few years ago and compared to most of the world, the west gives you some of the greatest freedoms ever seen to man - the US, Canada and Western Europe are parts of the world where you could truly be yourself - such freedoms and to an extent responsibility (depending on where you are), are what attracted to me to moving to the west.*

## Ethical Balances

Our findings clearly demonstrated that, amongst the extreme conspiracy theories – COVID-19 is a hoax, a biological weapon, caused by 5G; that masks are part of a government plan to create a subservient citizenry; that Bill Gates wants to microchip everyone – there were clear concerns pertaining to issues of rights and freedoms, particularly the right to freedom of expression, and especially as it relates to interference by the government. We cannot simply dismiss such concerns as unwarranted (Amnesty International, 2021).

This qualitative analysis was part of a project sponsored by the Canadian government's Minister of Heritage and Digital Citizenship Cooperation Program, as part of our longer-term goal to develop an artificial intelligence (AI) tool to assist in identifying and responding to misinformation on social media (Cartwright et al., 2019). Such a project causes us to consider unique ethical issues, due to our need to balance the harm of COVID-19 misinformation with people's rights to both privacy and freedom, made more germane by the fact that the project was undertaken on behalf of the government rather than for a social media platform. Thus, we must explore multiple ethical issues with an eye to balancing potential harms: the ethical considerations of conducting qualitative content analysis on social media data is only a starting point (Zimmer, 2010).

We must consider not only the potential actions of our own government, but also, examine the potential for contributing to the creation of precedents, as authoritarian governments have used the excuse of preventing misinformation in order to enact censorship of dissenting views (and, in Russia's case, to literally hide its commission of war crimes from its citizens) (Izadi & Ellison, 2022). To address the ethical situation properly, we must contemplate not only the harms created by COVID-19 misinformation spread by real people, but also, the instrumental use of COVID-19 misinformation by hostile foreign actors as part of ongoing foreign influence campaigns intended to sow distrust in government, media, and other authorities in order to foster polarization and weaken Western democracies (Matthews et al., 2021).

## Preventing Harm vs. Freedom of Expression: Legislation and Regulation

### Social Media Platforms

Despite widespread discussion of potential government regulation of misinformation on social media, no overarching international law has emerged. Instead, national governments have enacted their own piece-meal regulations around COVID-19 misinformation on social media (Bayer et al., 2021). Social media companies have made rules as well, and are currently the primary players that are publicly involved in monitoring and removing COVID-19 misinformation (Biggs, 2021). Social media companies – so-called "private actors" – are regulating what can and cannot be said on their platforms. Two positions emerge: (a) that private actors should not be permitted to take a controlling position in relation to human rights, as opposed to (b) private actors own the platforms that users are speaking on, and therefore have both the right and the responsibility to control content (Jorgensen & Zuleta, 2020). A case in point would be world-renowned entrepreneur Elon Musk's on-again, off-again offer to purchase Twitter, with his promise to restore "free speech," his open invitation to Donald Trump to return to the fold, and his proclamation that it was "morally wrong" to ban Donald Trump from the platform (Siddiqui & De Vycnk, 2022). In this case – assuming that he was to proceed with his purchase of Twitter, which is by no means assured – Elon Musk would be setting himself up as the arbiter of free speech and morality.

In the past, social media giants like Twitter and Facebook have been widely criticized for refusing to remove misinformation and out-and-out foreign disinformation from their platforms (Durkee, 2021; Tsesis, 2017). Social media platforms are, in most nations, unregulated, unlike broadcast and print media, which are held to standards and can face both reprimands and reputational damage (Allington et al., 2020). Social media platforms have claimed (so far with considerable success) that they should not be subject to regulation, because they are not making statements themselves, merely hosting statements made by others, for which they are not responsible (Allington et al., 2020; Gisondi et al., 2022). Additionally, many of the major social media platforms such as Twitter, Facebook, Instagram, and YouTube are headquartered in the United States, where they enjoy the protection of provisions of section 230 of the U.S. Communications Decency Act, which state: "No provider or user of an interactive computer service shall be treated as the publisher or speaker of any information provided by another information content provider" (47 U.S.C. § 230). To express it differently, social media platforms cannot be held accountable for content that is posted by users.

Furthermore, these social media platforms are corporations, not governments, and thus are not subject to same requirements as governments when it comes to protecting freedom of speech; instead, they can and do impose their own corporate policies from time-to-time (without having to respond to allegations of undue censorship) (Douek, 2021; Jørgensen & Zuleta, 2020). More recently, Twitter and Facebook have instead come under fire for removing misinformation, because they both fact-checked, warned about, and even removed what they regarded as COVID-19 misinformation – most infamously, posts by former President Trump (Rupar, 2021). They then de-platformed him altogether following his unsubstantiated claims that the 2020 U.S. Presidential election was stolen from him and the ensuing attack on the U.S. Congress by his supporters, thereby driving many of his followers on social media to "alternative" social media sites such as Telegram and Parler (Gilmore, 2022; Schulze, 2020).

Currently, Twitter removes COVID-19 misinformation "when it is confirmed to be false or misleading by subject-matter experts, such as public health authorities" (Roth & Pickles, 2020), whereas Facebook removes "false vaccine claims" (Ndiaye, 2021) and prohibits advertising if it contains "deceptive, false, or misleading claims like those relating to the effectiveness or characteristics of a product or service," including health claims pertaining to COVID-19 (Meta Business Help Center, 2022). How effectively these social media platforms do this and the standards that they apply when determining that a post is "misleading" is open to debate, but to this day, removal of misinformation by social media platforms, or even attempts to counter misinformation via fact-checking and warnings of inaccurate claims are met with cries of censorship and abuse of power – similar to the narratives revealed in our content analysis (Biggs, 2021; Radu, 2020). On the other hand, the seeming failure of social media platforms to adequately remove misinformation is greeted with demands to do more (Durkee, 2021; Radu, 2020). It could be said that they're damned if they do, and damned if they don't – yet it cannot be denied that social media platforms are the main vector of the spread of COVID-19 misinformation (Gisondi et al., 2022). With the ever-present issues and harms, governments have begun to consider more seriously the possibility of entering the fray of monitoring and directly addressing and curtailing COVID-19 misinformation on social media (Harrison, 2021; Radu, 2020). Notwithstanding the various actions taken by social media platforms to address misinformation, often under pressure from governments, the governments themselves are facing increasing pressure to address social media misinformation via legislation, raising questions about governmental restrictions on freedom of expression (Bayer et al., 2021).

## Governments

The United Nations' Universal Declaration on Human Rights states that "everyone has the right to freedom of opinion and expression," including the right to "impart information and ideas through any media…regardless of frontiers" (UN General Assembly, 1948). Freedom of speech – or, in Canada, freedom of expression – is enshrined in the Canadian Charter of Rights and Freedoms (1982), which states that individuals have the right to "freedom of thought, belief, opinion and expression, including freedom of the press and other media of communication." However, Charter rights may be limited if such limitation is "demonstrably justified in a free and democratic society" (Department of Justice, 2021). Therefore, in Canada, freedom of expression is not absolute: there are limits, and there are laws against libel, hate speech and harassment. Justification of limits is determined by the test from *R v. Oakes*: first, the goal of the limitation must be sufficiently important, and the method used to attain it must be proportionate. Second, there must be: a rational connection between the limitation and the goal; minimal impairment of rights or freedoms (only limiting the freedom as much as necessary to achieve the goal); and there must be a final balance between the harm the limitation causes and the good created by the limitation (Department of Justice, 2021). Basically, it is justifiable to limit a freedom in order to prevent serious harm. This test appears logical from an ethical standpoint, in that it demands justification for imposing limits when trying to balance harm.

The Online Streaming Act, previously known as Bill C-11, became legislation (an Act of Parliament) on June 22, 2022. Although this Act is largely intended to bring online content into line with requirements applied to other broadcast mediums in Canada – e.g., requirements for Canadian content– it has created great consternation with claims that it will restrict freedom of expression by increasing the regulatory power of the Canadian Radio-television and Telecommunications Commission (Bolongaro, 2021). Nonetheless, the Online Streaming Act has potential value, as it creates a means for Canadian regulators to exert control over foreign disinformation being streamed in Canada (Danks, 2022). A prime example might be the Russian-sponsored news outlet Russia Today, which– despite many EU nations and social media companies fully removing it from their airways and platforms – has only been removed from television in Canada, but still remains accessible online (Patel & Nuttall, 2022).

Our research team (in the course of other multi-year "disinformation" research undertaken on behalf of the Canadian defense department) has conducted extensive background research into and qualitative analysis of the messaging on Russia Today, and can state categorically that this "news" outlet unabashedly pushes out precisely the type of Kremlin-authorised propaganda referred to earlier in this chapter as an exemplar of state-organised, state-funded disinformation. And unlike most media outlets in Western nations, the "journalists" who work for these Russian government news outlets rarely if ever depart from the official government line, unless they have complete disregard for their own personal safety and the safety of their family, friends, and colleagues. We need look no further than the well-documented instances of Russian journalists who have been imprisoned or killed as a consequence of their failure to toe the official government line (Committee to Protect Journalists, 2022; Reporters Without Borders, 2022), not to mention the Russian government's recent introduction of a law against publishing what they describe as "false information" about the actions of Russian forces in Ukraine, with a possible sentence of 15 years in prison, causing 150 journalists to flee Russia in the two week period following their invasion of Ukraine (Human Rights Watch, 2022). The Russian example is particularly relevant, not only as it relates to direct disinformation from state-sponsored sources (much of it, at the present, relating to Russia's invasion of Ukraine), but also as it relates to significant harm that must go into our ethical balance: Russia's use of COVID-19 misinformation on social media as part of its ongoing foreign interference campaigns (European Union, 2022; Matthews et al., 2021).

## COVID-19 Misinformation: Weapon for Foreign Interference vs. Excuse for Censorship

Russian foreign interference campaigns frequently use misinformation and conspiracies (including, those about COVID-19) that originate from "real people"; instead of creating disinformation from whole cloth, Russia often amplifies existing misinformation, using it for its own political ends (Johnson & Marcellino, 2021). Even if a post was made by a real person, who truly believes it, the content of that post may itself originate in deliberately-created foreign disinformation; on the other hand, Russian state-sponsored media, like Russia Today, will often promote fake news and conspiracies that originated in misinformation (Matthews et al., 2021; Myers & Thompson, 2022). In addition to creating its own false media, Russia has provided funding to media which spreads false information that Russia finds useful. Russia hires real people (e.g., freelance writers) to write articles that hit key points; alternatively, Russia provides funding (sometimes hidden) to pre-existing domestic misinformation media (Johnson & Marcellino, 2021; Matthews et al., 2021). While Western media may use similar techniques when it comes to hiring journalists and freelance writers who subscribe to or are willing to support their political leanings, and/or may even fire journalists who refuse to "get with the program" – as Fox News did when they fired Chris Stirewalt when he correctly predicted Donald Trump's 2020 loss in Arizona (Sullivan, 2022) – they are somewhat more circumspect in their approach, given that their misdeeds can be widely reported and ridiculed (without fear) by other news outlets, and that (fortunately) the governments of Western "democratic" nations have yet to embark on a program of arresting, imprisoning and sometimes killing journalists who do not support the current political leader(s) and their administrations.

Canada plays an unfortunate part in COVID-19 misinformation – one of the most influential purveyors of COVID-19 misinformation is a Canadian website, Global Research, which is recognised as a Russian disinformation proxy (U.S. Department of State Global Engagement Center, 2020). Russia has used COVID-19 misinformation as part of its foreign interference campaigns against western democracies such as Canada, the United States, Australia, Romania, among others (Biggs, 2021; Bruns et al., 2020; Johnson & Marcellino, 2021; Magdin, 2020; Matthews et al., 2021). Russia has wielded COVID-19 misinformation in foreign interference (disinformation) campaigns worldwide, using COVID-19-based conspiracies and anger to foment distrust in governments, science, and the mainstream media, while encouraging division and chaos, all as part of its efforts to divide, undermine, and weaken Western democracy (Bentzen, 2020; Johnson & Marcellino, 2021; Matthews et al., 2021).

Beyond weakening Western democracies, Russia has seemingly used COVID-19 misinformation on social media in an attempt to bolster and justify its invasion of Ukraine, while also using this misinformation to create suspicion and extreme distrust of international organizations such as NATO, the UN and the EU (Buziashvilli, 2022; Johnson & Marcellino, 2021; Magdin, 2020; Matthews et al., 2021; Scott, 2022). By using COVID-19 misinformation to paint these international organizations as being shadowy, tyrannical, and elitist, with mainstream media acting as their servants, Russia has created an environment where people are susceptible to believing Russian narratives and denials of atrocities (Buziashvilli, 2022; European Union, 2022; Myers & Thompson, 2022). In Canada, for instance,

Telegram channels which previously hosted discussions of the so-called "freedom convoy" protests against COVID-19 mandates are now filled with pro-Russia, anti-Ukraine disinformation (Gilmore, 2022). Thus, we encounter a new concern to add to our ethical balance: do hostile foreign governments have the same right to freedom of expression that our own citizens and journalists enjoy when it comes to our Western media?

An easy question to answer, one might think. However, we must also be aware of the potential danger from governments such as these, and our potential for empowering their repression – as well as creating precedents for the future of our own nations (Amnesty International, 2021; Bleyer-Simon, 2021). Authoritarian governments have seized upon the excuse of "preventing disinformation" to enact harsh censorship of independent media and even of social media (Bayer et al., 2021; Bleyer-Simon, 2021; Harrison, 2021). As noted above, since invading Ukraine, Russia has viciously tightened its restrictive hold, banning any references to "war" or "invasion" under threat of 15-year prison sentences (Izadi & Ellison, 2022; Troianovski, 2022). Using the excuse of preventing harmful information, Russia has forced the shutdown of all independent media, and banned the majority of social media platforms, cutting many Russians off from anything other than official government propaganda (Izadi & Ellison, 2022; Waters, 2022). This is the authoritarianism and complete loss of a voice (other than the government's voice) that our research findings indicated many people feared (Harrison, 2021). It is understandable, therefore, that most Western democracies have shied away from such strong anti-misinformation measures. There is always a possibility that governmental restriction on social media speech could create a precedent for the authoritarian censorship of dissent (Bleyer-Simon, 2021).

## The Final Balance?

Justification for removing or suppressing speech should be about balance. While we have probed various ethical dilemmas in great depth, we ultimately concluded that certain restrictions on freedom of expression were justified – or balanced out – by taking into consideration the prevention of harm. COVID-19 misinformation is harmful in and of itself, as it encourages the spread of the virus and the fostering of political polarization (Gisondi et al., 2022; Pennycook et al., 2020). It can also be harmful in other ways, for example, when it is deliberately deployed by hostile nations as part of foreign interference campaigns, as Russia has done (Johnson & Marcellino, 2021; Matthews et al., 2021). Social media is powerful, and with power comes responsibility. The right to freedom of speech is not a blank cheque. While our findings show that users were deeply concerned with freedom, censorship, and control, we have also presented examples in this chapter of authoritarian governments unjustifiably censoring their citizens and media under the guise of "combatting disinformation." It is our hope that citizens, academics, community leaders and politicians alike can take part in assuring that both governments and companies meet reasonable standards, and together strive to achieve a balance between rights and harms. Our ongoing wrangling with ethical dilemmas as part of our own research can be viewed as part of this effort.

## References

Abiantoro, D., & Kusumo, D. S. (2020). Analysis of web content quality information on the Koseeker website using the web content audit method and ParseHub tools. *8th International Conference on Information and Communication Technology (ICoICT)*, 2020, 1-6. https://doi.org/10.1109/ICoICT49345.2020.9166396

Ahmed, W., Seguí, F. L., Vidal-Alaball, J., & Katz, M. S. (2020). Covid-19 and the "film your hospital" conspiracy theory: Social network analysis of Twitter data. *Journal of medical Internet research, 22*(10), e22374. https://preprints.jmir.org/preprint/22374

Allington, D., Duffy, B., Wessely, S., Dhavan, N., & Rubin, J. (2020). Health-protective behaviour, social media usage, and conspiracy belief during the COVID-19 public health emergency. *Psychological Medicine, 51*(10), 1763–1769. https://doi.org/10.1017/S003329172000224X

Alwan, N. A., Burgess, R. A., Ashworth, S., Beale, R., Bhadelia, N., Bogaert, D., Dowd, J., Eckerle, I., Goldman, L. R., Greenhalgh, T., Gurdasani, D., Hamdy, A., Hanage, W. P., Hodcroft, E. B., Hyde, Z., Kellam, P., Kelly-Irving, M., Krammer, F., Lipsitch, M., McNally, A., ... Ziauddeen, H. (2020). Scientific consensus on the COVID-19 pandemic: We need to act now. *Lancet (London, England), 396*(10260), e71–e72. https://doi.org/10.1016/S0140-6736(20)32153-X

Archer, S. (2020). 5 failings of the Great Barrington Declaration. *Queen's Gazette*. https://www.queensu.ca/gazette/stories/5-failings-great-barrington-declaration

Article 19, *United Kingdom (England and Wales)*. (2018). *Responding to 'hate speech.'* www.article19.org/wp-content/uploads/2018/06/UK-hate-speech_March-2018.pdf

Amnesty International. (2021). *Silenced and misinformed: Freedom of expression in danger during COVID*. https://www.amnesty.org/en/documents/pol30/4751/ 2021/en/

Bayer, J., Katsirea, I., Batura, O., Holznagel, B., Hartmann, S., & Lubianiec, K. (2021). *The fight against disinformation and the right to freedom of expression*. https://www.europarl.europa.eu/RegData/etudes/STUD/2021/695445/IPOL_STU(2021)695445_EN.pdf

Bentzen, N. (2020). *COVID-19 foreign influence campaigns: Europe and the global battle of narratives*. https://www.europarl.europa.eu/RegData/etudes/BRIE/2020/649367/EPRS_BRI(2020)649367_EN.pdf.

Berghel, H. (2017). Lies, damn lies, and fake news. *Computer, 50*(2), 80-85. https://doi.ieeecomputersociety.org/10.1109/MC.2017.56

Bernard, R., Bowser, G., Sullivan R., & Gibson-Fall, F. (2020). Disinformation and epidemics: Anticipating the next phase of biowarfare. *Health Security, 19*(1), 1-12. http://dx.doi.org/10.1136/bmjgh-2020-004206

Biggs, T. (2021). Twitter expands efforts in AI-assisted war on COVID fake news. *Sydney Morning Herald*. http://www.smh.com.au/technology/twitter-s-expands-efforts-in-ai-assisted-war-on-covid-fake-news-20210714-p589oa.html

Bleyer-Simon, K. (2021). Government repression disguised as anti-disinformation action: Digital journalists' perception of COVID-19 policies in Hungary. *Intellect Limited 2021 Journal of Digital Media & Policy, 12*(1), 159–176. https://doi.org/10.1386/jdmp_00053_1

Bolongaro, K. (2021). Trudeau's party passes bill to regulate social media, streaming. *Bloomberg*. https://www.bloomberg.com/news/articles/2021-06-22/trudeau-s-party-passes-bill-to-regulate-social-media-streaming

Breiman, L. (2001). Random forests. *Machine Learning, 45*, 5-32. https://link.springer.com/content/pdf/10.1023/A:1010933404324.pdf

Bruns, A., Harrington, S., & Hurcombe, E. (2020). 'Corona? 5G? or both?': The dynamics of COVID-19/5G conspiracy theories on Facebook. *Media International Australia, 177*(1), 12–29. https://doi.org/10.1177/1329878X20946113

Buziashvilli, E. (2022). *Kremlin media used claims of Ukraine creating a dirty bomb to justify invasion.* DFRLab. https://medium.com/dfrlab/kremlin-media-used-claims-of-ukraine-creating-a-dirty-bomb-to-justify-invasion-3c8bd6b45884

Caddell, A. (2022). The MOU says everything you need to know about the truckers protest. *The Hill Times.* www-hilltimes-com.proxy.lib.sfu.ca/2022/02/02/the-mou-says-everything-you-need-to-know-about-the-truckers-protest/341596

*Canadian Charter of Rights and Freedoms,* s8, Part 1 of the *Constitution Act,* 1982, being Schedule B to the Canada Act 1982 (UK), c 11, 1982.

Cartwright, B, Weir, G. R. S., & Frank, R. (2019). Fighting disinformation warfare with artificial intelligence: Identifying and combating disinformation attacks. *Tenth International Conference on Cloud Computing, GRIDS, and Virtualization,* May 2019, 67-72.

Centers for Disease Control and Prevention (2022). *COVID data tracker.* https://covid.cdc.gov/covid-data-tracker/

Committee to Protect Journalists (2022). 82 Journalists and media workers killed in Russia: Between 1992 and 2022 / motive confirmed or unconfirmed. https://cpj.org/data/killed/europe/russia/

Comstock, G. (2012). *Research ethics: A philosophical guide to the responsible conduct of research.* Cambridge University Press.

*Criminal Code,* RSC 1985, c C-46, s 318(1)(a), 1985.

Department of Justice. (2021). *Section 1 – Reasonable limits.* Government of Canada. https://www.justice.gc.ca/eng/csj-sjc/rfc-dlc/ccrf-ccdl/check/art1.html

Desai, S., Mooney, H., & Oehrli, J. A. (2019). *"Fake news," lies and propaganda: How to sort fact from fiction.* https://guides.lib.umich.edu/fakenews

Donahue, K. C. (2021). American far right ideologies have spread to Europe. *Social Anthropology, 28*(2), 344-346. https://doi-org.proxy. lib.sfu.ca/10.1111/1469-8676.13054

Douek, E. (2021). The free speech blind spot: Foreign election interference on social media. In J. D. Ohlin & D. B. Hollis (Eds.), *Defending democracies* (pp. 265-292). Oxford University Press.

Drake, A. (2022). So-called "Freedom Convoy" is a symptom of a deeply unequal society: How Ottawa police treat White protesters compared to others including Black and Indigenous people reveals an entrenched Canadian double standard. Policy Options. How Ottawa police treat White protesters compared to others including Black and Indigenous people reveals an entrenched Canadian double standard. https://policyoptions.irpp.org/magazines/february-2022/so-called-freedom-convoy-is-a-symptom-of-a-deeply-unequal-society/

Durkee, A. (2021). Biden says Facebook, tech platforms are "killing people" by spreading misinformation on COVID vaccines. *Forbes*. https://www.forbes.com/sites/alisondurkee/2021/07/16/biden-says-facebook-tech-platforms-are-killing-people-by-spreading-misinformation-on-covid-vaccines/?sh=dfda29e39f09

European Union. (2022). *Disinformation about Russia's invasion of Ukraine - Debunking seven myths spread by Russia*. https://www.eeas.europa.eu/delegations/china/disinformation-about-russias-invasion-ukraine-debunking-seven-myths-spread-russia_en

Gilmore, R. (2022). 'Freedom convoy' forums find new focus: Disinformation about Russia-Ukraine war. *Global News*. https://globalnews.ca/news/8659667/ukraine-russia-convoy-misinformation-conspiracy/

Gisondi, M. A., Barber, R., Faust, J. S., Raja, A., Strehlow, M. C., Westafer, L. M., & Gottlieb, M. (2022). A deadly infodemic: Social media and the power of COVID-19 misinformation. *Journal of Medical Internet Research, 24*(2), 1–13. https://doi.org/10.2196/35552

Gosselin-Malo, E. (2022). Canada's "Freedom Convoy": A far right protest, explained. *Italian Institute for International Political Studies*. https://www.ispionline.it/en/pubblicazione/canadas-freedom-convoy-far-right-protest-explained-33192

Government of Canada (2022). *COVID-19 daily epidemiology update*. https://health-infobase.canada.ca/covid-19/epidemiological-summary-covid-19-cases.html

Hall, M., Frank, E., Holmes, G., Pfahringer, B., Reutemann, P., & Witten, I. H. (2009). The WEKA data mining software: An update. *ACM SIGKDD explorations newsletter, 11*(1), 10-18. https://doi.org/10.1145/1656274.1656278

Harrison, R. (2021). Tackling disinformation in times of crisis: The European Commission's response to the COVID-19 infodemic and the feasibility of a consumer-centric solution. *Utrecht Law Review, 17*(3), 18–33. https://doi.org/10.36633/ULR.675/METRICS/

Heilferty, C. M. (2011). Ethical considerations in the study of online illness narratives: A qualitative review. *Journal of Advanced Nursing, 67*(5), 945-953. doi: 10.1111/j.1365-2648.2010.05563.x

Howard, J., Huang, A., Li, Z., Tufekci, Z., Zdimal, V., van der Westhuizen, H. M., ... & Rimoin, A. W. (2021). An evidence review of face masks against COVID-19. *Proceedings of the National Academy of Sciences, 118*(4), e2014564118. https://doi.org/10.1073/pnas.2014564118

Hudson, D. L. (2019). Free speech or censorship? Social media litigation is a hot legal battleground, *ABA Journal*. http://wwwr.abajournal.com/magazine/article/social-clashes-digital-free-speech

Human Rights Watch. (2022). Russia criminalizes independent war reporting, anti-war protests: 'Discrediting' armed forces, calling to end the war, backing sanctions become crimes. https://www.hrw.org/news/2022/03/07/russia-criminalizes-independent-war-reporting-anti-war-protests

Intelligence and Security Committee. (2020). *Russia: Presented to Parliament pursuant to section 3 of the Justice and Security Act 2013.* https://assets.documentcloud.org/documents/6999013/20200721-HC632-CCS001-CCS1019402408-001-ISC.pdf

Izadi, E., & Ellison, S. (2022). Russia's independent media, long under siege, teeters under new Putin crackdown. *The Washington Post,* Mar 4, 2022. https://www.washingtonpost.com/media/2022/03/04/putin-media-law-russia-news/

Jankowski, N. W. (2018). Researching fake news: A selective examination of empirical studies. *Javnost-The Public, 25*(1-2), 248-255. https://doi.org/10.1080/13183222.2018.1418964

Johnson, C., & Marcellino, W. (2021). *Bad actors in news reporting: Tracking news manipulation by state actors.* RAND Corporation. https://doi.org/10.7249/RRA112-21

Johnson, S. (2021, June 7). Spat at, abused, attacked: Healthcare staff face rising violence during COVID. *The Guardian*. https://www.theguardian.com/global-development/2021/jun/07/spat-at-abused-attacked-healthcare-staff-face-rising-violence-during-covid

Jørgensen, R. F., & Zuleta, L. (2020). Private governance of freedom of expression on social media platforms. *Nordicom Review, 41*(1), 51–67. https://doi.org/10.2478/nor-2020-000351

Judiciary of Scotland (2018). *PF v Mark Meecham,* 2018. http://www.scotland-judiciary.org.uk/8/1962/PF-v-Mark-Meechan

Kertscher, T. (2021). No, a vaping demo doesn't prove that masks don't work against COVID-19. *POLITIFACT, The Poynter Institute.* https://www.politifact.com/factchecks/2021/feb/08/facebook-posts/no-vaping-demo-doesnt-prove-masks-dont-work-agains/

Kitchin, H.A. (2002). The Tri-Council on cyberspace: Insights, oversights, and extrapolations. In W.C. Van den Hoonaard (Ed.), *Walking the tightrope: Ethical issues for qualitative researchers* (pp. 160-173). University of Toronto Press.

Knazan, B. (2016). *R. v. Elliott,* vol. [2016] ONCJ 310, 2016.

Krause, N. M., Freiling, I., Beets, B., & Brossard. D. (2020). Fact-checking as risk communication: The multilayered risk of misinformation in times of COVID-19. *Journal of Risk Research, 23*(7-8), 1052-1059.

Kshetri, A., & Voas, J. (2017). The economics of 'fake news.' *IEEE Computer Society, 19*(6), 8-12. https://doi.org/10.1109/MITP.2017.424145

Lazer, D. M. J., Baum, M. A., Benkler, Y., Berinsky, A. J., Greenhill, K. M., Menczer, F., Metzger, M. J., Nyhan, B., Pennycook, G., Rothschild, D., Schudson, M., Sloman, S. A., Sunstein, C. R., Thorson, E. A., Watts, D. J., & Zittrain, J. L. (2018). The science of fake news. *Science, 359*(6380), 1094–1096.

Liaw, A., & Wiener, M. (2002). Classification and regression by randomForest. *R news, 2*(3), 18-22.

Lindlof, T. R., & Taylor, B. C. (2002) *Qualitative communication research methods* (2nd ed.). Sage Publications.

Loebach, J., & Madigan, R. (2015). *Collecting social media data for qualitative research (Research Short Series #2).* Young Lives Research Lab, University of Prince Edward Island.

Magdin, R. (2020). Disinformation campaigns in the European Union: Lessons learned from the 2019 European Elections and 2020 Covid-19 infodemic in Romania. *Romanian Journal of European Affairs, 20*(2), 49-61.

Malik, K. (2018, March). The 'Nazi pug': giving offence is inevitable and often necessary in a plural society. *The Guardian*. www.theguardian.com/commentisfree/2018/mar/25/being-offensive-should-not-be-illegal-in-society-that-defends-free-speech

Mancosu, M., & Vegetti, F. (2020). What you can scrape and what is right to scrape: A proposal for a tool to collect public Facebook data. *Social Media + Society, 6*(3), 1–11. https://doi.org/10.1177/2056305120940703

Matthews, M., Migacheva, K., & Brown, R. A. (2021). *Superspreaders of malign and subversive information on COVID-19: Russian and Chinese efforts targeting the United States*. RAND Corporation.

McLaren, P. (2022). Some thoughts on Canada's 'Freedom Convoy' and the settler colonial state. *Educational Philosophy and Theory, 54*(7), 867-870. doi: 10.1080/00131857.2022.2051478

Mei, J., & Frank, R. (2015, August). *Sentiment crawling: Extremist content collection through a sentiment analysis guided webcrawler*. IEEE/ACM International Conference on Advances in Social Networks Analysis and Mining.

Meta Business Help Center. (2022). Advertising policies related to Coronavirus (COVID-19). https://www.facebook.com/business/help/1123969894625935?id=434838534925385

Meyers, J. B., Dishart, E., & Morgan, R. (2022). *Canada's legal disinformation pandemic is exposed by the "freedom convoy."* The Conversation. https://theconversation.com/canadas-legal-disinformation-pandemic-is-exposed-by-the-freedom-convoy-176522

Mian, A., & Khan, S. (2020). Coronavirus: the spread of misinformation. *MBC Medicine, 18*(89), 1-2. https://doi.org/10.1186/s12916-020-01556-3

Mieriņa, I., & Koroļeva, I. (2015). Support for far right ideology and anti-migrant attitudes among youth in Europe: A comparative analysis. *Sociological Review, 63*(S2), 183-205. https://doi.org/10.1111/1467-954X.12268

Minister of Canadian Heritage. (2020-2021). Bill C-10. An Act to amend the Broadcasting Act and to make related and consequential amendments to other Acts.

Moreno, M. A., Fost, N. C., & Christakis, D. A. (2008). Research ethics in the MySpace era. *Pediatrics, 121*(1), 157-160. doi: 10:1542/peds.2007-3015

Mueller, R. S. (2019). *Report on the investigation into Russian interference in the 2016 presidential election* (pp. 1–448). http://www.justsecurity.org/wp-content/uploads/2019/04/Muelller-Report-Redacted-Vol-II-Released-04.18.2019-Word-Searchable.-Reduced-Size.pdf

Myers, S. L., & Thompson, S. A. (2022, March 20). Truth is another front in Putin's war. *The New York Times.* https://www.nytimes.com/2022/03/20/world/asia/russia-putin-propaganda-media.html

National Intelligence Council. (2021). *Foreign threats to the 2020 US federal elections.* https://www.dni.gov/files/ODNI/documents/assessments/ICA-declass-16MAR21.pdf

Ndiaye, A. (2021). Together against Covid-19 misinformation: A new campaign in collaboration with the WHO. https://www.facebook.com/formedia/blog/together-against-covid-19-misinformation-a-new-campaign-in-partnership-with-the-who

O'Connell, O. (2022). Soup kitchen harassment to confederate flags: Controversial moments at Canadian trucker convoy protest. *Independent.* https://www.independent.co.uk/news/world/americas/canada-trucker-protest-convoy-freedom-b2004613.html

OECD. (2020). Combatting COVID-19 disinformation on online platforms. *OECD Policy Responses to Coronavirus (COVID-19),* OECD Publishing. https://www.oecd.org/coronavirus/policy-responses/combatting-covid-19-disinformation-on-online-platforms-d854ec48/

Owoeye, K., & Weir G.R.S. (2018). Classification of radical Web text using a composite-based method. *IEEE International Conference on Computational Science and Computational Intelligence.* https://pure.strath.ac.uk/ws/portalfiles/portal/86519706/Owoeye_Weir_IEEE_2018_Classification_of_radical_web_text_using_a_composite_based.pdf. Accessed: 13 August 2020

*Packingham v. State of North Carolina,* 137 S. Ct. 1730, No. 15-1194, 582 US __, 198 L. Ed. 2d 273 - Supreme Court, 2017.

Pedregosa, F., Varoquaux, G., Gramfort, A., Michel, V., Thirion, B., Grisel, O., Blondel, M., Prettenhofer, P., Weiss, R., Dobourg, V., Vanderplas, J., Passos, A., Cournapeau, D., Brucher, M., Perrot, M., & Duchesnay, E. (2011). Scikit-learn: Machine learning in Python. *The Journal of Machine Learning Research, 12*, 2825-2830.

Pennycook, G., McPhetres, J., Zhang, Y., Lu, J. G., & Rand, D. G. (2020). Fighting COVID-19 misinformation on social media: Experimental evidence for a scalable accuracy-nudge intervention. *Psychological Science, 31*(7), 770–780. https://doi.org/10.1177/0956797620939054

Posetti, J., & Bontcheva, K. (2020). *DISINFODEMIC: Deciphering COVID-19 disinformation*. The United Nations Educational, Scientific and Cultural Organization. https://en.unesco.org/covid19/disinfodemic/brief1

Prasad, R. R. (2020). *Media freedom and COVID-19*. International Press Institute. https://www.international.gc.ca/world-monde/issues_development-enjeux_developpement/human_rights-droits_homme/policy-orientation-covid-19.aspx?lang=eng

Radu, R. (2020). Fighting the 'infodemic': Legal responses to COVID-19 disinformation. *Social Media and Society*, *6*(3). https://doi.org/10.1177/2056305120948190

Reporters Without Borders. (2022). Russian military court sentences Crimean journalist to 19 years in prison. https://rsf.org/en/russian-military-court-sentences-crimean-journalist-19-years-prison

Rokach, L., & Maimon, O. (2008). *Data mining with decision trees: Theory and applications.* World Scientific Publishing.

Roth, Y., & Pickles, N. (2020). Updating our approach to misleading information. https://blog.twitter.com/en_us/topics/product/2020/updating-our-approach-to-misleading-information

Rubin, R. (2022). When physicians spread unscientific information about COVID-19. *JAMA*, Feb 16, 2022. https://jamanetwork.com/journals/jama/fullarticle/2789369

Rupar, A. (2021, July 9). Trump's Twitter and Facebook ban is already working. Here's how we know. *Vox*. https://www.vox.com/2021/1/16/22234971/trump-twitter-facebook-social-media-ban-election-misinformation-zignal

Schulze, H. (2020). Who uses right-wing alternative online media? An exploration of audience characteristics. *Politics and Government, 8*(3), 6-18. https://doi.org/10.17645/pag.v8i3.2925

Scott, M. (2022). As war in Ukraine evolves, so do disinformation tactics politico. *Politico.* https://www.politico.eu/article/ukraine-russia-disinformation-propaganda/

Shane, S., & Mazzetti, M. (2018) The plot to subvert an election: Unraveling the Russian story so far. *The New York Times.* https://www.nytimes.com/interactive/2018/09/20/us/politics/russia-interference-election-trump-clinton.html

Sharkey, S., Jones, R. A., Smithson, J., Hewis, E., Emmens, T., Ford, T,. & Owens, C. (2011). Ethical practice in internet research involving vulnerable people: lessons from a self-harm discussion forum study (SharpTalk). *Journal of Medical Ethics, 37*(12), 752-758.

Siddiqui, F., & De Vycnk, G. (2022). Elon Musk's deal to buy Twitter is in peril: Talks with investors have cooled in recent weeks and Musk's camp believes it can't confirm Twitter's claims about spam accounts. *Washington Post,* July 7, 2022. https://www.washingtonpost.com/technology/2022/07/07/elon-musk-twitter-jeopardy/

Smith, G. D., Ng, F., & Li, W. H. C. (2020). COVID-19: Emerging compassion, courage and resilience in the face of misinformation and adversity. *Journal of Clinical Nursing, 29* (9-10), 1425-1428.

Spinello, R. A. (2017). *Cyberethcis: Morality and law in cyberspace*. Jones & Bartlett Learning.

Sullivan, M. (2022). Chris Stirewalt lost his job at Fox News. But he knows he was right. The politics editor behind the Arizona call in 2020 that enraged Trump brought his journalism bona fides to the House Jan 6. hearing. *The Washington Post,* June 13, 2022. https://www.washingtonpost.com/media/2022/06/13/chris-stirewalt-fox-news-jan-6-hearing-trump-arizona/

StatCan COVID-19: (2021). *Data to insights for a better Canada: COVID-19 vaccine willingness among Canadian population groups.* https://www150.statcan.gc.ca/n1/en/pub/45-28-0001/2021001/article/00011-eng.pdf?st= vpGfk0q0

Suarez-Lledo, V., & Alvarez-Garcia, J. (2021). Prevalence of health misinformation on social media: Systematic review. *Journal of Medicine Internet Research, 23*(1), 1-17. https://doi.org/10.2196/17187

Tandoc Jr, E. C., Lim, Z. W., & Ling, R. (2018). Defining "fake news" A typology of scholarly definitions. *Digital Journalism, 6*(2), 137-153. https://doi.org/10.1080/21670811.2017.1360143

Troianovski, A. (2022). Russia takes censorship to new extremes, Stifling War Coverage. *New York Times.* https://www.nytimes.com/2022/03/04/world/europe/russia-censorship-media-crackdown.html

Tsesis, A. (2017). Social media accountability for terrorist propaganda. *Fordham Law Review, 86*(2), 605–632. https://ir.lawnet.fordham.edu/flr/vol86/iss2/12/

UN General Assembly. (1948). *Universal declaration of human rights.* http://www.un.org/en/udhrbook/pdf/udhr_booklet_en_web.pdf

*United States v. Internet Research Agency LLC,* Case 1:18-cr-00032-DLF. (2018). The United States District Court for the District of Columbia, February 26, 2018. www.justice.gov/file/1035477/download

U.S. Department of State Global Engagement Center. (2020). *GEC special report: Pillars of Russia's disinformation and propaganda ecosystem.* https://www.state.gov/russias-pillars-of-disinformation-and-propaganda-report/

Velásquez, N., Leahy, R., Restrepo, N. J., Lupu, Y., Sear, R., Gabriel, N., Jha, O. K., Goldberg, B., & Johnson, N. F. (2021). Online hate network spreads malicious COVID-19 content outside the control of individual social media platforms. *Nature: Scientific Reports, 11*(11549). https://doi.org/10.1038/s41598-021-89467-y

Vosoughi, S., Roy, D., & Aral, S. (2018). The spread of true and false news online. *Science, 359*(6390), pp. 1146-1151. https://www.science.org/doi/10.1126/science.aap9559

Walker, J. (2018). *Hate speech and freedom of expression: Legal boundaries in Canada.* Library of Parliament. https://lop.parl.ca/sites/PublicWebsite/default/en_CA/ResearchPublications/201825E

Walker, S., Mercea, D., & Bastos, M. (2019). The disinformation landscape and the lockdown of social platforms. *Information, Communication & Society, 22*(11), 1531–1543. https://doi.org/10.1080/1369118X.2019.1648536

Waters, N. (2022). *'Exploiting cadavers' and 'faked IEDs': Experts debunk staged pre-war 'provocation' in the Donbas.* Bellingcat. https://www.bellingcat.com/news/2022/02/28/exploiting-cadavers-and-faked-ieds-experts-debunk-staged-pre-war-provocation-in-the-donbas/

Weir, G. R. S. (2007). The posit text profiling toolset. *12th Conference of Pan-Pacific Association of Applied Linguistics,* pp. 106-109. https://www.researchgate.net/publication/228740404_The_Posit_Text_Profiling_Toolset

Weir, G. R. S. (2009, July). Corpus profiling with the Posit tools. *Proceedings of the 5th Corpus Linguistics Conference.* http://citeseerx.ist.psu.edu/viewdoc/download?doi=10.1.1.159.9606&rep=rep1&type=pdf

Weir, G., Frank, R., Cartwright, B., & Dos Santos, E. (2016). Positing the problem: Enhancing classification of extremist web content through textual analysis. *International Conference on Cybercrime and Computer Forensics (IEEE Xplore).* https://www.researchgate.net/publication/310499613_Positing_the_problem_enhancing_classification_of_extremist_web_content_through_textual_analysis

Weir, G., Owoeye, K., Oberacker, A., & Alshahrani, H. (2018). Cloud-based textual analysis as a basis for document classification. *International Conference on High Performance Computing & Simulation (HPCS),* 672-676. https://ieeexplore.ieee.org/document/8514415

WHO (2022). *Coronavirus (COVID-19) dashboard.* https://covid19.who.int/

Wilson, S. L., & Wiysonge, C. D. (2020). Social media and vaccine hesitancy. *BMJ Global Health, 5*(10), 1-7. https://doi.org/10.1089/hs.2020.0038

World Health Organization (2021). *WHO Coronavirus (COVID-19) Dashboard.* https://covid19.who.int/

Yang, K.-C., Pierri, F., Hui, P.-M., Axelrod, D., Torres-Lugo, C., Bryden, J., & Menczer, F. (2021). The COVID-19 infodemic: Twitter versus Facebook. *Big Data & Society, 8*(1), 1–16. https://doi.org/10.1177/20539517211013861

Zajko, M. (2016). Telecom responsibilsation: Internet governance, surveillance, and new roles for intermediaries." *Canadian Journal of Communication, 41*(1), 75-93. https://doi.org/10.22230/cjc.2016v41n1a2894

Zimmer, M. (2010). "But the data is already public": On the ethics of research in Facebook. *Ethics and Information Technology, 12*(4), 313–325. https://doi.org/10.1007/s10676-010-9227-5

Zimmer, M. (2018). Addressing conceptual gaps in big data research ethics: An application of contextual integrity. *Social Media + Society, 4*(2), 1–11. https://doi.org/10.1177/2056305118768300

Zulkarnine, A. T., Frank, R., Monk, B., Mitchell, J., & Davies, G. (2016, September). Surfacing collaborated networks in dark web to find illicit and criminal content. *2016 IEEE Conference on Intelligence and Security Informatics (ISI).* https://ieeexplore.ieee.org/document/7745452

# ELEMENTS OF PROPAGANDA IN THE WESTERN WORLD'S POLITICAL, PUBLIC HEALTH, AND MEDIA NARRATIVES OF 2020-2022

**Oliver Hirsch[1] and Claus Rinner[2]**

**Abstract:** In this chapter, we briefly review foundational contributions to the study of propaganda along with examples of the use of propaganda techniques in medicine in the past. We then illustrate and discuss elements of propaganda found in communications from government, public health administration, and the mainstream media during the COVID-19 pandemic from 2020 to early 2022. The examples are drawn from Germany, Canada, and other countries in the Western World. They include elements of simplification and faulty analogies, emotional appeals and scapegoating, and manipulating numbers. We discuss the use of propaganda from an ethical perspective with particular attention to fear narratives, the weakness of the underlying evidence, and the use of moral appeals. We conclude that the use of propaganda techniques to support the COVID-19 pandemic response was unethical, since the broad scope and uniformity of the response measures were not sufficiently established by scientific evidence or by the facts on the ground.

## Introduction

Ellul (1965) views propaganda as a broad societal phenomenon closely linked to technological advances. While discussing the difficulty of defining "propaganda", Ellul refers to the "aim to indoctrinate" (p. xi). Colloquially, propaganda can be viewed as a biased form of communication geared towards influencing the recipients without their awareness. It has been further characterized as a persuasive attempt to change attitudes and behaviors by limiting freedom and promoting obedience (Taylor & Kent, 2014). Propaganda is thus regarded as a special form of unethical communication (Jowett & O'Donnell, 2018). In the context of ethical challenges with respect to the COVID-19 pandemic, we

---

[1] FOM University of Applied Sciences, Siegen, Germany.

[2] Professor, Toronto Metropolitan University in Toronto, Ontario, Canada.

identify elements of propaganda techniques according to Conserva (2003) as they were used by governments and media worldwide to press people into compliance with pandemic response measures.

The field of propaganda is inevitably associated with the standard works of Bernays and Kocks (2019), Le Bon (2018), and Meerloo (2015). If one reads Edward Bernays' book, published in 1928, today, some of his formulations read like conspiracy theories. He argues that purposeful manipulation of the behaviour and attitudes of the masses is an essential component of democratic societies and that organisations working in secret are directing the processes of society; these are the real governments in the country, he states (Bernays & Kocks, 2019, p. 19).

According to Bernays, propaganda should be described more positively as "public relations". Harmonious cooperation between politicians and the press is the best way to censor information for effective propaganda. Similarly, Le Bon (2018) assumes that the masses are easily influenced and gullible. The masses are incapable of distinguishing the personal from the factual and can slip into psychotic states. Critical reflection is then no longer possible. The masses think in images and are receptive to religious dogmas. Therefore, the rulers only need to repeat their messages over and over again as assertions without substantiating them. This has the best effect, since the masses are unwilling and unable to weigh up arguments logically (Le Bon, 2018).

Meerloo (2015) created the additional term "menticide", the killing of one's own mind. This is an organised system of psychological intervention and abuse of justice through which the desired conformity can be imposed on opposition members. Their confessions are then used as propaganda to exert constant psychological pressure on the population. The aim is to create confusion so that no one can distinguish truth from lies. The core strategy of menticide is to destroy all hope, all anticipation, all belief in a future. The modern ways of mass communication bring the entire world into one's living room on a daily basis, there is hardly any retreat from the constant verbal and visual assaults on the psyche (Meerloo, 2015). Propaganda intends to change the attitudes and/or the behaviour of people who are not aware that they are in a situation where they are supposed to be given information or instructions (Sell, 1977).

Lasswell (1950) highlights that propaganda can contain words, gestures, pictures, and written characters. In a totalitarian society, rulers seek to monopolise communication, use the language of orders, and employ ceremonies and rituals to influence the population. Attempts are made to create a climate of insecurity so that the population develops an increased need to be protected from danger. For this reason, increasingly strong propaganda is developed that denigrates opponents (Lasswell, 1950).

In earlier work, Belbin (1956a, 1956b) reported that some subjects could describe and recognize propaganda they were exposed to, but this had no measurable effect on their behaviour. Other subjects were affected in their behavior but were not able to describe the propaganda they were confronted with. The decisive variable was previous experience with the material. Therefore, such techniques as pre-teaching, where topics that will be taken up again in the future are mentioned again and again in advance, are important to create familiarity. In this way, propagandistic messages can be anchored in the behaviour of as many people as possible.

An application example showed that safety propaganda should not involve horror without offering proper solutions as this evokes defence mechanisms. Furthermore, it should not be negative, because this can lead to wrong ways of acting (Sell, 1977). However, this contrasts with the current fear propaganda in the media around COVID-19 and consequently raises questions about its function, which we aim to discuss in this chapter.

## Propaganda in Medicine

Trimble (2021) warns in one of his editorials in the *Ulster Medical Journal* about the dangers of propaganda. He mentions the Scientific Pandemic Influenza Group on Behaviour (SPI-B), which has deliberately generated fear in Great Britain so that the population will comply with the government's draconian measures. Trimble also warns against an "over-organised" society in the sense of Aldous Huxley, in which the population is controlled. Education is no protection against propaganda. In fact, intellectuals are the most susceptible to propaganda because they process large amounts of information. Several terms have been proposed in this context: Propaganda-based medicine, arrogance-based medicine or eminence-based medicine (Isaacs & Fitzgerald, 1999; Mariotto, 2000) are concepts that stress the departure from an empirical basis denying any pluralistic scientific debate.

Propaganda in medicine can be found in areas where one would not initially expect it. For example, Penston (2011) criticises that only the relative risk reduction (16%) and not the absolute risk reduction (0.1%) in bowel cancer mortality is given for bowel cancer screening programmes. This is reminiscent of the presentation of the trial results on vaccine efficacy against COVID-19, as discussed in the following section. Furthermore, ghost-written articles by pharmaceutical companies are published in medical journals reporting supporting findings of clinical trials for their drugs (Jowett & O'Donnell, 2018). Evidence based medicine is regarded as an illusion because medicine is dominated by large pharmaceutical companies that tend to suppress negative trial results and the reporting of adverse events. Critics of these companies are often rejected by journals and face the potential destruction of their careers (Jureidini & McHenry, 2022).

Individuals who are critical of the current COVID-19 vaccinations are often labelled with the term "vaccine hesitant", which has a psychopathological component implying that the decision to vaccinate is the only correct decision A "vaccine hesitant" person is often colloquially called "anti-vaxxer" referring to a controversy that already existed about smallpox vaccination. Criticism of additives in smallpox vaccination was called "anti-vaccination propaganda" (Antivaccination, 1898). As early as 100 years ago, data from medical experts were cited that suggested that the disease had been overdramatised in its significance in the Western world (Millard, 1923). This argumentation was vehemently opposed by others, who spoke of "anti-scientific propaganda" and "pseudo and unscientific cults" (Frandsen, 1926, p. 336). The author does however concede that scientific knowledge is never complete and must always be revised and updated in light of new findings (Frandsen, 1926).

Another critical case in the context of medical propaganda is the thalidomide scandal. Thalidomide had been widely advertised since 1958 and prescribed against morning sickness in pregnant women. In 1961-1962, however, there were increasing suspicions that newborns with malformations were linked to the mother's ingestion of thalidomide. This proved to be true and the Grünenthal company had to face a huge scandal. The resulting malformations in the affected children were presented as tragic and unavoidable. However, it had been clear at an early stage that thalidomide can cause peripheral neuritis and has teratogenic potential, but this was hardly noticed (Dally, 1998). At that time, the scientific opinion was that the placenta was impermeable to harmful substances, so that contrary findings were ignored. According to Dally, this cognitive bias then led to the catastrophic developments.

In 2016, Wildner took a critical look at propaganda and nudging in medicine. With reference to Bernays, he notes that public health campaigns for health education have similarities to propaganda. Wildner (2016) mentions nudging, which is a gentle, persistent, and unconscious pressure towards adopting desired behaviours and stems from behavioural economics. He emphasizes the transparency of such methods and the possibility of free counter-decision-making. Furthermore, valid, transparent, and relevant information should be made available, and the population should be enabled to understand this information and make informed decisions through measures to increase health literacy. Public, critical discussion, participatory involvement, accountability of policy-makers and the opportunity for political participation should also be essential components of public health decisions (Wildner, 2016).

Previously, Fava (2002) criticized that the pharmaceutical industry and academic medicine form an unhealthy alliance that selectively reports clinical research, occupying leading roles in journals, medical associations and nonprofit research organizations and marginalizing those with different evidence based views. He explicitly refers to this as propaganda. Fava (2001) also presented several investigations that found clear conflicts of interest by authors in the *Journal of the American Medical Association* and the *New England Journal of Medicine* in studies that support certain drugs. He showed the close links between the World Health Organization (WHO) and the pharmaceutical industry, and criticised that industry-sponsored reviewers in scientific journals prevent the publication of critical articles that doubt the effectiveness of certain drugs. Regarding the long-term use of antidepressants he further criticizes that few controlled trials were performed, their efficacy overemphasized, and the effects of non-pharmacological treatments neglected (Fava, 2002, 2021). Dalrymple (2019) also examined the content of the *New England Journal of Medicine* over the course of a year and came to the conclusion that it was dominated by political correctness, as if censorship was at work, and by massive conflicts of interest regarding involvement with the pharmaceutical industry.

Gambrill and Reiman (2011) propose a Propaganda Index for reviewing problem framing in articles and manuscripts. The index consists of 32 yes/no items in seven categories: nature of the problem, and claims regarding effectiveness of interventions; prevalence; significant distress and adverse effects; course without treatment; under-diagnosis; and undertreatment. The authors are stressing the problem of flawed peer review regarding the medicalization of problems, exaggerating mild concerns as being serious, and claiming underdiagnosis and undertreatment. By applying the Propaganda Index in their empirical study on randomized controlled trials on social anxiety disorder participants were able to discover more propaganda indicators. Further empirical investigation of the propaganda index was recommended.

Cohn (2020) argues that the flu pandemic 1918-20 was a plague of compassion and triggered the greatest wave of volunteerism in any pandemic or epidemic. On the other hand, he reports about draconian punishments in the United States during this pandemic like coughing or sneezing in public as a criminal offence, imposing limitations in shops, mask mandates, and forbidding children to visit each other. Restrictions were promoted using propaganda posters. In contrast to this seemingly positive picture, distrust, violence, and scapegoating are elements of the current declared pandemic. It is said that blaming was always used to make mysterious and devastating diseases comprehensible (Nelkin & Gilman, 1988).

## Propaganda during the COVID-19 Pandemic

The COVID-19 pandemic response was arguably impacted by numerous blunders in public policy. In Germany, the Heilmittelwerbegesetz (Drug

Advertising Act) prohibits advertising prescription drugs, which also includes vaccinations. However, by promoting mobile vaccinations at McDonald's or at IKEA stores, "late-night vaccination parties", etc. the German government arguably broke its own law (Bahner, 2021). Similarly, promising gifts to those willing to be vaccinated is unethical and allowing teenagers to get vaccinated without parental consent is reckless, when the same teenagers require parental consent to go on school trips or get a tattoo.

Furthermore, authorities constantly emphasized that the mRNA vaccines are safe and effective (Baden et al., 2021; Dagan et al., 2021; Polack et al., 2020), yet emerging studies are being ignored when they show the opposite. An alarming level of serious adverse event reports was observed for the COVID-19 vaccines in comparison to influenza vaccines in the European Database of Suspected Adverse Drug Reaction (EudraVigilance) and the Vaccine Adverse Events Reporting System (VAERS) from 2020 to October 2021 (Montano, 2021). Considerable waning of vaccine efficacy was also reported after 4-6 months (Chemaitelly et al., 2021; Nordström et al., 2022). Vaccinated people are just as contagious as unvaccinated people and can equally contribute to the spread of the disease (Singanayagam et al., 2022; Wilder-Smith, 2022). Consequently, the COVID-19 vaccination campaign can be considered as misleading advertising according to the law (Bahner, 2021, pp. 375–379).

In the remainder of this section, we illustrate and discuss propaganda techniques employed by government, public health administration, and the mainstream media during the COVID-19 pandemic from 2020 to early 2022. Based on Conserva's (2003) seminal work, the following examples drawn from Germany, Canada, and other countries in the Western World include elements of simplification and faulty analogies, emotional appeals and scapegoating, and manipulating numbers.

## Simplification and faulty analogies

From the onset of the Western world's pandemic response, mobility restrictions, social distancing, and face masks were mandated to slow the spread of SARS-Cov2. Each of these population-wide measures were based on simplistic assumptions. More than two years after the start of "two weeks to flatten the curve", the Brownstone Institute has collected over 400 studies indicating "that mask mandates, lockdowns, and school closures have had no discernible impact [on] virus trajectories" (Alexander, 2021, para. 2). The simplification of respiratory virus transmission, infection, and illness processes in public health propaganda slogans such as "my mask protects you" worked well to engage the public, yet these non-pharmaceutical interventions did not have tangible effects on the progress of the pandemic (Bundgaard et al., 2021; Spira, 2022). Until now there are 18 meta-analyses on the use of face masks of which 5 are inconclusive, 3 critical, and 9 showing limited evidence. The meta-analysis with the highest degree of quality comes to the conclusion that there is uncertainty regarding the use of face masks (Jefferson et al., 2020). Studies in favor of face masks were highly controversial (Abaluck et al., 2021) or were based on simulations which made incorrect assumptions hardly corresponding to real life situations (Cheng et al., 2021). In addition, face masks entail unpredictable harms (Fögen, 2022; Kisielinski et al., 2021; Kisielinski & Wojtasik, 2022; Sukul et al., 2022).

In another simplification and faulty analogy, Bavaria's Premier Markus Söder equated the daily COVID-19 death count with a daily airplane crash (Welt, 2020), ignoring the multi-week delays in many death reports and the proportionality with the regular mortality (2,750 every day in Germany). Equally simplistic was the catchphrase that "vaccines are [the] only way out of [the] pandemic" e.g., from Canada's Prime Minister Trudeau (Rabson, 2021, headline).

The mRNA products available for COVID-19 vaccination themselves are wrongly likened to, or compared with, traditional vaccines such as the polio vaccine (Drillinger, 2021). This faulty analogy is meant to promote confidence in the novel mRNA technology. However, the COVID-19 vaccines contain new ingredients and are still in the midst of medium- and long-term trials, while the coronavirus as a respiratory virus is transmitted in very different ways than, for example, the poliovirus. The pharma industry is well aware of the value of faulty analogies, as exemplified by the headline "Bayer executive: mRNA shots are 'gene therapy' marketed as 'vaccines' to gain public trust" (Bingham, 2021).

## Emotional Appeals and Scapegoating

Using the term "hero" for nurses coping with the burden of disease is problematic, as it implies that all health professionals must behave heroically, which could have negative consequences for them (Cox, 2020). Heroism implies a voluntary commitment with an acknowledgement of personal risk to help others. However, an application of this "hero" narrative to all individuals in this occupational group fails to recognise that the commitment to sacrifice oneself is limited. The "hero" narrative can be a convenient tool for politicians to distract from their own failures. However, using militaristic metaphors in connection with the pandemic risks shifting responsibility from the individual to the government which was not intended (Schnepf & Christmann, 2022). For example, the "Clap for Carers" campaign in Great Britain, which initially appeared to be a grassroots initiative, showed clear signs of a propaganda campaign organised by the government, which was then discontinued due to controversy (Dodsworth, 2021).

A different type of "hero" was evoked in a campaign by the German federal government. Using the hashtag #besondereHelden ("special heroes"), everyday citizens were presented as "heroes" in short video clips (e.g., https://www.youtube.com/watch?v=UH1757U0aeg) for the accomplishment of "courageously bumming around" at home and "doing nothing" in order to "collectively" combat viral spread. In a related campaign with the hashtag #wirbleibenzuhause ("we stay home"), prominent German artists contributed video snippets appealing to the population to interrupt SARS-CoV-2 transmission by staying at home. Similar campaigns were undertaken e.g., in the United Kingdom ("Stay home, protect the NHS, save lives"). The simplified appeals combine a message of empowerment (being a "hero") and morality (saving others). Interestingly, the UK's appeal to protect the national health care system has been criticized as reversing the duty of care between government and citizens.

In an example of a reverse accusation of using propaganda, Italian physicians were disciplined for "anti-vaccination propaganda" (Day, 2020). Punishments ranged from warnings to two-month suspensions. These doctors were denounced by other doctors and by citizens. They were accused of denying scientific evidence, even though numerous studies and datasets now question the safety and efficacy of COVID-19 vaccines (Chemaitelly et al., 2021; Montano, 2021; Nordström et al., 2022; Singanayagam et al., 2022; Wilder-Smith, 2022). These studies, the continued volatility of the situation, and recent work demonstrating mechanisms of possible toxicity of the vaccines (Seneff et al., 2022), and increased risks of adverse events (Karlstad et al., 2022; Patone et al., 2022; Sun et al., 2022) should be enough to allow for an open dialogue in the medical community. Unfortunately, similar disciplinary measures against doctors who doubt the prevailing public health narrative have been taken in Austria, Germany, and Canada, up to and including the withdrawal of the licence to practise medicine.

Surveillance tools such as machine-learning have been proposed to find propaganda on the topic of COVID-19 on social media such as Twitter (Khanday et al., 2020). However, the authors assume a simple, binary understanding of propaganda, which does not do justice to the complexity of the topic (Trimble, 2021). The selection and classification criteria remain unclear, and the result was limited to the scope of messages. The impact of these parameters results in the danger that everything that does not conform to the respective government narrative will be labelled as propaganda.

A recent example of scapegoating can be drawn from a speech by German President Frank-Walter Steinmeier. His remarks at a round table discussion on "Hate and Violence in Times of Pandemic - Experiences and Reactions" (Steinmeier, 2022) must be considered historically unique. He referred to participants of the Monday walks against the government's Corona measures as "enemies of the state" (para. 7) and, in a dehumanising manner, as "all the rest" (para. 5). He is clearly in violation of his neutrality requirement. Other world leaders are on record with similar scapegoating statements such as French President Emmanuel Macron confessing "The unvaccinated, I really want to piss them off. And so we're going to continue doing so until the end. That's the strategy" (FRANCE 24, 2022, para. 3); U.S. President Joe Biden claiming "We are looking at a winter of severe illness and death for the unvaccinated -- for themselves, their families and the hospitals they'll soon overwhelm" (Malloy & Vazquez, 2021, para. 3); and

Italian Prime Minister Mario Draghi's statement that "The unvaccinated are not part of our society" (Radio Genova, 2022).

Similarly, Canada's Prime Minister Justin Trudeau went on record calling unvaccinated people "racist" and "misogynistic", asking whether leaders should "tolerate these people" (Ivison, 2022, para. 3). The comments were made during a tense fall 2021 election campaign, in which Trudeau increasingly targeted "the unvaccinated" and promoted divisive policies such as vaccination mandates and passports in order to score points against the more lenient conservative party. Trudeau continued this approach after the inconclusive election, most recently by aggravating Canadian truck drivers with a vaccine mandate for the lucrative cross-border transportation with the U.S. The resulting Freedom Convoy 2022 protests in Ottawa generated two distinct narratives, one of tremendous suffering of local residents under an alt-right occupation of the city's downtown core, the other of a peaceful, inclusive celebration of freedom and democracy comparable to a winter carnival or Canada Day in winter.

## Manipulating Numbers

Propaganda is often based on the presentation and interpretation as well as the omission of data. In Germany, so-called "incidences" were used for decisions on restrictions. The incidence is supposed to represent new COVID-19 infections in the past seven days extrapolated to 100,000 inhabitants. However, these figures did not refer to a representative population sample as necessary, but were susceptible to unsystematic testing strategies. Apart from this, it should be emphasised that the SARS-CoV-2 PCR test has to be considered an "imperfect gold standard" (Kohn et al., 2013, p. 1201). This is an epidemiological term which implies that the criterion against which other tests are validated has itself questionable quality criteria. The PCR test fails to distinguish active infection from non-infectious probes when processed at high Cycle threshold (Ct) values. Ct values higher than 25-30 signal a low viral load but there is no standardized procedure leading to high numbers of false positive results and a pseudovalidation regarding other measures like rapid on-site testing (Gniazdowski et al., 2020; Hirsch et al., 2022; Stang et al., 2021; Surkova et al., 2020). It can even show positive results many weeks after the initial infection in the absence of evidence for viral replication (Zhang et al., 2021) which clearly argues against basic quality criteria.

Focacci et al. (2022) found that the presentation of the crude mortality rate (CMR) elicited the highest willingness to follow the preferences of policy makers. It should be said that the classification of deaths as primarily caused by COVID-19 is now considered highly controversial, and there is strong evidence that the death figures with respect to COVID-19 should be considered significantly inflated. In Great Britain, for example, it was announced that only about 10% of the deaths had COVID-19 as the sole diagnosis (Otter, 2022). In the United States, the Centers for Disease Control (CDC) stated on March 2nd, 2022: "For over 5% of these deaths, COVID-19 was the only cause mentioned on the death certificate. For deaths with conditions or causes in addition to COVID-19, on average, there were 4.0 additional conditions or causes per death" (CDC, 2022, para. 5). According to von Wachter, corona death counts are not based on even a halfway decent causal analysis. The most serious error, he says, is that every death in which the SARS-CoV-2 test is positive is labelled a death caused by COVID-19 infection. In reality, the danger of SARS-CoV-2 must be assessed on the basis of cases in which one can be as certain as possible that no other factors are involved. But in the weakened state that patients with several pre-existing conditions were in, if SARS-CoV-2 had not spread to them, another virus could have done the same, e.g., influenza A or another coronavirus (Wachter, 2020). Armstrong (2021) showed that in April 2020 new rules to classify COVID-19 on death certificates were introduced. Previously, COVID-19 had the same status as pneumonia or respiratory failure as the final endpoint in the causal chain of events leading to death on the basis of other underlying conditions. From April 2020, COVID-19 had to be the underlying cause, and therefore, the causal chain of events was changed. Any long-term, chronic conditions were then moved to Part II of the Death Certificate as 'contributing' causes which resulted in the inflation of COVID-19 deaths.

The case fatality rate (CFR), which indicates the number of deaths in relation to the number of people with the disease, again depends on the definition of a COVID-19 case. If this is based only on a positive SARS-CoV-2 test, then this parameter is also questionable. According to the authors, the CFR should be used to increase public understanding and consent to public life restrictions. The Infection Fatality Rate (IFR), which represents the proportion of infected deaths, was the parameter that elicited the least willingness to comply with measures such as mask-wearing and social distancing. Therefore, the authors advise against presenting this to the population (Focacci et al., 2022). It is thus clear that the authors are only concerned with getting the population to follow government orders by presenting metrics without questioning the evidence base of these orders. This is to be seen as an example of unethical research.

Communicating benefits and costs of medical procedures is challenging and subject to legal considerations, as outlined by Freeman (2019). While the author recommends "Never give just relative risks (and be careful with just absolute risks)" (p.120), the mRNA vaccine trial results were reported exclusively in terms of relative risk reduction. For example, the Pfizer/BioNTech trial found a Relative Risk Reduction (RRR) of 95%, which keeps being peddled by public health officials and the media, while its absolute risk reduction was below 1% (Brown, 2021; Olliaro et al., 2021). By boosting vaccine efficacy in this manner, a reporting bias occurs that does not allow the public to adequately assess the true effect of the treatment and make an informed decision (Alsulamy et al., 2020).

## Discussion and Conclusion

Researchers have suggested that the ethics of propaganda may be subject to the moral positions of its author and their goals. For example, propaganda conducted by a democratic state may be considered "good" whereas propaganda conducted by a dictatorship would be seen as "bad" (Ellul, 1965). We think that this view is too simplistic, and the Corona crisis has illustrated that within a "good" state, individual actors and groups are using propaganda techniques for goals that are not sufficiently backed by evidence. While public health officials may have had noble goals, in resorting to propaganda techniques they over-stepped their competencies.

Who is to pass final judgement upon a crisis situation in order to trigger a unified public response? In the Western World, it was the health ministers or health bureaucrats who made far-reaching decisions on non-pharmaceutical interventions, health care procedures, and vaccination campaigns with little consultations of experts in other fields such as psychology, sociology, economics, or even a broader range of health scientists and medical practitioners. Some of the elements of propaganda used to support the adoption of these mandates were discussed in this chapter.

If we take a critical stance on the pandemic response, we also have to ask why the population in our liberal democracies has not been more sceptical. What is the role of an educated, generally well-informed citizenry in unquestioningly accepting the information they were fed by the mainstream media? The answer likely lies in the moral, virtue-signalling dimension briefly discussed earlier and in the existential power of fear narratives. Interestingly, though without in-depth analysis, the emotional appeals to solidarity work in different ways in the two countries that the authors are most familiar with. In Germany, the population tends to trust that authorities will do the right thing for the greater good. In Canada, people like to think of themselves as nice and considerate, so that public health messaging just had to present mandates in this light.

When it comes to the role of fear, anxiety and related disorders were the second highest risk factor for death among a large sample of hospitalized COVID-19 patients in the United States (Kompaniyets et al., 2021). One has to be cautious with respect to causality but there may be a subgroup of patients who were affected by the constant fear spread by governments and mainstream media. We know from neuropsychoimmunology that sustained fear significantly weakens the immune system making humans more susceptible to respiratory diseases. Anxiety might also be diagnosed before COVID-19 and was therefore not independently associated with death. There is even a COVID-19 anxiety syndrome discussed in the literature with avoidance, checking, worrying and threat monitoring around the disease (Albery et al., 2021). A special scale to measure this construct was published, which contains perseveration and avoidance of COVID-19-related threats and stimuli (Nikčević & Spada, 2020). There were significant correlations with generalized anxiety disorder and depression scores stressing the possible importance of the construct.

As far as this fear is generated and maintained using elements of propaganda techniques, these have to be rejected as unethical. Accurate information should be available to enable citizens to form their own opinion and make informed choices. What accurate means, however, seems to be defined by the authorities in charge of the pandemic response. Those who turn to alternative media are being ostracised or censored. This is reminiscent of the strictest ban on listening to the BBC radio programme in Germany during the Second World War.

Wenzel wrote a short perspective article in the *New England Journal of Medicine* that fits well with the present day despite the different context. In his view, unpleasant facts are often presented as "fake news" and fabrications as reality. Students already have to be taught critical analysis of research. Critical thinking does not fit into a tweet or a brief social media post. Reasoned doubt about what is read and heard should be rewarded, in Wenzel's view. Current knowledge is only ever a temporary state of affairs that needs to be continuously reviewed and further analysed (Wenzel, 2017). Propagating a single, static view of all aspects of a crisis situation is unwise and morally reprehensible.

## References

Abaluck, J., Kwong, L. H., Styczynski, A., Haque, A., Kabir, M. A., Bates-Jefferys, E., Crawford, E., Benjamin-Chung, J., Raihan, S., Rahman, S., Benhachmi, S., Bintee, N. Z., Winch, P. J., Hossain, M., Reza, H. M., Jaber, A. A., Momen, S. G., Rahman, A., Banti, F. L., . . . Mobarak, A. M. (2022). Impact of community masking on COVID-19: A cluster-randomized trial in Bangladesh. *Science, 375*(6577), eabi9069. https://doi.org/10.1126/science.abi9069

Albery, I. P., Spada, M. M., & Nikčević, A. V. (2021). The COVID-19 anxiety syndrome and selective attentional bias towards COVID-19-related stimuli in UK residents during the 2020-2021 pandemic. *Clinical Psychology & Psychotherapy, 28*(6), 1367–1378. https://doi.org/10.1002/cpp.2639

Alexander, P. E. (2021, November 30). *More than 400 studies on the failure of compulsory Covid interventions (lockdowns, restrictions, closures).* Brownstone Institute. https://brownstone.org/articles/more-than-400-studies-on-the-failure-of-compulsory-covid-interventions/

Alsulamy, N., Lee, A., Thokala, P., & Alessa, T. (2020). What influences the implementation of shared decision making: An umbrella review. *Patient Education and Counseling,* Aug 11, Online ahead of print. https://doi.org/10.1016/j.pec.2020.08.009

Antivaccination Propaganda. (1898). *British Medical Journal,* 2(1960), 246–247.

Armstrong, D. (2021). The COVID-19 pandemic and cause of death. *Sociology of Health & Illness, 43,* 1614–1626. doi: 10.1111/1467-9566.13347

Baden, L. R., El Sahly, H. M., Essink, B., Kotloff, K., Frey, S., Novak, R., Diemert, D., Spector, S. A., Rouphael, N., Creech, C. B., McGettigan, J., Khetan, S., Segall, N., Solis, J., Brosz, A., Fierro, C., Schwartz, H., Neuzil, K., Corey, L.,... Zaks, T. (2021). Efficacy and safety of the mRNA-1273 SARS-CoV-2 vaccine. *The New England Journal of Medicine, 384*(5), 403–416. https://doi.org/10.1056/NEJMoa2035389

Bahner, B. (2021). *Corona-Impfung: Was Ärzte und Patienten unbedingt wissen sollten* (1. Auflage). Rubikon.

Belbin, E. (1956a). The effects of propaganda on recall, recognition, and behavior. II. The conditions which determine the response to propaganda. *British Journal of Psychology, 47*(4), 259–270. https://doi.org/10.1111/j.2044-8295.1956.tb00588.x

Belbin, E. (1956b). The effects of propaganda on recall, recognition, and behaviour. I. The relationship between the different measures of propaganda effectiveness. *British Journal of Psychology, 47*(3), 163–174. https://doi.org/10.1111/j.2044-8295.1956.tb00579.x

Bernays, E. L., & Kocks, K. (2019). *Propaganda: Die Kunst der Public Relations* (P. Schnur, Trans.) (Deutsche Erstausgabe, 9. Auflage). Orange-Press.

Bingham, J. (2021). *Bayer executive: mRNA shots are 'gene therapy' marketed as 'vaccines' to gain public trust.* LifeSiteNews. https://www.lifesitenews.com/news/bayer-executive-mrna-shots-are-gene-therapy-marketed-as-vaccines-to-gain-public-trust/

Brown, R. B. (2021). Outcome reporting bias in COVID-19 mRNA vaccine clinical trials. *Medicina (Kaunas, Lithuania), 57*(3). https://doi.org/10.3390/medicina57030199

Bundgaard, H., Bundgaard, J. S., Raaschou-Pedersen, D. E. T., Buchwald, C. von, Todsen, T., Norsk, J. B., Pries-Heje, M. M., Vissing, C. R., Nielsen, P. B., Winsløw,

U. C., Fogh, K., Hasselbalch, R., Kristensen, J. H., Ringgaard, A., Porsborg Andersen, M., Goecke, N. B., Trebbien, R., Skovgaard, K., Benfield, T., . . . Iversen, K. (2020). Effectiveness of adding a mask recommendation to other public health measures to prevent SARS-CoV-2 infection in Danish mask wearers: A randomized controlled trial. *Annals of Internal Medicine*. Advance online publication. https://doi.org/10.7326/M20-6817

Centers for Disease Control and Prevention. (2022, March 02). *Weekly updates by select demographic and geographic characteristics: Provisional death counts for Coronavirus disease 2019 (COVID-19).* https://web.archive.org/web/20220305164624/ https://www.cdc.gov/nchs/nvss/vsrr/covid_weekly/index.htm

Chemaitelly, H., Tang, P., Hasan, M. R., AlMukdad, S., Yassine, H. M., Benslimane, F. M., Al Khatib, H. A., Coyle, P., Ayoub, H. H., Al Kanaani, Z., Al Kuwari, E., Jeremijenko, A., Kaleeckal, A. H., Latif, A. N., Shaik, R. M., Abdul Rahim, H. F., Nasrallah, G. K., Al Kuwari, M. G., Al Romaihi, H. E., . . . Abu-Raddad, L. J. (2021). Waning of BNT162b2 vaccine protection against SARS-CoV-2 infection in Qatar. *The New England Journal of Medicine, 385*(24), e83. https://doi.org/10.1056/NEJMoa2114114

Cheng, Y., Ma, N., Witt, C., Rapp, S., Wild, P. S., Andreae, M. O., Pöschl, U., & Su, H. (2021). Face masks effectively limit the probability of SARS-CoV-2 transmission. *Science*. Advance online publication. https://doi.org/10.1126/science.abg6296

Cohen, D., & Carter, P. (2010). WHO and the pandemic flu "conspiracies". *BMJ (Clinical Research Ed.), 340*, c2912. https://doi.org/10.1136/bmj.c2912

Cohn, S. K. (2020). Social and institutional reactions to the influenza pandemic of 1918-20. *Medicine, Conflict, and Survival, 36*(4), 315–332. https://doi.org/10.1080/13623699.2020.1820165

Conserva, H. T. (2003). *Propaganda techniques*. 1st Books Library.

Cox, C. L. (2020). 'Healthcare heroes': Problems with media focus on heroism from healthcare workers during the COVID-19 pandemic. *Journal of Medical Ethics, 46*(8), 510–513. https://doi.org/10.1136/medethics-2020-106398

Dagan, N., Barda, N., Kepten, E., Miron, O., Perchik, S., Katz, M. A., Hernán, M. A., Lipsitch, M., Reis, B., & Balicer, R. D. (2021). Bnt162b2 mRNA Covid-19 vaccine in a nationwide mass vaccination setting. *The New England Journal of Medicine, 384*(15), 1412–1423. https://doi.org/10.1056/NEJMoa2101765

Dalrymple, T. (2019). *False positive: A year of error, omission, and political correctness in the New England Journal of Medicine*. Encounter Books.

Day, M. (2020). Covid-19: Italian doctors are disciplined for anti-vaccination propaganda. *BMJ (Clinical Research Ed.), 371,* m4962. https://doi.org/10.1136/bmj.m4962

Dodsworth, L. (2021). *A state of fear: How the UK government weaponised fear during the COVID-19 pandemic*. Pinter & Martin.

Drillinger, M. (2021, May 03). *We eradicated polio from the U.S. with vaccines. Can we do the same with COVID-19?* Healthline. https://www.healthline.com/health-news/we-eradicated-polio-from-the-u-s-with-vaccines-can-we-do-the-same-with-covid-19

Ellul, J. (1965). *Propaganda : The formation of men's attitudes*. Knopf.

Fava, G. A. (2001). Conflict of interest and special interest groups. The making of a counterculture. *Psychotherapy and Psychosomatics, 70*(1), 1–5. https://doi.org/10.1159/000056218

Fava, G. A. (2002). Long-term treatment with antidepressant drugs: The spectacular achievements of propaganda. *Psychotherapy and Psychosomatics, 71*(3), 127–132. https://doi.org/10.1159/000056279

Fava, G. A. (2021). *Discontinuing antidepressant medications*. Oxford University Press Incorporated.

Focacci, C. N., Lam, P. H., & Bai, Y. (2022). Choosing the right COVID-19 indicator: Crude mortality, case fatality, and infection fatality rates influence policy preferences, behaviour, and understanding. *Humanities and Social Sciences Communications, 9*(1), 1155. https://doi.org/10.1057/s41599-021-01032-0

Fögen, Z. (2022). The Foegen effect: A mechanism by which facemasks contribute to the COVID-19 case fatality rate. *Medicine, 101*(7), e28924. https://doi.org/10.1097/MD.0000000000028924

FRANCE 24. (2022, January 05). *Macron's vow to 'piss off' the unvaccinated sparks outrage*. FRANCE 24. https://www.france24.com/en/france/20220105-macron-says-he-wants-to-piss-off-france-s-unvaccinated

Frandsen, P. (1926). Anti-scientific propaganda. *California and Western Medicine, 25*(3), 336–338.

Freeman, A. L. J. (2019). How to communicate evidence to patients. *Drug and Therapeutics Bulletin, 57*(8), 119–124. https://doi.org/10.1136/dtb.2019.000008

Gambrill, E., & Reiman, A. (2011). A propaganda index for reviewing problem framing in articles and manuscripts: An exploratory study. *PloS One, 6*(5), e19516. https://doi.org/10.1371/journal.pone.0019516

Gniazdowski, V., Morris, C. P., Wohl, S., Mehoke, T., Ramakrishnan, S., Thielen, P., Powell, H., Smith, B., Armstrong, D. T., Herrera, M., Reifsnyder, C., Sevdali, M., Carroll, K. C., Pekosz, A., & Mostafa, H. H. (2020). Repeat COVID-19 molecular testing: Correlation of SARS-CoV-2 culture with molecular assays and cycle thresholds. *Clinical Infectious Diseases : An Official Publication of the Infectious Diseases Society of America, Oct 27,* Online ahead of print. https://doi.org/10.1093/cid/ciaa1616

Hirsch, O., Bergholz, W., Kisielinski, K., Giboni, P., & Sönnichsen, A. (2022). Methodological problems of SARS-CoV-2 rapid point-of-care tests when used in mass testing. *AIMS Public Health, 9*(1), 73–93. https://doi.org/10.3934/publichealth.2022007

Isaacs, D., & Fitzgerald, D. (1999). Seven alternatives to evidence based medicine. *BMJ (Clinical Research Ed.), 319*(7225), 1618. https://doi.org/10.1136/bmj.319.7225.1618

Ivison, J. (2022, January 04). John Ivison: Trudeau and other partisans should rein in the rage: Trudeau's 'misogynists and racists' outburst is ever more typical of the illiberal left — and of his government in particular. *National Post.* https://nationalpost.com/opinion/john-ivison-trudeau-and-other-partisans-should-rein-in-the-rage

Jefferson, T., Del Mar, C. B., Dooley, L., Ferroni, E., Al-Ansary, L. A., Bawazeer, G. A., van Driel, M. L., Jones, M. A., Thorning, S., Beller, E. M., Clark, J., Hoffmann, T. C., Glasziou, P. P., & Conly, J. M. (2020). Physical interventions to interrupt or reduce the spread of respiratory viruses. *The Cochrane Database of Systematic Reviews, 11,* CD006207. https://doi.org/10.1002/14651858.CD006207.pub5

Jowett, G. S., O'Donnell, V. (2014). *Propaganda and persuasion*. Sage.

Jureidini, J., McHenry, L. B. (2022). The illusion of evidence based medicine. *British Medical Journal* 376, o702. http://dx.doi.org/10.1136/bmj.o702

Karlstad, Ø., Hovi, P., Husby, A., Härkänen, T., Selmer, R. M., Pihlström, N., Hansen, J. V., Nohynek, H., Gunnes, N., Sundström, A., Wohlfahrt, J., Nieminen, T. A., Grünewald, M., Gulseth, H. L., Hviid, A., & Ljung, R. (2022). Sars-CoV-2 vaccination and myocarditis in a nordic cohort study of 23 million residents. *JAMA Cardiology*. Advance online publication. https://doi.org/10.1001/jamacardio.2022.0583

Khanday, A. M. U. D., Khan, Q. R., & Rabani, S. T. (2020). Identifying propaganda from online social networks during COVID-19 using machine learning techniques. *International Journal of Information Technology : An Official Journal of Bharati Vidyapeeth's Institute of Computer Applications and Management, 13,* 115-122. https://doi.org/10.1007/s41870-020-00550-5

Kisielinski, K., Giboni, P., Prescher, A., Klosterhalfen, B., Graessel, D., Funken, S., Kempski, O., & Hirsch, O. (2021). Is a mask that covers the mouth and nose free from undesirable side effects in everyday use and free of potential hazards? *International Journal of Environmental Research and Public Health, 18*(8). https://doi.org/10.3390/ijerph18084344

Kisielinski, K. & Wojtasik, B. (2022). Suitability of Rose Bengal sodium salt staining for visualisation of face mask contamination by living organisms. *AIMS Environmental Science*, 9(2), 202-215

Kohn, M. A., Carpenter, C. R., & Newman, T. B. (2013). Understanding the direction of bias in studies of diagnostic test accuracy. *Academic Emergency Medicine, 20*(11), 1194–1206. https://doi.org/10.1111/acem.12255

Kompaniyets, L., Pennington, A. F., Goodman, A. B., Rosenblum, H. G., Belay, B., Ko, J. Y., Chevinsky, J. R., Schieber, L. Z., Summers, A. D., Lavery, A. M., Preston, L. E., Danielson, M. L., Cui, Z., Namulanda, G., Yusuf, H., Mac Kenzie, W. R., Wong, K. K., Baggs, J., Boehmer, T. K., & Gundlapalli, A. V. (2021). Underlying medical conditions and severe illness among 540,667 adults hospitalized with COVID-19, March 2020-March 2021. *Preventing Chronic Disease, 18,* E66. https://doi.org/10.5888/pcd18.210123

Lasswell, H. D. (1950). Propaganda and mass insecurity. *Psychiatry, 13*(3), 283–299. https://doi.org/10.1080/00332747.1950.11022781

Le Bon, G. (2018). *Psychologie der Massen* (R. Eisler, Trans.) (17. Auflage). Nikol Verlag.

Malloy, A., & Vazquez, M. (2021, December 16). *Biden warns of winter of 'severe illness and death' for unvaccinated due to Omicron.* CNN. https://edition.cnn.com/2021/12/16/politics/joe-biden-warning-winter/index.html

Mariotto, A. (2000). Alternatives to evidence based medicine. Propaganda based medicine is an alternative. *BMJ (Clinical Research Ed.), 321*(7255), 239.

Meerloo, J. (2015). *The rape of the mind: The psychology of thought control, menticide, and brainwashing*. Martino Publishing.

Millard, C. K. (1923). Vaccination propaganda and the medical profession. *British Medical Journal, 2*(3274), 564. https://doi.org/10.1136/bmj.2.3274.564

Montano, D. (2021). Frequency and associations of adverse reactions of COVID-19 vaccines reported to pharmacovigilance systems in the European Union and the United States. *Frontiers in Public Health, 9,* 756633. https://doi.org/10.3389/fpubh.2021.756633

Nelkin, D., & Gilman, S. L. (1988). Placing blame for devastating disease. *Social Research, 55*(3), 361–378.

Nikčević, A. V., & Spada, M. M. (2020). The COVID-19 anxiety syndrome scale: Development and psychometric properties. *Psychiatry Research, 292,* 113322. https://doi.org/10.1016/j.psychres.2020.113322

Nordström, P., Ballin, M., & Nordström, A. (2022). Risk of infection, hospitalisation, and death up to 9 months after a second dose of COVID-19 vaccine: A retrospective, total population cohort study in Sweden. *The Lancet, 399*(10327), 814–823. https://doi.org/10.1016/S0140-6736(22)00089-7

Olliaro, P., Torreele, E., & Vaillant, M. (2021). COVID-19 vaccine efficacy and effectiveness—the elephant (not) in the room. *The Lancet Microbe, 2*(7), e279-e280. https://doi.org/10.1016/S2666-5247(21)00069-0

Otter, S. (2022, January 22). The number of people who died of Covid-19 with no underlying health conditions revealed - as restrictions are scrapped: Figures show there have been a total of 175,256 Covid deaths. *Manchester Evening News.* https://www.manchestereveningnews.co.uk/news/uk-news/number-people-who-died-covid-22818253

Patone, M., Mei, X. W., Handunnetthi, L., Dixon, S., Zaccardi, F., Shankar-Hari, M., Watkinson, P., Khunti, K., Harnden, A., Coupland, C. A. C., Channon, K. M.,

Mills, N. L., Sheikh, A., & Hippisley-Cox, J. (2022). Risks of myocarditis, pericarditis, and cardiac arrhythmias associated with COVID-19 vaccination or SARS-CoV-2 infection. *Nature Medicine, 28*(2), 410–422. https://doi.org/10.1038/s41591-021-01630-0

Penston, J. (2011). Bowel cancer screening. Beware next wave of propaganda. *BMJ (Clinical Research Ed.), 342,* d3369. https://doi.org/10.1136/bmj.d3369

Polack, F. P., Thomas, S. J., Kitchin, N., Absalon, J., Gurtman, A., Lockhart, S., Perez, J. L., Pérez Marc, G., Moreira, E. D., Zerbini, C., Bailey, R., Swanson, K. A., Roychoudhury, S., Koury, K., Li, P., Kalina, W. V., Cooper, D., Frenck, R. W., Hammitt, L. L.,... Gruber, W. C. (2020). Safety and efficacy of the BNT162b2 mRNA Covid-19 vaccine. *The New England Journal of Medicine, 383*(27), 2603–2615. https://doi.org/10.1056/NEJMoa2034577

Rabson, M. (2021, May 04). *Trudeau says he is glad he got AstraZeneca, vaccines are only way out of pandemic.* The Canadian Press. https://www.cp24.com/news/trudeau-says-he-is-glad-he-got-astrazeneca-vaccines-are-only-way-out-of-pandemic-1.5413736

Radio Genova. (2022, February 15). *In Italy today 500 thousand unvaccinated citizens over 50 will be suspended from work and left without salary* [Tweet]. Twitter. https://twitter.com/RadioGenova/status/1493506165505990656

Schnepf, J., & Christmann, U. (2022). "It's a war! It's a battle! It's a fight!": Do militaristic metaphors increase people's threat perceptions and support for COVID-19 policies? *International Journal of Psychology : Journal International De Psychologie, 57*(1), 107–126. https://doi.org/10.1002/ijop.12797

Sell, R. G. (1977). What does safety propaganda do for safety? A review. *Applied Ergonomics, 8*(4), 203–214. https://doi.org/10.1016/0003-6870(77)90165-x

Seneff, S., Nigh, G., Kyriakopoulos, A. M., & McCullough, P. A. (2022). Innate immune suppression by SARS-CoV-2 mRNA vaccinations: The role of G-quadruplexes, exosomes, and MicroRNAs. *Food and Chemical Toxicology : An International Journal Published for the British Industrial Biological Research Association, 164,* 113008. https://doi.org/10.1016/j.fct.2022.113008

Singanayagam, A., Hakki, S., Dunning, J., Madon, K. J., Crone, M. A., Koycheva, A., Derqui-Fernandez, N., Barnett, J. L., Whitfield, M. G., Varro, R., Charlett, A., Kundu, R., Fenn, J., Cutajar, J., Quinn, V., Conibear, E., Barclay, W., Freemont, P. S., Taylor, G. P., . . . Lackenby, A. (2022). Community transmission and viral load kinetics of the SARS-CoV-2 delta (B.1.617.2) variant in vaccinated and unvaccinated individuals in the UK: a prospective, longitudinal, cohort study. *The Lancet Infectious Diseases*, 22(2), 183–195. https://doi.org/10.1016/S1473-3099(21)00648-4

Spira, B. (2022). Correlation between mask compliance and COVID-19 outcomes in Europe. *Cureus, 375*. https://doi.org/10.7759/cureus.24268

Stang, A., Robers, J., Schonert, B., Jöckel, K.-H., Spelsberg, A., Keil, U., & Cullen, P. (2021). The performance of the SARS-CoV-2 RT-PCR test as a tool for detecting SARS-CoV-2 infection in the population. *The Journal of Infection, 83*, 244-245. https://doi.org/10.1016/j.jinf.2021.05.022

Steinmeier, F. W. (2022). *Gespräch zu Hass und Gewalt in der Pandemie [Conversation on hate and violence in the pandemic]: Rede im Schloss Bellevue am 24. Januar 2022 [Speech at Bellevue Palace on January 24, 2022]*. https://www.bundespraesident.de/SharedDocs/Reden/DE/Frank-Walter-Steinmeier/Reden/2022/01/220124-Hass-Gewalt-Pandemie.html

Sukul, P., Bartels, J., Fuchs, P., Trefz, P., Remy, R., Rührmund, L., Kamysek, S., Schubert, J. K., & Miekisch, W. (2022). Effects of COVID-19 protective face-masks and wearing durations onto respiratory-haemodynamic physiology and exhaled breath constituents. *The European Respiratory Journal*. Advance online publication. https://doi.org/10.1183/13993003.00009-2022

Sun, C. L. F., Jaffe, E., & Levi, R. (2022). Increased emergency cardiovascular events among under-40 population in Israel during vaccine rollout and third COVID-19 wave. *Scientific Reports, 12*(1), 6978. https://doi.org/10.1038/s41598-022-10928-z

Surkova, E., Nikolayevskyy, V., & Drobniewski, F. (2020). False-positive COVID-19 results: Hidden problems and costs. *The Lancet Respiratory Medicine, 8*(12), 1167–1168. https://doi.org/10.1016/S2213-2600(20) 30453-7

Taylor, M., Kent, M.L. (2014). Dialogic engagement: Clarifying foundational concepts. *Journal of Public Relations Research, 26*(5), 384–398.

Trimble, M. (2021). Propaganda. *The Ulster Medical Journal, 90*(3), 133–134.

Wachter, D. von (2020). A philosophic investigation of the new Coronavirus. *The Beacon: Journal for Studying Ideologies and Mental Dimensions, 3*(1), 10910203. https://doi.org/10.55269/thebeacon. 3.010910203

Welt. (2020, November 25). *„Todeszahlen sind so hoch, als würde jeden Tag ein Flugzeug abstürzen", sagt Söder.* Welt. https://www.welt.de/politik/deutschland/article220993632/Markus-Soeder-Todeszahlen-so-hoch-als-wuerde-jeden-Tag-ein-Flugzeug-abstuerzen.html

Wenzel, R. P. (2017). Medical education in the era of alternative facts. *The New England Journal of Medicine, 377*(7), 607–609. https://doi.org/10.1056/NEJMp1706528

Wilder-Smith, A. (2022). What is the vaccine effect on reducing transmission in the context of the SARS-CoV-2 Delta variant? *The Lancet Infectious Diseases, 22*(2), 152–153. https://doi.org/10.1016/S1473-3099(21)00690-3

Wildner, M. (2016). Propaganda, nudging, information [Not Available]. *Gesundheitswesen (Bundesverband der Arzte des Offentlichen Gesundheitsdienstes (Germany)), 78*(6), 357–358. https://doi.org/10.1055/s-0042-109289

Zhang, L., Richards, A., Barrasa, M. I., Hughes, S. H., Young, R. A., & Jaenisch, R. (2021). Reverse-transcribed SARS-CoV-2 RNA can integrate into the genome of cultured human cells and can be expressed in patient-derived tissues. *Proceedings of the National Academy of Sciences of the United States of America, 118*(21). https://doi.org/10.1073/pnas.2105968118

# PART TWO

# COVID-19 management: Whose duties, whose rights?

# BALANCING THE RIGHTS OF THE INDIVIDUAL WITH THE 'COMMON GOOD' - ETHICAL AND POLICY FRAMEWORKS FOR COVID-19 PANDEMIC MANAGEMENT

**Michael Tomlinson**[1]

**Abstract:** The ethics literature is broadly favourable to governments using their coercive powers to impose mandatory lockdowns and vaccinations in response to dangerous pandemics. The world's governments had established plans for managing the periodic influenza pandemics based on a model or quarantining symptomatic individuals, but in 2020 they transitioned to confining the entire population of their countries for the interim period until vaccines became available, without considering policy options more broadly. This might be justified through a utilitarian appeal to 'the greatest good of the greatest number', but in calculating this, ethicists and governments tend to ignore the potential harms arising from lockdowns and assume that all vaccines are safe and effective for all individuals. Until possible harms are estimated and weighed in the balance against possible benefits in each individual case, mandates cannot be considered.

**Keywords:** SARS-CoV-2, COVID-19, lockdowns, vaccination, ethics

## Introduction

There have been a number of influenza epidemics and pandemics over the last hundred years, and there has been broad continuity in the approach governments have taken to managing them when they occur and to plan for future pandemics. However, the SARS-CoV-2 virus which causes COVID-19 was seen as a 'novel' virus and it was assumed that the world's populations would have minimal pre-existing immunity to it. As the death toll mounted in urbanised countries of Europe and the Americas in early

---

[1] Chair, Human Research Ethics Committee, National Institute of Integrative Medicine, Hawthorne, Australia

2020, governments were persuaded that 'novel' strategies were needed to counteract this grave threat. Some of these new strategies raised ethical issues more than those experienced during earlier pandemics.

## Pandemic Management Models

Governments had previously laid the foundations for their responses to future pandemics which would include surveillance, the deployment of 'non-pharmaceutical interventions' (NPIs) designed to mitigate the impact of pandemics and the development and deployment of vaccines to protect the population and reduce the impact of a pandemic further.

This overall model can be seen in the United States of America's *Pandemic Influenza Plan* (USA, 2017), and also in the World Health Organisation's *Global Influenza Strategy 2019-2030* (WHO, 2019a).

These plans are based on the model of seasonal influenza in which there would be recurring waves of influenza, which would "cause severe disease annually", with epidemics from time to time, and pandemics at unpredictable intervals (WHO, 2019b, p. 2). Despite differences in terminology, both documents essentially recommended mitigation strategies that would reduce the burden of disease but would not attempt to eliminate a virus that was expected to recur indefinitely.

The arrival on the world scene of SARS-CoV-2 caused a much higher level of concern than seasonal influenza, as it was assumed that the world population would have little or no pre-existing immunity and therefore the novel virus could cause extreme levels of mortality. Extreme levels of mortality were seen as likely by the Imperial College London (ICL) COVID-19 Response Team. Their influential *Report 9: Impact of non-pharmaceutical interventions (NPIs) to reduce COVID-19 mortality and healthcare demand of 16 March 2020* (Ferguson et al., 2020) recommended 'suppression' instead of mitigation, for at least 18 months 'until a vaccine becomes available' (p. 2).

By September of that year, Doshi (2020) pointed to a number of studies that indicated the need for a rethink about the lack of pre-existing immunity (p. 2):

> With public health responses around the world predicated on the assumption that the virus entered the human population with no pre-existing immunity before the pandemic, serosurvey data are leading many to conclude that the virus has, as Mike Ryan, WHO's head of emergencies, put it, "a long way to burn."
>
> Yet a stream of studies that have documented SARS-CoV-2 reactive T cells in people without exposure to the virus are raising questions about just how new the pandemic virus really is, with many implications.

The Imperial College Response Team used statistical modelling to project various scenarios and concluded that there would be 'approximately 510,000 deaths in GB and 2.2 million in the US' if no control measures were introduced. These figures were frightening but had no bearing on the choice they asked governments to make between mitigation or suppression. Figure 2 in their report shows in graphical form the projected effect of various combinations of mitigation strategies on the requirement for critical care intensive care unit (ICU) beds in the United Kingdom. The most successful of these strategies is shown (p. 8) as resulting in demand for ICU beds peaking at below 100 per 100,000 of population, a strategy consisting of: 'case isolation, home quarantine and social distancing of those aged over 70'. The recommended strategy was one which combined case isolation, social distancing of the entire population and either household quarantine or school and university closure. Yet Figure 3A showed the projected curve for this strategy peaking at a much higher level of just under 300 ICU beds per 100,000 of population.

The report does not explain why the team recommended a suppression strategy that was projected to result in peak demand for ICU beds around three times higher than the most successful mitigation strategy.

A critical assumption that the team made here without justification was that it would be necessary to reduce contact outside the home by 75% not only for symptomatic people, but also for asymptomatic people as well, over the interim period. The report does not discuss why confining all asymptomatic people would be necessary. There was an unspoken assumption that a vaccine would either end the pandemic or greatly reduce mortality.

To reduce outside contacts by 75% over the whole population it would be necessary to reduce mobility by that amount, which could only be achieved by governments using their coercive powers to impose 'stay at home' orders, preventing people from leaving their homes except for certain specified reasons (such as to exercise or to buy essential food and supplies). Backing this up were public health campaigns which presented the virus as a universal risk to everyone, whereas COVID-19 mortality in fact increases exponentially by age (Levin et al., 2020).

Most governments followed the recommendations of the ICL Team, abandoned traditional selective strategies and turned towards universal strategies in the first instance, with the most severe restrictions often referred to as 'lockdowns'. Definitions of 'lockdowns' vary in the literature, but for the purposes of this chapter we will use the ICL concept of drastic restriction of personal freedom of movement for the whole population, which was achieved through a mix of policies including public health campaigns and stay-at-home orders.

It had been common in previous epidemics to place symptomatic individuals in quarantine for short periods until they were no longer symptomatic. But never before had governments placed their entire population in quasi-quarantine for months at a time, including the vast majority of individuals who were entirely healthy and displaying no symptoms of the disease. Once vaccines did become available in 2021, governments believed it was imperative to vaccinate the entire population of all countries and so resorted to coercive methods again.

## Ethical Principles and Public Health Frameworks

To understand whether these restrictions on basic freedoms can be justified, we need to consider the interaction of public health policy with ethical and human rights frameworks. We need to consider how the most relevant generic principles interact with the specific and particular nature of the COVID-19 pandemic and of the first generation of COVID-19 vaccines. What principles of ethical conduct can potentially be used to support the government strategies, and are those principles relevant to all pandemics and all vaccines, or do they need to be tailored to the circumstances of particular pandemics and particular vaccines?

The relationship between these various factors and frameworks can be seen within the context of a decision sequence or tree, in which the government decision maker proceeds through a series of decision gates to formulate a plan or a program. Although explicit ethical principles form only one component of this sequence, the decision will not be ethically defensible unless each of these decision gates is negotiated correctly.

The starting point needs to be defining what the objectives of a program should be, the outcomes that are designed to be achieved or the nature of the problem that you are trying to solve (Schofield, 2001). Having decided what the objectives are, agencies then need to consider the most plausible options for achieving those objectives. Which strategies are the most likely to achieve the objectives given the evidence available? Here policymakers need to ensure that not only have they considered the evidence, but they have derived logically compelling conclusions from it, without falling into error in the way we have seen in the Imperial College Report 9. How likely is it that the chosen strategies are going to achieve the policy objective? Will the benefits exceed the costs (in human lives, health and wellness, not just the financial costs)? Are the restrictions ethically justifiable and compatible with human rights? Is there a way of achieving the objective without infringing human rights?

Once decision-makers start to consider using the coercive power of the state, they then need to consider the principles of classical liberalism and the need for checks and balances against the overreaching use of state power. Finally, if it is decided to use executive power to make a decision binding on everyone, certain legal tests need to be applied.

In formulating public policy during the outbreak of a pandemic, policy makers should have recourse to established frameworks which enable the widest possible view. The aggregate population health perspective (APHP) referred to by Reddy (2020) aims to reduce the burden of disease in similar terms to the ICL Report 9 and the U.S. *Pandemic Influenza Plan 2017*. However, the APHP framework entails a much wider scope than developing a strategy for an individual disease or pandemic at a point in time:

> First, it is concerned with mortality and morbidity from all sources and not merely from one source. All deaths matter, so to speak.
>
> Second, APHP does not seek to minimise deaths, but rather to maximise population health (or to minimise ill health, as the case may be). (p. 2)

Reddy goes on to derive several inferences from these axioms, including that the adverse effects of interventions need to be weighed in the balance and that alternative strategies need to be considered. Would investing in interventions in completely different areas of preventative health (e.g., nutritional support) raise the average number of life years of a population more than limiting the spread of the pandemic? The medium- and long-term effects of interventions need to be considered as well as the short-term effects.

In the case of COVID-19, Reddy (2020, pp. 5-6) advocates the use of 'smart' policies, such as focussing on the protection residents of aged care homes where at least 40% of deaths occurred in developed countries such as England during the first wave of the pandemic (Schultze et al., 2022), and differentiating interventions according to the needs of world regions (which vary greatly in susceptibility to COVID-19 because of variations in population age profile and urbanisation).

World governments never considered these issues, and never considered the potential of focused strategies targeting the groups at highest risk instead of universal strategies aimed at the entire population of the world. This was a major failure at the first decision gate leading to ethically unacceptable consequences, as the adverse effects of the decline in economic activity that was caused largely by lockdowns (and the associated public health campaign about the dangers of the virus) were thrown disproportionately on to the global poor, leading to increased inequality both within and between countries (World Bank, 2022).

Other strategic options should have been considered, including the deployment of a public health campaign to prevent symptomatic people leaving home, or systematically rolling out immune support nutrients such as vitamin D to nursing homes. Governments imposed lockdowns and (with the pharmaceutical companies) made investments of billions of dollars in the development of novel vaccines with no track-record of effectiveness or safety, while Vitamin D was neglected, despite the fact that it *did* have an acknowledged track-record in reducing respiratory infections (Martineau et al., 2017).

The closure of borders and the major restrictions on circulation within and between countries led to a disproportionate burden being placed on the poorer strata of each country and on the poorer regions of the world. For example, the World Bank projected that 97 million people would be thrown into extreme poverty in 2020. While they expected the economies of the poorer regions to recover, they also expect the after-effects of the downturn in 2020 to continue (Mahler et al., 2020).

These adverse effects are not purely economic (which would be difficult to weigh against the loss of lives through disease). For example, unemployment and poverty have a known adverse effect on health and specifically on mortality (Allen, 2021). The economic impacts are usually attributed to the pandemic itself, but the reductions in circulation of people and trade resulted primarily from the countermeasures.

The principles invoked in the ethical literature on mandatory public health measures essentially revolve around trade-offs: 'it should be a balance between all relevant harms and benefits that matters' (Dawson, 2011). But the authors and the governments do not weigh the potential harms enough in the balance to ensure that the trade-offs are favourable.

Dahlquist and Kugelberg (2021) note that 'public officials typically must offer a combination of normative and empirical reasons when they justify policies'. The policies must be justifiable in principle, and they must have good reason to believe they are likely to succeed in practice. In the case of coercive policies, these must be founded in general principles or normative reasons 'that every reasonable citizen could endorse or share'. But they ask (p. 1): 'is it permissible to implement policies justified with empirical claims that some reasonable citizens disagree with?' The normative principles are the subject of this chapter, while the empirical claims are discussed in a later chapter.

Dahlquist and Kugelberg (2021) also note that most political philosophers believe it is acceptable if there is a clear 'scientific consensus' that the policies are effective, but that this is a problematic test to pass in the early stages of a pandemic. The existence of the Great Barrington Declaration and the John Snow Memorandum clearly shows that there was no such consensus in 2020 (Alwan et al., 2020; Kulldorff et al., 2020).

Dahlquist and Kugelberg (2021) maintain the concept should be adapted and propose a requirement that there should be a 'negative consensus', i.e., that there is no scientific consensus at the time that the proposed measures are *not* effective. As they acknowledge, this allows for the initial adoption of measures (such as deep cleaning and disinfection of public spaces) that are later found to be ineffective.

But Dahlquist and Kugelberg (2021) do not address the scenario where the effectiveness of measures is fiercely contested by opposing groups of experts.

Their negative consensus model also does not engage with the scenario where measures violate individual rights or may cause major harms.

## Application of ethical principles to pandemic mandates

The discussion is more advanced in the case of vaccine mandates than in the case of the NPIs. Only a few governments went as far as the Austrian government in passing legislation to enable vaccination mandates for the entire population, but others put in place mandates for entering workplaces and hospitality venues, effectively shutting the unvaccinated out of society in an unprecedented way. Governments have assumed an overriding imperative to vaccinate the entire population of every country without making out a compelling case for universality.

Universal vaccination is often considered necessary in the ethics literature to create 'herd immunity' (the collective immunity of a whole population), resulting in elimination of the disease. Rare side effects would indeed be a small price to pay for population immunity.

But herd immunity is not always attainable through vaccines which do not always conform to the stereotype presented in the ethics literature, and are situated along a spectrum of harms, benefits and effectiveness. At one end of this spectrum, smallpox vaccination has been so effective that the disease has actually been eliminated. The measles vaccine may only have to be taken once, and produces long-lasting (even lifetime) immunity and protection against transmission to others.

At the other end of the spectrum in terms of effectiveness, the influenza vaccines are given annually, and vary in their effectiveness from year to year. And adverse effects can be severe. According to Miller et al. (2015), the 1976 U.S. swine flu vaccine 'was estimated to have caused approximately one Guillain–Barré syndrome case per 100,000 persons vaccinated, resulting in 53 deaths' (p. 2). This establishes a precedent showing that severe harms can possibly be caused by a vaccine, even deaths.

This brings into play the principle of 'non-maleficence' – governments must ensure that their policies do not cause undue harm (Varkey, 2021, p. 18). The effectiveness and safety of each individual vaccine need to be considered on a case-by-case basis. The more effective (especially in preventing transmission) and the less harmful they are, the stronger the case for inducing a population to be vaccinated, and the converse is also true.

Some writers invoke the need to provide for the 'common good' or the 'public good', both in the case of NPIs and vaccination. For example, in referring to herd immunity as a 'common good' Rus and Groselj (2021) make use of analogies:

> Usual examples of common goods are drinking water, food safety, clean air, etc. Their features are that they are non-excludable and non-rival, which means that nobody can be excluded from their benefits and new subjects do not diminish their availability. (p. 7)

Dawson (2011) expresses it well:

> A public good is a good that cannot be created by any individual alone: it takes collective efforts. It cannot be broken down into individual goods and distributed among the members of a population. All benefit in a population, if it exists.

But the analogy between herd immunity and common goods like drinking water breaks down insofar as the provision of clean water does not entail the possibility of causing any harms unlike vaccination, which it is accepted can produce vaccine injury. And, as we have noted above, while some vaccines may be capable of bringing about herd immunity, others (for example the influenza vaccines) are not.

So, although policymakers certainly need to consider the possibility of overall population benefits, they need to weigh these and the individual benefits against possible harms. This means that utilitarian ethics is the more relevant framework for the mandatory provision of both vaccination and NPIs, using the test of which strategy produces the greatest good for the greatest number of people.

Consistent with this, Reddy (2020) writes of the need to calculate and compare the number of quality adjusted life years (QALYs) to be gained from the alternative policy options, but it is also necessary to balance the lives to be gained against the lives that might be lost. A full utilitarian calculus would include all these positive and the negative factors - credits must greatly outweigh debits.

It would theoretically be possible to make a utilitarian defence of vaccines even if they caused some deaths using the model of the well-known 'trolley problem'. This is a philosophical thought experiment in which a decision-maker could throw a lever to save five people instead of only one from a runaway trolley on railway tracks (D'Olimpio, 2016), But health agencies do not allow any treatment or vaccine that is known to cause deaths, and this is not likely to change.

Ethical discussions of lockdowns prioritise collective interests just as the vaccination advocates do, for example: 'policy assessment and analysis must progress at the level of the group, rather than the individual' (John & Curran, 2021, p. 6). But they only consider the benefits to individuals and the benefits to society.

The ethical frameworks used for both vaccination and lockdown mandates must allow for the possibility of severe adverse effects such as the adverse effects of lockdowns on poverty and the consequential impact of unemployment and poverty on mortality referred to above.

Other studies have warned of the unintended consequences of ill patients avoiding doctors and appointments with hospitals. For example, Mansfield et al. (2021) found:

> Primary care contacts for almost all conditions dropped considerably after the introduction of population wide restrictions. The largest reductions were observed for contacts for diabetic emergencies...depression... and self-harm. (p. 1)

They also found a significant reduction in contacts for anxiety, eating disorders, obsessive-compulsive disorder, self-harm, severe mental illness, stroke transient, ischaemic attack heart failure, myocardial infarction, unstable angina, venous thromboembolism and asthma exacerbation. Deoni et al. and the RESONANCE Consortium (2021) also found that lockdowns and the closure of kindergartens and schools were 'significantly and negatively affecting infant and child development'.

Public health agencies have an ethical obligation to undertake due diligence in each pandemic to ensure that severe adverse effects of their measures are identified and considered, and also an obligation to ensure that they avoid the worst-case scenario in which harm is caused to individuals or classes of individuals without contributing to the common good.

## Individual Rights

*The International Covenant on Civil and Political Rights* (UN, 1976) includes a right to freedom of movement, and the Universal Declaration on Bioethics and Human Rights includes a right to personal autonomy for individuals to make their own decisions while respecting the autonomy of others. Some rights are regarded as inviolate or 'non-derogable' but other rights may be suspended during the period of the pandemic states of emergency.

Ethicists argue that both general lockdowns and universal vaccination are justifiable because people have a moral obligation to help each other in times of crisis, a line of argument that has great appeal to the public.

However, there are many moral obligations that are not enforced by law. Once governments consider using the coercive power of the state to promote vaccinations or NPIs, or any policy that potentially causes harm, additional justifications are needed, as these decisions introduce a political dimension that goes beyond moral obligations. The need to demonstrate that the measures do in fact help others becomes paramount.

A key reference point is 'On Liberty' published in 1859 by the utilitarian philosopher John Stuart Mill. Mill famously made a distinction between measures designed to protect an individual, and measures designed to stop that individual from harming others. The state should use its power only to prevent third-party harms:

> The only part of the conduct of anyone, for which he is amenable to society, is that which concerns others. In the part which merely concerns himself, his independence is, of right, absolute. Over himself, over his own body and mind, the individual is sovereign. (p. 18)

This distinction is generally brushed aside by contemporary ethicists and political philosophers writing on vaccination or lockdowns, and the rights of the individual are regarded as only one consideration to be weighed in the balance with others, and then quickly discarded.

This devaluing of individual rights is a regrettable trend. It ignores Mill's central contention, that the public (in the form of a government) cannot necessarily be trusted to make the right decisions about the interests of everyone: 'the strongest of all the arguments against the interference of the public with purely personal conduct, is that when it does interfere, the odds are that it interferes wrongly, and in the wrong place' (p. 158). Governments may make mistakes in the utilitarian calculus, in estimating the overall balance of benefits and harms. And they will naturally favour across-the-board strategies that might not be in the interests of every individual.

It is for this reason that individual rights must continue to have a special status when governments want to use their coercive power. The bar must be raised high when considering measures that are likely (based on consideration of the available evidence) to cause major harm. The evidence of benefits needs to be at a higher level than for measures (such as decontamination) that impose only financial costs. And the restrictive measures should only be put in place for a few weeks, at the most, as the epidemic wave rises.

NPIs were often justified on the basis of the 'precautionary principle', i.e., that the state had to take action to avert the possibility of future harms (from the pandemic) even if it was not certain they would eventuate. But the same principle should apply to the harms that may arise from government measures – these should be minimised as much as possible.

## Conclusion

Faced with a mounting death toll from COVID-19, governments were stampeded into abandoning traditional methods for mitigating pandemics and adopted new and untried measures that imposed extreme limitations on individual liberties. They believed that these limitations on individual liberty were necessary to maintain the common good. But the traditional concept of the common good does not take into consideration the severe harms that can result from lockdowns and sometimes from vaccination. The effects of lockdowns on economic interests were well understood and it was not considered ethically justified to trade off lives for prosperity. But their potential adverse effects on health and wellbeing (in both the short and long term) should also have been considered and weighed in the balance.

Governments could try and justify their policies on the basis that more lives would be saved than the lives lost. But in practice they have never acknowledged that their public health measures could cause any lives to be lost, which is a form of ethical bad faith. Governments have not been open about the fact that they are trading off current lives they believe will be saved against future lives that will probably be lost.

New principles need to be considered when framing public health policy, for example: the greater the harms potentially caused by a policy, then the higher the level of evidence needs to be that benefits will outweigh harms, and the greater the need for a consensus of scientific opinion in support. And the greater the violation of individual rights, the more the benefit to third parties must be evident rather than uncertain.

And rather than accepting any measure where the trade-off between benefits and harms might be at all positive, they should adapt the central objective of all traders, who aim to buy low and sell high. Governments should seek to implement pandemic policies that maximise their return on investment in terms of quality-adjusted life years. They should take an optimising approach to their public health decisions and adopt a mix of policies that are likely to save the maximum number of lives and cause the least number of lives to be lost. They should maximise the benefits and minimise the harms including the violations of individual rights.

To guard against the risk of governments making decisions that inflict harm on them. Individuals should remain sovereign over their own bodies and should not be usurped by their governments.

## References

Alwan, N. A., Burgess, R. A., Ashworth, S., Beale, R., Bhadelia, N., Bogaert, D., Dowd, J., Eckerle, I., Goldman, L. R., Greenhalgh, T., Gurdasani, D., Hamdy, A., Hanage, W. P., Hodcroft, E. B., Hyde, Z., Kellam, P., Kelly-Irving, M., Krammer, F., Lipsitch, M.,... Ziauddeen, H. (2020). Scientific consensus on the COVID-19 pandemic: We need to act now. *Lancet, 396*(10260), 671-672. https://doi.org/10.1016/S0140-6736(20)32153-X

Dahlquist, M., & Kugelberg, H. D. (2021). Public justification and expert disagreement over non-pharmaceutical interventions for the COVID-19 pandemic. *Journal of Medical Ethics.* https://doi.org/10.1136/medethics-2021-107671

Dawson, A. (2011). Vaccination ethics. In A. Dawson (Ed.), *Public health ethics: Key concepts and issues in policy and practice* (pp. 143-153). Cambridge University Press. https://doi.org/10.1017/CBO9780511862670.009

Deoni, S., Beachemin, A., & Da Sa, V. (2021). Impact of the COVID-19 pandemic on early child cognitive development: Initial findings in a longitudinal observational study of child health. *medRxiv*. https://doi.org/10.1101/2021.08.10.21261846

D'Olimpio, L. (2016). The trolley dilemma: Would you kill one person to save five? https://theconversation.com/the-trolley-dilemma-would-you-kill-one-person-to-save-five-57111 (Accessed: 18 February 2022).

Doshi, P. (2020). Covid-19: Do many people have pre-existing immunity? *BMJ, 370*. https://www.bmj.com/content/370/bmj.m3563

Ferguson, N., Laydon, D., Nedjati-Gilani, G., Imai, N., Ainslie, K., Baguelin, M., Bhatia, S., Boonyasiri, A., Cucunuba, Z., Cuomo-Dannenburg, G., Dighe, A., Dorigatti, I., Fu, H., Gaythorpe, K., Green, W., Hamlet, A., Hinsley, W., Okell, L. C., van Elsland, S.,... & Ghani, A. C. (2020). Report 9: Impact of non-pharmaceutical interventions (NPIs) to reduce COVID19 mortality and healthcare demand. *Imperial College London, 10*(77482). https://www.imperial.ac.uk/media/imperial-college/medicine/sph/ide/gida-fellowships/Imperial-College-COVID19-NPI-modelling-16-03-2020.pdf

John, S. D., & Curran, E. J. (2021). Costa, cancer and coronavirus: Contractualism as a guide to the ethics of lockdown. *Journal of Medical Ethics*. https://doi.org/10.1136/medethics-2020-107103

Kulldorff, M., Gupta, S., & Bhattacharya, J. (2020). Great Barrington Declaration. https://gbdeclaration.org/ (accessed 31 March 2022).

Mahler, D., Yonsan, N., Lakner, C., Aguilar, R., & Wu, H. (2021). Updated estimates of the impact of COVID-19 on global poverty: Turning the corner on the pandemic in 2021? https://blogs.worldbank.org/opendata/updated-estimates-impact-covid-19-global-poverty-turning-corner-pandemic-2021 (Accessed: 16 February 2022).

Martineau, A. R., Jolliffe, D. A., Hooper, R. L., Greenberg, L., Aloia, J. F., Bergman, P., Dubnov-Raz, G., Esposito, S., Ganmaa, D., Ginde, A. A., Goodall, E. C., Grant, C. C., Griffiths, C. J., Janssens, W., Laaksi, I., Manaseki-Holland, S., Mauger, D., Murdoch, D. R., Neale, R.,... & Camargo, C. A. (2017). Vitamin D supplementation to prevent acute respiratory tract infections: Systematic review and meta-analysis of individual participant data. *BMJ, 356*. https://dx.doi.org/10.1136/bmj.i6583

Mill, J., S. (2011). *On liberty*. Project Gutenberg. (Original work published 1859). https://www.gutenberg.org/files/34901/34901-h/34901-h.htm

Miller, E., Moro, P., Cano, M, & Shimabukuro, T. (2015). Deaths following vaccination: What does the evidence show? *Vaccine, 33*(29), 3288-3292. https://www.ncbi.nlm.nih.gov/pmc/articles/PMC4599698/

Reddy, S. G. (2020). Population health, economics and ethics in the age of COVID-19. *BMJ Global Health, 5*(7), e003259. https://doi.org/10.1136/bmjgh-2020-003259

Rus, M. & Groselj U. (2021) Ethics of vaccination in childhood - A framework based on the four principles of biomedical ethics. *Vaccines, 9*(2), 113. https://doi.org/10.3390/vaccines9020113

Schofield, J. (2001). Time for a revival? Public policy implementation: A review of the literature and an agenda for future research. *International Journal of Management Reviews, 3*(3), 245-263. https://doi.org/10.1111/1468-2370.00066

United Nations (UN). (1976). *International covenant on civil and political rights*. https://www.ohchr.org/en/professionalinterest/pages/ccpr.aspx.

United States of America (USA). (2017). *Pandemic influenza plan 2017.* Department of Health and Human Services. *Update*. https://www.cdc.gov/flu/pandemic-resources/national-strategy/index.html

Varkey, B. (2021). Principles of clinical ethics and their application to practice. *Medical Principles and Practice, 30*(1), 17-28. https://doi.org/10.1159/000509119

World Bank. (2022). *Global economic prospects, January 2022.* https://doi.org/10.1596/978-1-4648-1758-8

World Health Organisation (WHO). (2019a). *Global influenza strategy 2019-2030.* World Health Organisation. https://www.who.int/publications /i/item/9789241515320

World Health Organisation (WHO). (2019b). *Non-pharmaceutical public health measures for mitigating the risk and impact of epidemic and pandemic influenza.* World Health Organisation. https://www.who.int/publications/i/item/non-pharmaceutical-public-health-measuresfor-mitigating-the-risk-and-impact-of-epidemic-and-pandemic-influenza

# SCIENCE CENSORSHIP, PUBLIC POLICY AND THE RULE OF LAW: A CRITICAL REVIEW

**Christiaan W. J. M. Alting von Geusau**[1]

**Abstract:** In this chapter we analyze the interplay between government, (social) media and the scientific community during the COVID-19 pandemic. Both the reality of a global health emergency and ideological attitudes have shaped public policy and the way in which we think about what a proper pandemic response is or should be. In this process, the need for political action that is firmly grounded in scientific evidence has at times been confused with the politicization of science for ideological reasons. This in turn has led in our liberal democratic societies to an atmosphere where freedom of speech, academic freedom and an open scientific debate have been limited, even leading to the censorship or cancelling of some of the world's most renowned scientists and doctors. In this chapter we will argue that ultimately, such developments lead to the regression of science and the weakening of the rule of law, which is the foundation of liberal democracies in the West.

## 1. Introduction

> Pride blinds us to our own blindness, and there is no pride sweeter to the taste, and so enslaving, as the illusion of superior knowledge. This is especially true when one has a great deal invested emotionally in one's own theory. (O'Brien, 1996, p. 338)

The claim to superior knowledge and a great deal of emotional investment in the implementation of far-reaching public health policies purportedly grounded in science, have been hallmarks of the COVID-19 response of governments and the media the world over. An illustrative example is how on 19 March 2020, Prime Minister Jacinda Ardern of New Zealand, at an impromptu press conference on the emerging COVID-19 pandemic, made

---

[1] Rector and Professor of Law and Education, Katholische Hochschule ITI, Trumau, Austria

the blunt statement that "we will continue to be your single source of truth," (BFD, 2020), referring to what in her view was the proper source of information as compared to information coming from alternative social media and the internet not sourced by her government. These words by a senior political leader of a Western liberal democracy could easily be taken out of context and used for political purposes to dismiss an opponent. The statement is related to a journalist's question concerning rumors of a lockdown being imposed in New Zealand at the time. Yet if one reads the verbatim quote and the subsequent parliamentary debate cited in the official publication of the New Zealand parliament (Oral Questions – Questions to Ministers, 2 Sept. 2020), it becomes clear that the intended message of this public statement by the government leader seems somewhat broader: when it comes to the COVID-19 response, only trust information provided by the government and dismiss the rest as probably false, no matter what the source is.

This small and easily overlooked incident illustrates a problem that we have seen unfolding globally since the outbreak of the COVID-19 pandemic in 2020: governments, with the help of most of the major (social) media outlets, either openly claiming, or suggesting by their way of handling the situation, that they are the sole arbiters of (scientific) truth where it comes to the question of what the right sort of response to the health crisis is. Not only the Chinese communist dictatorship through its infamous shaming and silencing of whistleblower doctor Li Wenliang, who exposed COVID-19 to the world, engaged in this behavior (Nie & Elliott, 2020), but also some Western governments and media organizations went down a similar path. One of the direct consequences of this rather undemocratic and not very progressive attitude has been that those manifold equally knowledgeable scientists, doctors and other medical and legal experts that are not amongst the very small group of people advising governments and the World Health Organization (WHO), such as for example world renowned academics Dr. Jay Bhattacharya (Professor of Medicine at Stanford University), Dr. Peter McCullough (a widely published epidemiologist and cardiologist), Dr. Martin Kulldorf (epidemiologist, biostatistical experts and former Professor of Medicine at Harvard University) or Dr. Luc Montagnier (Nobel Prize in Medicine), have at best been ignored and at worst were censored or otherwise silenced, no matter their senior status or stellar academic reputation and wealth of knowledge and published peer-reviewed research. How did this situation come about?

There is of course no question that in situations of national or global health emergencies governments and international organizations must act and often need to do so fast without the time that is normally available to investigate and debate at length what the full range of possible options is and how these are supported by the science and relevant experience of earlier crises. At the same time, the political pressure to act fast can also lead to a distorted understanding of how a government should respond in such emergency situations and a negation of the full spectrum of available and relevant science. For example, at the very beginning of the COVID-19 pandemic, Western countries were looking with puzzlement and alarm at the draconian lockdown measures that were being imposed by Chinese government authorities and that are being imposed again now in 2022 in major cities such as Shanghai. Until the beginning of March 2020, most Western countries and the World Health Organization (WHO) rejected the idea of lockdowns as an acceptable and effective instrument for pandemic management, then suddenly changed course in March of that same year, ultimately leading to half of the world population being in lockdown by April 2020. This was whilst the science on the instrument of lockdowns had, in the meantime, not substantially changed. Magness and Earle note in the *Wall Street Journal* in December 2021, referencing a series of authoritative pre-pandemic WHO and other relevant studies: "Yet before March 2020, the mainstream scientific community, including the World Health Organization, strongly opposed lockdowns and similar measures against infectious disease." (Magness & Earle, 2021, para. 1). Furthermore, in the months and two years that followed, an impressive body of additional science was published that confirmed this long-standing notion about the ineffectiveness and serious multi-faceted drawbacks and unintended negative consequences of lockdowns (Alexander, 2020; Herby et al., 2022). Why was this specific evidence after March 2020 largely ignored by many governments and the media the world over, whilst citing as alternative evidence far fewer and only recently published scientific studies and "speculative and untested epidemiological models" (Magness & Earle, 2021, para. 10) that now spoke in favor of lockdowns? Was it ignored because it was a novel virus that was suddenly hospitalizing and killing many people, whilst political and health leaders did not know how to handle the situation due to a lack of clinical experience? Was reverting to lockdowns an act of helplessness in the face of an unprecedented public health crisis with no ready alternative solutions and little in the way of experience?

Respected scientific voices and publications that were critical of these lockdown measures were in turn, as of March 2020, regularly silenced and censored. A striking example is that of the internationally highly respected (now former) Harvard Professor of Medicine, epidemiologist, and bio-statistician Dr. Martin Kulldorff, who in April 2020 wrote an article titled "COVID-19 Counter Measures Should be Age Specific" and published it on his LinkedIn page, since no medical journal at the time was willing to publish his contribution critical of lockdown measures, this in itself being a sign of self-censorship by medical journals. Then, at the end of January 2022, any mention of this article and the whole LinkedIn profile page of Kulldorff suddenly disappeared. It took a widely circulated article on the Brownstone Institute website (Tucker, 2022) protesting this turn of events to have Kulldorff's profile and article fully restored. It was not the first time this happened to him. In February 2021, Facebook, without warning or prior communication deleted the official page of the Great Barrington Declaration, an October 2021 statement signed by himself and two equally internationally renowned infectious disease epidemiologists and public health scientists from the University of Oxford (Gupta) and Stanford University (Bhattacharya), in which they proposed a science-based alternative approach to nationwide lockdowns and that has in the meantime been co-signed by close to a million people from around the globe, many of them medical professionals (see https://gbdeclaration.org/). As was revealed at the end of 2021 (Magness & Harrigan, 2021), senior U.S. Government officials in late 2020 participated in an effort to instigate "a devastating published take down" of the scientifically argued premises of the Great Barrington Declaration. Also, Gupta and Bhattacharya, tenured professors at Oxford and Stanford, were heavily censored whilst undergoing defamatory attacks in the media (Bhattacharya, 2022). Even established medical journals are not free from the "fact-checkers" and censors of the social media conglomerates. This also affects those respected publications that would write supportive of government COVID-19 policies and that for example published heavy criticism of the same authors of the Great Barrington Declaration (Gorski & Yamey, 2021). For example, it took a December 2021 open letter (Godlee & Abbasi, 2021) published by the incoming and current editors-in-chief of the *British Medical Journal* (*BMJ*) to Mark Zuckerberg, CEO of Meta, to draw public attention to the shocking fact of Facebook censoring a *BMJ* peer-reviewed article that reported on proven irregularities in one of the main COVID-19 vaccine trials (Thacker, 2021). Kamran Abbasi, the *BMJ*'s current editor in chief, did not mince his words when asked to comment on this incident:

> We should all be very worried that Facebook, a multibillion-dollar company, is effectively censoring fully fact checked journalism that is raising legitimate concerns about the conduct of clinical trials. Facebook's actions won't stop The BMJ doing what is right, but the real question is: why is Facebook acting in this way? What is driving its world view? Is it ideology? Is it commercial interests? Is it incompetence? Users should be worried that, despite presenting itself as a neutral social media platform, Facebook is trying to control how people think under the guise of 'fact checking'. (Godlee & Abbasi, 2021)

These are just some of many examples (see reference to the website Censortrack below) of censorship and cancelling of respected scientists and journals with sound professional records, yet who have had the audacity to question the official government or WHO line on COVID-19 response and consequently seem to have been singled out for heavy-handed intervention by mostly the major social media platforms. The American website censortrack.org documents such cases and until February 9$^{th}$, 2022, recorded 808 cases of specific censorship by (social) media regarding COVID-19 related topics (Vazquez & Pariseau, 2022). In a modern liberal democratic society, where science and technology drive much of what we do and is promoted as such, it is imperative that, also in crisis situations where many lives are at stake, full scientific and government transparency is guaranteed, as well as a generous willingness for critical assessment, public debate, and the possibility to revisit previous conclusions and change course where necessary. As Kulldorff noted, "[s]cience is about rational disagreement, the questioning and testing of orthodoxy and the constant search for truth." (Kulldorf, 2021). It is this search for truth that seems often to have been lost during the COVID-19 crisis and around the related public health responses instigated by elected and appointed political and civil leaders and communicated by (social) media outlets. Both the specific nature of this health emergency, as well as political considerations, seem to have caused this. Therefore, the role of science in the democratic process of governance, especially in times of grave crisis, needs to be re-assessed in light of the question how science relates to lawmaking?

## What is the role of science in a democratic society?

Science in a liberal democratic society has the role of informing us on the complicated and ever-changing realities of human life and nature. Science should assist us in making informed and responsible decisions in many areas of life, of which health and medicine are some of the most important. They pertain to the well-being of individual citizens, communities, nations and humanity as a whole. Hence, good science is paramount to sound public policy and lawmaking. The most important indicator of "good science" is that it always remains open to public scrutiny and discussion. In this context we need to understand that a public health norm that has been decided and implemented by a democratically elected government or its agencies, mostly upon the advice of expert committees, is not the same as there being scientific consensus on the subject matter that this norm seeks to regulate. To apply this vital distinction to the COVID-19 crisis: the fact that a government or the WHO decides to respond to COVID-19 by recommending or implementing mask mandates, lockdowns and vaccine mandates, each of these measures limiting fundamental rights and freedoms of individual citizens, does not automatically mean that there is scientific consensus as to the necessity, effectiveness and thus justifiability of these public health norms. According to Abbasi (2020) "[p]oliticians often claim to follow the science, but that is a misleading oversimplification. Science is rarely absolute. It rarely applies to every setting or every population" (para. 7). Kulldorf (2020) adds that "[a]cademics backing lockdown (or any major theory) ought to welcome challenges, knowing – as scientists do – that robust challenge is the way to identify error, improve policy and save lives." (para. 1).

In situations of a public health emergency as we have seen developing globally since 2020, it is understandable, as was already noted above, that governments must take tough decisions and often must do so fast to try to contain the spread and the negative public health effects of a highly contagious virus. Knowing that science plays such a vital role in guiding political leaders to take these difficult decisions, the danger of science being used in a selective and biased way is real as elected officials seek to find acceptable arguments for the far-reaching and unpleasant public health responses they have decided on. For example: the fact that fear scenarios were being used to nudge populations into accepting lockdowns or other COVID-19 measures (Dodsworth, 2021) and that these measures were based on only one specific interpretation of science, did not therefore make that science the only truth and the actions based on that (including the use of fear) necessarily justifiable. Abbasi (2020) points out the challenge in such situations, where he states that:

> [s]cience is a public good. It doesn't need to be followed blindly, but it does need to be fairly considered. Importantly, suppressing science, whether by delaying publication, cherry picking favorable research, or gagging scientists, is a danger to public health, causing deaths by exposing people to unsafe or ineffective interventions and preventing them from benefiting from better ones. (para. 13)

In a liberal democratic society, all knowledgeable and reasonable voices need to be heard where science has the role of providing the necessary arguments both in favor and against certain public health decisions that affect the individual citizen. This is especially important for those measures that limit the exercise of fundamental rights and freedoms and thus have a negative effect on the rule of law that is based on a fragile system of equilibrium between state authority and individual liberty and responsibility. It is not for the state to make medically relevant choices for its citizens, rather it has a duty to offer its citizens, without coercion, the best available options to protect themselves and allow them to help their communities to responsibly do the same. Science communicated and openly debated in a transparent and balanced way, whilst always acknowledging the fact that it is a process and not an endpoint in finding out the truth about the realities of human life and nature, will help citizens to make informed decisions that are the right ones for them and for their communities. This in turn will build the public trust that is necessary in a democratic society to convince the general population to accept state authority in general and to also actively support the public health policies implemented, especially if in times of great physical danger this might lead to a temporary inability to fully enjoy one's constitutional rights and freedoms. If science is not applied in this democratic manner, it quickly becomes politicized, and risks being rejected by ever more citizens as a trustworthy source of knowing. The question that begs itself here is why relatively few doctors, other medical experts and lawyers have really engaged in a robust public debate on the science and legal implications in connection with the COVID-19 measures implemented by the WHO and governments around the word since 2020? Were they afraid for their careers, and if so, what would have caused such fear, and was the resulting silence justified? Were doctors and hospitals free in choosing the treatment protocols that they deemed best for their patients, and if not, why did they not have this freedom? Was all relevant and peer-reviewed scientific research sufficiently made available and communicated to those making policy and those treating patients whilst trying to mitigate the (deadly) effects of the pandemic? If not, why not?

We have seen a dynamic at work since the beginning of 2020 whereby few governments and major media outlasts have been willing to bring to the fore that the science on most of the public health measures implemented in response to COVID-19 is not settled but still very much in development, as science usually is. This has led, as already stated above, to government and media not sufficiently informing the public on important data, new studies and conclusions by experienced and respected scientists and academics that at times have been at odds with official policy. This could for example be observed again when Twitter in March 2022 censored the widely respected British epidemiologist Carl Heneghan who had written an article in the Mail on Sunday about an Oxford University study published by the prestigious medical journal *The Lancet* (COVID-19 Excess Mortality Collaborators, 2022). The study, referenced by the censored article, explained with clear data how the conclusion was warranted that the actual COVID-19 death toll in Great Britain might be lower than was initially reported by official sources and the media. Twitter however thought it had a better grip on the science and intervened to block Heneghan. In a liberal democratic society based on the rule of law, openness, freedom, personal responsibility and solidarity are the pillars of an ordered and prosperous society. When government and media suppress or deliberately ignore relevant scientific information and opinions pertaining to public health, especially in times of a severe health crisis, they undermine the trust that is the foundation for the functioning of that society. They also throttle the disagreement and debate that is necessary to come to new hypotheses and potentially better solutions to thew problems at hand.

## Science censorship and the limitation of rights in times of crisis

When in times of national or international emergency science is being extensively cited by democratically elected leaders and their unelected experts to justify far-reaching public health measures that limit the exercise of the fundamental rights and freedoms of its citizens, the state needs to act with great care and maximum restraint, whilst strictly abiding by the legal principle of proportionality. This principle, when correctly applied to government action, ensures that whatever measure is taken, it has been carefully weighed so as to assure that under the circumstances no other measure could have been taken that would have been less invasive and yet achieve the same, a comparable or otherwise acceptable result. If a government wishes to apply the principle of proportionality, it thus requires a transparent and unbiased relationship with and application of the supporting science and independence from conflicting commercial interests. The first step in such a process would be, especially in a liberal democratic society, that the state and the media responsible for informing the citizens of that state, guarantee full disclosure and freedom of expression without which, as we noted above, science cannot function. Jeffrey Singer (2022) points out how during COVID-19 a relatively small group of experts has been exerting disproportionate influence over their peers and thereby "establish an orthodoxy enforced by a priesthood. If anyone, expert or otherwise, questions the orthodoxy, they commit heresy. The result is groupthink, which undermines the scientific process."

There exists no constitution or law in democratic societies that would give the state or its unelected health experts the authority to generally suspend rights and freedoms in times of emergency. What legal systems and human rights treaties of Western liberal democracies do permit is for the state alone to restrict the execution of these rights, but only when strictly limited in time and under clearly defined circumstances as regulated by a law approved by the legislature. This in turn would only be possible when doing so is in the immediate and compelling interest of protecting public health and safety and no acceptable alternative options are available. These limitations cannot however lead to such fundamental rights and freedoms losing their inalienable character within the system of the rule of law and international human rights principles and treaties. One example of such a provision can be found in the European Convention on Human Rights. It states in article 10 (highlighting CAvG):

> 1. Everyone has the right to freedom of expression. This right shall include freedom to hold opinions and **to receive and impart information and ideas without interference by public authority** and regardless of frontiers. (...)
>
> 2. The exercise of these freedoms, since it carries with it duties and responsibilities, **may be subject to such formalities, conditions, restrictions or penalties as are prescribed by law and are necessary in a democratic society, in the interests of national security, territorial integrity or public safety, for the prevention of disorder or crime, for the protection of health or morals**, for the protection of the reputation or rights of others, for preventing the disclosure of information received in confidence, or for maintaining the authority and impartiality of the judiciary.

To arrive at the point where the execution of the right to freedom of expression – also within the scientific community - may be limited, a very high bar of justification needs to be met. In the case of the COVID-19 pandemic, the justification for the state or the (social) media to suppress the imparting of certain medical information as well as scientific interpretations that do not correspond with the information and conclusions that are used to provide the argumentation for certain public health interventions, needs to be able to convincingly (beyond reasonable doubt) show that proceeding otherwise would cause an immediate clear and present danger to the health of the general population or parts thereof. In the case of lockdowns for example, one could now conclude, thanks to the meta study published by Herby et al. (2022) from John Hopkins University in January and May 2022, that it was wholly justified for European and American scientists like those quoted above to question the efficacy of lockdowns in the beginning of and throughout the pandemic. Yet the website Censortrack.org has documented over 800 instances of censorship, silencing and cancelling by social media between March 17, 2020, and February 3, 2022 of scientists, doctors, medical journals, elected officials and journalists (Vazquez & Pariseau, 2022) who did not follow the conclusions and interpretations proposed by the WHO and most national governments.

Niemiec (2020, pp. 1-2) of the Uppsala University *Centre for Research Ethics and Bioethics* deals extensively with the question of censorship of science in the purported interests of combatting "medical misinformation" in times of a health emergency. She points out that the categories used by social media for removing "objectionable content" are far broader than those listed within the legal frameworks of liberal democratic societies. Niemiec also observes that content moderation is often politically biased and that the moderating platforms are themselves not immune to commercial interests. She goes on to explain that social media removing medical information or scientifically argued opinions simply because they contradict what national health authorities or the WHO say is problematic:

> (...) who exactly defines and how which information is deemed to be false or harmful? And can we rely on these judgements? One of the authoritative sources that all three major social media platforms mention in their policies on COVID-19 is the WHO. It is an established and influential organization, yet it may make mistakes, including in the context of handling epidemics. (p. 2)

We have seen during the past two years that indeed the WHO is not unerring, and neither are national public health authorities, like the United States' Centers for Disease Control and Prevention (CDC). An example is the fact that in 2020 and 2021, public health officials the world over understandably and enthusiastically declared that the newly launched COVID-19 vaccines were largely going to stop infection and transmission, referring to scientific data to prove this (Choi, 2021). These same officials had to admit only some months later in the summer of 2021 that this was unfortunately not the case and hence the data used previously seems not to have been accurate (Mascarenhas & Maxouris, 2021). Niemiec (2020) observes: "[c]onstructive critique, questioning of evidence and opinions of scientists and policymakers are thus necessary to identify and correct potential errors and to prevent them from being propagated" (p. 2).

This is the reason why in a liberal democratic society, where so much depends on the trust of the governed in their leaders and the institutions shaping and implementing public policy, it is of vital importance that when science is used to explain and then to encourage adherence to far-reaching public health measures, the way in which science is applied remains transparent and is always open to further scrutiny, public debate and the inclusion of alternative viewpoints that are also rooted in science. A real failure of such transparency and democratic due process can be observed through the fact that the European Commission refuses until today to disclose the contracts between Pfizer and the European union (EU) on the production, effects and distribution of COVID-19 vaccines, even not allowing the duly elected members of the European Parliament to gain access to these contracts.

Assembly Bill 2098, that is currently working its way through the California Legislature, is another example of a problematic state intervention in the dissemination of medical science and the practice of medicine itself. It seeks to combat what is deemed to be "misinformation" or "disinformation" and seems to propose punishment for medical practitioners who provide information to their patients that is not approved by the state:

> 2270. (a) It shall constitute unprofessional conduct for a physician and surgeon to disseminate or promote misinformation or disinformation related to COVID-19, including false or misleading information regarding the nature and risks of the virus, its prevention and treatment; and the development, safety, and effectiveness of COVID-19 vaccines.

Who defines what is "misinformation" and "disinformation"? The proposed law does not clearly define this and leaves it open to broad interpretation by state medical boards. Should this be the exclusive role of the state and its institutions, aided by media outlets? Or do we want a broad public debate rooted in science and continued research amongst peers who should have full access to all relevant evidence collected both by the scientific community and the relevant government agencies? Is it the exclusive prerogative of the state, especially in times of health emergencies, to interpret science? Here we come back to what was noted already above: science in a liberal democratic society is a process, not an endpoint. It requires constant questioning of the already accepted interpretations, conclusions and measures, in order that better interpretations, conclusions and measures might be put forth. This is especially important where it concerns medical science: it is about the health and well-being of individual people. Where human life is at stake, science can never be "settled" if further (lifesaving) improvements or corrections can still be made. Ultimately, as the *British Medical Journal* stated, "[w]hen good science is suppressed, people die" (Abbasi, 2020). I would like to add to this: when good science is suppressed, democracy and progress also die.

## Conclusion

Taking into consideration the process described above, it is likely that as a result self-censorship has been, and continues to be, the most widespread form of suppression of science during the COVID-19 pandemic. Wherever externally imposed censorship by certain actors in society has become the norm under the label of "protecting public health" and "fighting misinformation", the logical result has been that most of those who were already censored, or those who fear to be censored, will prefer to avoid such a situation and its (possibly career-ending) consequences by not publishing research and conclusions they would have otherwise published, or by toning down or adapting their writings in such a way as not to fall under the hammer of censorship. We all know that ultimately, this does not serve the interests of public health and it certainly does not save lives. Public health too, even when it is threatened by a pathogen that causes overflowing hospitals and much death, needs freedom of speech and a robust scientific discourse. In the words of the Canadian psychoanalyst Jordan Peterson, during a November 2021 lecture at Cambridge University:

> Free speech is not just another freedom or right among many. It is certainly not viewpoint diversity or anything like that. It is the mechanism by which we generate conceptions that allow us to organize our experience in the world. It is that mechanism. And more than that, it is the mechanism that

> allows us to reformulate and criticize those conceptions which when they become outdated and sterile, to dissolve them into the chaos that we have to contend with while it is occurring and then to reanimate in a new form so that we can move into the future. (Peterson, 2022)

For a democratic society based on the rule of law and that prides itself in its liberal ideals and the seemingly unstoppable achievements of science and technology, censorship and other suppression of free speech and scientific investigation is a tragic and dangerous development. It will undoubtedly lead to a serious undermining of science itself and of human progress in general. When a society is no longer capable or willing to deal with differing insights in times of crisis and beyond, whilst it cancels those views that do not fit into a specific narrative that has been chosen to be the exclusively acceptable way of looking at the situation with the unassailable argument "to keep everybody safe", tyranny is not far around the corner. As C.S. Lewis put it strikingly:

> Of all tyrannies, a tyranny sincerely exercised for the good of its victims may be the most oppressive... those who torment us for our own good will torment us without end for they do so with the approval of their own conscience. (Lewis, 2014, p. 234)

Assuredly less presumption of the superiority of our knowledge, a greater willingness to listen to fellow human beings with equally carefully researched yet differing insights and interpretations, and a healthy dose of modesty in our dealings with science as an argument for public policy could avert such a tyranny and instead strengthen democracy and the rule of law. In such a constellation, the inalienable dignity of every human being is taken into consideration as the starting point. A human being that by its very nature is capable of living in freedom and taking responsibility, whilst carefully weighing all interests involved, also those of the larger community. Here we should never scare away from the simple fact that contradiction and debate is the flip side of democracy, no less so in times of crisis where much is at stake. The history of Western civilization and its impressive achievements tells us that this will with certainty lead to better science and further enlightened progress for humanity. This is something we all desire and can thus together strive for.

## References

Abbasi, K. (2020). Covid-19: Politicisation, "corruption," and suppression of science. *BMJ, 371*(m4425). https://doi.org/10.1136/bmj.m4425

Alexander, P. E. (2021). More than 400 studies on the failure of compulsory Covid interventions (lockdowns, restrictions, closures). Brownstone Institute. https://brownstone.org/articles/more-than-400-studies-on-the-failure-of-compulsory-covid-interventions/

BFD. (2020, May 15). *Jacinda Ardern – "We will continue to be your single source of truth"* [Video]. YouTube. https://youtu.be/ENEUktOrQV8

Bhattacharya, J. (2022). *A warning from Shanghai.* Common Sense. https://www.commonsense.news/p/a-warning-from-shanghai?s=r

California Legislature, 2021 – 2022 Regular Session, Assembly Bill No. 2098, introduced by Assembly Member Low. https://leginfo.legislature.ca.gov/faces/billTextClient.xhtml?bill_id=202120220AB2098

Choi, J. (2021). *Fauci: Vaccinated people become 'dead ends' for the coronavirus.* The Hill. https://thehill.com/homenews/sunday-talk-shows/553773-fauci-vaccinated-people-become-dead-ends-for-the-coronavirus/

Coombes, R., & Davies, M. (2022). Facebook versus BMJ: When fact-checking goes wrong. *BMJ, 376.* https://doi.org/10.1136/bmj.o95

COVID-19 Excess Mortality Collaborators. (2022). Estimating excess mortality due to the COVID-19 pandemic: A systematic analysis of COVID-19-related mortality, 2020-21. *The Lancet, 399*(10334), 1513-1536. https://doi.org/10.1016/S0140-6736(21)02796-3

Dodsworth, L. (2021). *A state of fear: How the UK government weaponised fear during the Covid pandemic.* Pinter & Martin.

European Convention on Human Rights, Council of Europe. https://www.echr.coe.int/Documents/Convention_ENG.pdf

Godlee, F., & Abbasi, K. (2021). Rapid response: Open letter from the BMJ to Mark Zuckerberg. *BMJ, 375.* https://doi.org/10.1136/bmj.n2635

Gorski, D., & Yamey, G. (2021). Covid-19 and the new merchants of doubt. *The BMJ Opinion*. https://blogs.bmj.com/bmj/2021/09/13/covid-19-and-the-new-merchants-of-doubt/

Herby, J., Jonung, L., & Hanke, S. H. (2022). A literature review of the effects of lockdowns on COVID-19 mortality. *Studies in Applied Economics, 200*. https://sites.krieger.jhu.edu/iae/files/2022/01/A-Literature-Review-and-Meta-Analysis-of-the-Effects-of-Lockdowns-on-COVID-19-Mortality.pdf

Kulldorff, M. (2020). COVID-19 counter measures should be age specific. LinkedIn. https://www.linkedin.com/pulse/covid-19-counter-measures-should-age-specific-martin-kulldorff?trk=public_profile_ article_view

Kulldorff, M. (2021). *Covid, lockdown and the retreat of scientific debate*. The Spectator. https://www.spectator.co.uk/article/covid-lockdown-and-the-retreat-of-scientific-debate

Lewis, C. S. (2014). *God in the dock: Essays on theology and ethics*. W. Hooper (Ed.). Wm. B. Eerdmans Publishing.

Magness, P. W., & Earle, P. C. (2021). The fickle 'science' of lockdowns. *The Wall Street Journal*. https://www.wsj.com/articles/lockdown-science-pandemic-imperial-college-london-quarantine-social-distance-covid-fauci-omicron-11639930605

Magness, P. W., & Harrigan, J. R. (2021). *Fauci, emails, and some alleged science*. American Institute for Economic Research. https://www.aier.org/article/fauci-emails-and-some-alleged-science/

Mascarenhas, L., & Maxouris, C. (2021). *Fully vaccinated people who get a breakthrough infection can transmit the virus, CDC chief says*. CNN. https://www.cnn.com/2021/08/05/health/us-coronavirus-thursday/index.html

Nie, J. B., & Elliott, C. (2020). Humiliating whistle-blowers: Li Wenliang, the response to Covid-19, and the call for a decent society. *Journal of Bioethical Inquiry, 17*(4), 543–547. https://doi.org/10.1007/s11673-020-09990-x

Niemiec E. (2020). COVID-19 and misinformation: Is censorship of social media a remedy to the spread of medical misinformation? *EMBO reports, 21*(11), e51420. https://doi.org/10.15252/embr.202051420

O'Brien, M. D. (1996). *Father Elijah: An apocalypse*. Ignatius Press.

Oral Questions — Questions to Ministers (2020). https://www.parliament.nz/en/pb/hansard-debates/rhr/document/HansS_20200902_050580000/1-question-no-1-prime-minister

Peterson, J. B. (2021). *Why free speech is the antidote to our problems* [Video]. YouTube. https://youtu.be/T1B_QH0mR7M

Powell, M. (2022). Twitter bans Oxford academic who shared this Mail on Sunday article - but allows anti-vax rants amid fears over new 'online safety' powers letting tech giants censor legitimate journalism. *Daily Mail*. https://www.dailymail.co.uk/news/article-10655577/Twitter-bans-Oxford-academic-shared-MoS-article-allows-anti-vax-rants.html

Singer, J. A. (2022). Against scientific gatekeeping. *Reason*. https://reason.com/2022/04/03/against-scientific-gatekeeping/

Thacker, P. D. (2021). Covid-19: Researcher blows the whistle on data integrity issues in Pfizer's vaccine trial. *BMJ, 375*. https://doi.org/10.1136/bmj.n2635

The Rule of Law is defined as "a principle of governance in which all persons, institutions and entities, public and private, including the State itself, are accountable to laws that are publicly promulgated, equally enforced and independently adjudicated, and which are consistent with international human rights norms and standards." https://www.un.org/ruleoflaw/what-is-the-rule-of-law/

Tucker, J. A. (2022). *Kulldorff deleted: Famed epidemiologist and early opponent of lockdowns banned by LinkedIn*. Brownstone Institute. https://brownstone.org/articles/kulldorff-deleted-famed-epidemiologist-and-early-opponent-of-lockdowns-banned-by-linkedin/

Vasquez, J., & Pariseau, G. (2022). *Study: CensorTrack documents over 800 cases of Big Tech censoring COVID-19 debate*. #FreeSpeech America. https://censortrack.org/study-censortrack-documents-over-800-cases-big-tech-censoring-covid-19-debate

# THE SOCIAL CONTRACTS WE DIDN'T SIGN: VIEWING COVID-19 TECHNOLOGIES AS DETERMINISTIC EXTENSIONS OF THE STATE TO UNDERSTAND AND MITIGATE ISSUES

**Ashley Metz[1], Vurain Tabvuma[2]**

**Abstract:** During the COVID-19 pandemic, governments deployed various technologies that caused controversy. While technical concerns about privacy and data management have been discussed in the literature, we propose that governments have unwittingly faced a deeper issue that we can investigate with theoretical tools from ethics and technology studies. From this perspective, we discuss debates about three types of COVID-19 technologies: track and trace apps, data models and vaccine QR codes. We theoretically suggest that privacy concerns are tensions manifested from deeper discomfort with the idea that the state signs social contracts on citizen's behalf, which brings an implicit fear of technological determinism. This thought experiment can help us better understand people's fears. In response, governments can find ways to encourage constructive iteration whereby citizens are able to negotiate these new social contracts democratically. At the same time, the notion that people are upset by this breach brings into focus larger issues than technical concerns.

This chapter is based in part on ideas developed during a study of the Dutch track and trace app, funded by ZonMw, the Dutch organization for health research and care innovation.

The COVID-19 pandemic has given rise to, or accelerated the use of, many new *technologies*, defined as functional artifacts or techniques[3] - from new medicines, to the widespread adoption of online conferencing and work

---

[1] Assistant Professor, Tilburg University, Netherlands

[2] Associate Professor, St. Mary's University, Halifax, Nova Scotia, Canada

[3] Technology is defined by the Cambridge Dictionary as "the methods for using scientific discoveries for practical purposes, especially in industry" (https://dictionary.cambridge.org/dictionary/english/technology)

facilitation tools, to various apps and models. In this chapter, we use three basic categories of technologies as exemplars for investigating the challenges and issues related to deploying new technology by governments responding to a crisis: track and trace apps, data models and vaccine passports. These technologies promised advanced solutions to pandemic management. Track and trace apps were deployed to mitigate the spread of disease. Data models were used to bolster political- and scientific-decision making. Vaccination passports have been required to cross borders and for readmission into social life. However, these technologies have also received extensive criticism from experts and citizens (Demeyer et al., 2020; Singer, 2020), especially related to functionality, effectiveness, and human rights issues such as privacy (Cho et al., 2020; Dar et al., 2020; Luciano, 2020). In this chapter, we offer an additive explanation to contextualize general concerns and provide a broader basis for thinking about technologies deployed in crisis. We propose that issues with and concerning distrust of COVID-19 technologies can be understood by analyzing these technologies' placement vis-à-vis the standard social contracts citizens abide by.

The concept of the social contract helps us to understand the relationship between individuals and governing parties, such as the state (Gauthier, 1986; Hampton, 1968). Accordingly, citizens agree to abide by laws because they believe that doing so is in their interest. Social contract theory has been translated from its origins in philosophy across fields, including to studies of business and of technology, including how privacy can be understood as a social contract (Kruikemeier et al., 2020; Martin, 2016, 2021).

We propose that when usage is viewed as involving additional unintentional contracts, technologies can be seen as extensions or instruments of the state. This thought experiment could help us better understand people's fears. It is possible that, rather than fearing actual technical privacy concerns regarding data use today, people mostly fear the overreaches of the state, and what may happen when technologies adopted in a crisis become established and irreversible, but not consensually, coupled with the social contracts they hold. To better understand technology as instruments of the state, its potential consequences, and thus to potentially surface unconscious fears, we turn to the technological determinism theoretical perspective, which identifies technologies as political actors that can shape social relations (Dafoe, 2015; Winner, 1977, 1980).

The chapter proceeds as follows. First, we provide an overview of social contract theory and technological determinism and explain how they apply to COVID-19 technologies. Next, we outline three different types of COVID-19 technologies: track and trace apps, data models, and vaccine passports; and discuss their implicit social contracts and issues, if perceived as deterministic. Lastly, we explain how this thought experiment can help policymakers manage technologies in crises.

## Social Contracts

Variations of social contract theories date back to Socrates (Plato, 1981) and later Plato's Republic (1968), and have been adapted for different settings such as economics and business (Dunfee & Donaldson, 1995), media (Merrill, 2011; Ward, 2005) and technology (Fogel & Nehmad, 2009; Kruikemeier et al., 2020; Martin, 2016)[4]. In general, the social contract relates to the arrangements between parties such as a state and its citizens. Citizens, consumers, or users enter into an informal, consensual agreement or contract with their state, businesses, technology firms respectively, involving mutual expectations. One chooses to engage with the powerful body and abide by its laws or rules, knowing that what one obtains in return serves one's interests.

The Hobbesian view of social contracts holds that people are self-interested, but rational, and choose to relinquish certain freedoms to the state because it serves their interests (Hampton, 1986). People are motivated to accept rules and laws, "first because we are vulnerable to the depredations of others, and second because we can all benefit from cooperation with others" (Narveson, 1988, p. 148). Here, we focus on

---

[4] Social contract theory, according to Thomas Hobbes, is understood as, "the method of justifying political principles or arrangements by appeal to the agreement that would be made among suitably situated rational, free, and equal persons" (Lloyd & Sreedhar, 2020).

Hobbes' self-interested perspective, which underpins the notion of consent-based contracts, as opposed to justice-based contracts promoted by Rawls' ideas of social contracts based on distributed justice and equal rights (Rawls, 1999). Hobbes' social contracts are agreements to live together and accept authority in order to avoid a hypothetical State of Nature, in which people live in uncertainty, fear, and distrust of one another as self-interested, equal members with limited resources, who are constantly on the verge of threat. For Hobbes, a social contract must include two pieces: 1). a set of laws or rules people agree to follow, and 2). An enforcement mechanism and repercussions for non-abiders. Gauthier (1986) later argues that enforcement is not necessary because rationality is enough to agree to cooperate and to follow through. If people are rational, they will cooperate to maximize their own gain - "constrained maximizers," rather than, "straightforward maximizers" (Man in a state of Nature; Gauthier, 1986, p. 167). When what others do can influence one's own outcome, it is rational to be cooperative and constrain the maximization of one's own benefits and follow the given rules.

In a technology setting, such as the internet, social contracts in the form of rules and their enforcement exist to maintain harmony between individuals, such as seller's rankings on eBay.com (Snyder et al., 2006). Between technology users and technology providers there is an implicit social contract about information exchange (Fogel & Nehmad, 2009; Martin, 2016). Users' perceptions of the contract can vary regarding the extent of their risk perceptions and privacy concerns (Kruikemeier et al., 2020), which can vary by community (Martin, 2012). Social contracts with Big Data are yet unclear (Herschel & Miori, 2017). The notion of privacy as a social contract with technology firms places emphasis on the negotiation and acceptability of norms about the information shared, who it is shared with, and how it is used (Martin, 2012, 2016).

In studies that apply social contract theory to technology, users negotiate their requirements and enter into contracts with technology providers, or decline to use the technology. Though governments may mediate this relationship through regulation, they do not dictate the use of the technology. At the same time, users abide by terms, such as providing personal data, under the internalized assumption that it is in their rational self-interest, and their adherence is enforced.

In classic discussions, social contracts exist between people and their governments or users and their technologies. Theoretically, a social contract is between *two* parties, whether applied to political or technological settings. However, many COVID-19 technologies rearrange and complicate existing dyadic relationships. While people maintain a social contract with the state – agreeing implicitly to abide by governmental rules under the assumption that doing so is in the ultimate service of one's own wellbeing, people separately maintain social contracts with technologies – such as a user agreeing to the terms of service for Google Maps - agreeing to terms and conditions, and relinquishing control over data, in exchange for services they believe benefit them. Governments are expected to enforce social contracts in cases where technologies do not respect nor adhere to social contracts (such as the Cambridge Analytica and Facebook data scandal), adding further nuance to the didactic relationship between users and technologies. The government's ability and willingness to respond to such social contract breaches influences rational self-interested users' subsequent beliefs about the social contract their level of trust in both technologies and government.

COVID-19 technologies have required people to adhere to new social contracts with technologies that are dictated by the state without necessarily agreeing that the services proffered by those technologies are in their best interest. Though they may in some cases agree that their adherence to the rules of the technology is in their rational self-interest, they are still sometimes enforced externally, as in the case of track and trace apps in certain countries, and vaccine passports. To better contextualize this, we draw on theory used to understand the political role of technology, *technological determinism*.

## COVID-19 Technologies as Political Actors

Different perspectives of technology focus on the level of agency we have over technology or it has over us (Dafoe, 2015; Martin & Freeman, 2004). *Technological determinism* (Dafoe, 2015; Winner, 1977, 1980) holds that technology is political and shapes social relations. *Social essentialism* suggests that technology is neutral and tools are interpreted in social interactions, while *technology-in-practice* (Orlikowski, 1991, 2005) builds on a structuration view (Giddens, 1979) to refer to a constructivist, dialectic relationship between technology and its users. Over time, it has become fashionable to dismiss technological determinism as 'incorrect,' but as Dafoe's work to 'reclaim' it from a critical position articulates how doing so misses many important questions about the degree, scope, and context of human agency (Dafoe, 2015). Here, we adhere to this perspective to attend to the situations in which technologies can be understood to have deterministic properties - they are understood to potentially shape society.

Within this view, *technological politics* (Winner, 1980, 1986) refers to the idea that technologies are inscribed with intentions, including biases towards political structures, which influence others. In one famous example, overpasses in Long Island were designed to be too low for buses to move under them, and thus prevent lower income people from traveling to the public parks there. The bridges served the function of transport over the highway, while also being used to enhance power and privilege. The choice to use a technology, therefore is, "similar to legislative acts or political foundings that establish a framework for public order that will endure over many generations" (Winner, 1980, p. 128). Technological determinism features prominently in studies of military technologies. Notable examples include the creation of killing machines that inventors would later regret, including machine guns (Ellis, 1975) and Alfred Nobel's dynamite (Schultz, 2013). Three important ways technological determinism manifests can be summarized as normative, nomological, and consequential (Bimber, 1994; Dafoe, 2015):

1. **Normative** implies that "technology tells us how the world should be," and, may thus imply no need to debate its ethics. Norms of efficiency and productivity are prized in society, and society consequentially adopts scientific decisions (Bimber, 1994: 1).
2. **Nomological**, in which technology, along with natural laws, lead to "only one possible course of social change" (Bimber, 1994, p. 83). Society changes in response to technologies. In the science and

technology literature, this form of technological determinism is referred to as the "technological imperative," (Aldrich 1972; Hickson et al., 1969, p. 387- 388), a belief that a technology must be further developed and deployed to achieve goals, and will influence organizations and people. Eventually, technologies' own logic drives their evolution, separate from human agency (Winner, 1977), having a life of their own that is not restricted by social concerns. In other words, a system gains inertia that perpetuates itself following a sunk cost logic by which future decisions are constrained based on prior decisions to invest in assets or upfront costs (Dafoe, 2015; Hughes, 1987), and thus what is inscribed in technology replicates and advances.

3. **Consequential (Unintended consequences)**, occur because foreseeing and intending all consequences would not be possible under the assumption that technology is not considered a social process in this perspective. At the time of their design, people are ignorant of the consequences of their decisions, which can cause unexpected effects. In the famous example, while trying to ensure safe handling of nitroglycerin, Alfred Nobel invented dynamite, making it possible to transport the explosive to both mines that unearthed materials necessary for modern computing, and for war (Halasz, 1959).

## COVID-19 Technologies as Deterministic Extensions of the State

By combining ideas from social contract theory and technological determinism, we can view COVID-19 technologies as deterministic extensions of the state, which can give us context for understanding the issues they face. In this section, we outline three different COVID-19 technologies. Viewing technology from a technological determinism perspective, wherein technology is political, we apply the normative, nomological and consequential dimensions of three COVID-19 technologies to organize and contemplate issues, underlying fears, and possible mitigation strategies.

**Overview of technology types discussed**

| | Generic decisions supported by COVID-19 technologies |
|---|---|
| **Track and trace apps** | • Quarantine regulations based on proximity to infected persons<br>• Quarantine regulations based on own infection, including 'electronic fence' |
| **Data models** | • Lockdown and social distancing decisions<br>• Orders of supplies<br>• Vaccine timing and guidance |
| **Vaccine passports** | • Decisions to allow travel and event attendance<br>• Decision to enable access without full knowledge of immunity dynamics<br>• Separation of groups into mobile and non-mobile |

## Track and Trace COVID-19 Apps

Across the globe, approximately 52 countries launched COVID-19-related mobile apps for tracing and tracking infected people and/or visitors (Council of Europe, 2020). Apps brought the pandemic-management strategy of contact tracing to the digital world by alerting users if they had been in the proximity of a person who later tested positive for the virus. Contact tracing mobile applications could be understood as promising tools to overcome human error in contact tracing and to increase the pace of the contact tracing process while requiring fewer resources (Ahmed et al., 2020; Chen et al., 2020). Apps have been found to be useful for notifying larger amounts of people more efficiently, which does reduce infections slightly (Rodríguez, Graña & Alvarez-León, et al., 2021; Wymant, 2021), but faced scalability, privacy, adaptability challenges (Metz, 2022; Shahroz et al., 2021).

The *social contract* between citizens and track and trace apps involves relinquishing one's own health status data and whereabouts in return for knowledge from the collective about health data that could matter for oneself. A rational actor would conceivably accept track and trace technology, believing that other rational actors would as well, and the individual as well as the group would be better off. In some countries, apps were also used to enforce quarantine requirements. Especially in Asia, track and trace apps were used to decide where users could go and what they could do based on where their phones had been (Nageshwaran et al., 2021). Enforcement elsewhere did not happen automatically, however, not only due to the irrationality of actors, but their concerns and discomfort about being asked to abide by rules without fully understanding or agreeing with the benefits. For example, focus group data from the UK (Williams, Armitage, Tampe & Dienes, 2020) and survey data from the Netherlands (Metz, 2022) found that people had misconceptions about the extent of technical privacy infringement.

*Normatively,* track and trace apps make several judgments. First, they assume that automated, and 'efficient' tracking and tracing is a preferred method. While they may be faster and possibly more accurate than manual track and trace efforts, their image of efficiency may suggest that they can achieve more than they actually can, and consequentially, result in a disproportionate allocation of resources to developing, tinkering with, marketing and studying technologized solutions. For example, with limited uptake, their effectiveness is questionable.

In addition, apps presuppose that people should avoid infections. While this may be the best course of action with certain diseases for certain people, by focusing on developing the most efficient, effective tracing technologies, productive discussion about the benefits of natural immunity development could be inhibited.

*Nomologically,* if tracing apps continue in use as is, they could perpetuate disjointed efforts, if not well-integrated already. For example, from preliminary population and expert survey data, we found that individuals in South Korea believed that their government used tracing apps as tools for one part of the country's overall pandemic response strategy, whereas respondents in the Netherlands and Canada believed tracing apps were disjointed pieces aiming to technically solve, and thus inhibited from solving, a much bigger, more complex social problem (Metz, 2022). Ideas around tracing could have been set in motion such that re-shaping their roles is increasingly difficult. Yet, better integration with health systems could lead to increased use of tracing for other diseases, such as STDs, that pose more personal risks.

*Consequentially,* understanding technologies as potentially deterministic highlights how there could be *unintended consequences* we cannot yet imagine, but which shape the new social reality. These unintended consequences could manifest in areas both related and unrelated to the COVID-19 response. For example, there could be unintended consequences in the form of using track and trace technology across wider social and economic activities.

## Data Models and Analysts

Models are not new for informing decisions in public policy; however, the COVID-19 pandemic accelerated their use and policymakers' reliance on them for decision-making. In one notable example, Boris Johnson implemented strict measures after a simulation predicted the health service would be overwhelmed with cases (Adam, 2020). Modeling involves mechanistic descriptions based on pathogen biology, transmission routes, host behavior, the natural history of infection and other information (Brooks-Pollock et al., 2021). Mathematical, statistical, and other types of disease modeling were used to predict infection spread (Wynants et al., 2020), mortality (Friedman et al., 2020) and the impact of social distancing, lockdown, and other measures. These models were useful to guide policymaking, though they depend not only on information about the disease itself, which is not always available, but good math and correct code. They were often wrong (Chin et. al., 2020; Eker, 2020; Ioannidis et al., 2020), but useful (Holmdahl & Buckee, 2020). Various studies have begun to investigate when, why and how models predict more accurately. In a study analyzing 242 peer-reviewed articles, the authors found that accuracy and precision varied significantly (Gnanvi et al., 2021), with one important factor for accuracy being the longer period of time covered.

*Social contracts* between individuals and data-driven models are slightly different from the other two COVID-19 technologies discussed here. Though models as technological tools used by policymakers are already understood as instruments of the state to fuel decision-making. In this case, models were behind the decisions, and thus regulations, governments made to mitigate and manage the pandemic, for which citizens were subjected, theoretically in exchange for their collective well-being. Without the government's actions, citizens in Hobbes' 'State of Nature' would simply get ill. The social contract holds when people believe they are better off in the care of the state and willingly abide by restrictions. Though myriad decisions can go poorly in emergencies, when decisions that harmed people were based on inaccurate models, there is a specific technology and its development process and deterministic properties that could be to blame.

*Normatively,* there is a risk that politicians and scientists rely on data models that seem efficient and rational when they are only as good as the information and assembly available. Inevitably, before details are known about a particular disease, even if all technicalities are perfect, models will be inaccurate and policy mistakes, economic effects and deaths may result. Additionally, technology can become decoupled from political accountability (Bimber, 1994), leaving politicians an easy scapegoat for poorly considered decisions or overreliance on unpredictable models. Shifting policymaking power more heavily to data analysts changes norms about where actionable information comes from. Another important norm involves the speed required for models in emergencies, which is at odds with the traditional months-long peer-review process (Brooks-Pollock et al., 2021). If norms of speedy modeling persist, there are risks that standards decrease as rigorous reviews are condensed. Likewise, the inherent speediness of the COVID-19 modeling technology reviews carry norms of open science, code release and reproducibility, which could continue.

*Nomological* - Due to the urgent need, models were built on existing frameworks. Future needs and speed requirements could perpetuate the reuse of existing components without allowing space for deconstruction and innovation. Reliance on established building blocks could also perpetuate biases and issues with those building blocks and discourage innovation. Furthermore, models can only simulate what they set out to simulate, but may encourage myopia around the issues they can answer. Institutionalization of model types could occur and perpetuate policy responses related to that model and the universe of information it relates to. This could occur at the risk of missing other pertinent information and alternatives. For example, focusing on hospitalization likelihood may continually lead to policy decisions to lockdown.

*Unintended consequences* could involve unforeseen collaboration effects based on new norms of open science, or conversely, the spread of inaccurate models and building blocks that are reused before faults are known. Secondly, myriad unintended consequences based on what is modeled or not modeled can occur. For example, the impact on youth mental health was not a major part of early models designed to help inform lockdown decisions. In addition, unforeseen consequences may result from the increased attention and need for more simple models. Models that can be published in academic journals are typically more complex, but less useful for decision-makers (Brooks-Pollock et al., 2021). The need for and use of simpler models in the COVID-19 pandemic might accelerate a shift in support of policy-relevance as a criterion for academic career advancement, in addition to, or instead of, only the reliance on academic publications.

## Vaccine Passports and Immunity Certificates

Deployed in apps with scannable QR codes, vaccine passports hold personal data and records of COVID-19 vaccination, infection status and recovery. In Europe, a standardized certificate system allows entry to other countries, if the regulations at the time allow (EU Digital, 2022) As one researcher noted, "This is not a passport aimed at restrictions, it is a Covid-era portable and limited medical record," (Davidson, 2021, p. 5). The unvaccinated invariably perceive them as gatekeepers, moderating travel and event attendance, while myriad stakeholders view them as tools to re-open society and begin to reverse damage from social isolation and lack of economic activity in tourism (Davidson, 2021; Voo et al., 2021).

However, rather than representing a rationalized ideal that politicians believe perpetuates efficiency or progressiveness, vaccine and immunity passports actually stretch scientific logic to a certain degree. Prior to their development, the WHO advised against immunity certifications because of the gap in knowledge about the dynamics and duration of immunity, in addition to the validity of tests (Voo et al., 2021). Its most recent briefing on COVID-19 immunity still states that, "the strength and duration of the immune responses to SARS-CoV-2 are not completely understood and currently available data suggests that it varies by age and the severity of symptoms," (WHO, 2021, p. 1). Policymakers who called for the creation of vaccine passports did so based on the available information that indicated reduced spread and mortality in vaccinated or recovered individuals, but they knew that a full picture of immunity duration and strength was impossible. Even today, we know that immunity is contingent on many individual factors as well as the particular variant that caused a prior infection and the particular variant circulating at the time.

Aside from their potential inefficacy in limiting the spread of certain variants, vaccine passports that restrict access to certain people, have also raised ethical concerns about inequitable access to testing and other class disparities. (Hall & Studdert, 2020).

*Normatively,* vaccine passports solidify views that vaccines and prior infection do confer immunity, while exact data are not yet known. Passports normalize check-ins and inclusion/exclusion.

*Nomologically,* the usage of vaccine passports could persist and evolve to collect increasing amounts of health information that can be used to determine a person's ability to do certain things.

*Unintended consequences* - Though passports enable movement and the opening of travel restrictions, they may impose as-yet unimaginable discrimination. If vaccine passports become more ubiquitous for other health data, they could be used to restrict people uniformly without taking into account individual differences, or they could be designed to account for specifics.

**Summary:** *Analyzing the potential future of COVID-19 technologies from a deterministic perspective*

| | Surfacing underlying fears and possible implications | | |
|---|---|---|---|
| | **Normative** | **Nomological** | **Consequential** |
| **Track and trace apps** | • Imply the most efficient way forward and take resources away from other efforts<br>• Presuppose that people should avoid infections, potentially inhibiting alternative or nuanced paths | • Focus on technical solution at expense of integration as part of larger strategy and re-shaping roles may become increasingly difficult<br>• Better integration with health systems could situate tracing apps as norms for many infectious diseases, ending privacy for public health benefits. | Policymakers may ensure tracking functions of technologies today are not abused, but we do not know how they will be used tomorrow and if they may restrict our movement. |
| **Data models** | • Shift in decision-making power toward mechanistic approaches that appear rational, but can easily fail<br>• Decoupling of accountability between modelers, models, and decision-makers<br>• Shift in speed expectations, potentially lowering standards<br>• This urgency could also solidify new norms about open science | • Reusing existing frameworks and building blocks to maintain speedy modeling could perpetuate bias and obstruct innovation<br>• Focus on sharpening and reusing existing models and model-able questions could direct focus on a narrow set of policy options | • Unforeseen collaboration effects based on new norms of open science<br>• Spread of inaccurate models and building blocks that are reused before faults are known<br>• Unintended effects of focus on what is modeled or not modeled (e.g., prioritizing lockdowns over youth mental health)<br>• Shift toward valuing policy-relevance in academic modeling contexts |
| **Vaccine passports** | • Solidify views that vaccines and prior infection do confer immunity, while immunity dynamics are not completely understood<br>• Normalize check-ins and inclusion/exclusion from activities | • Passports could persist and evolve to collect increasing amounts of health information and dictate further restrictions | • Passports may impose as-yet unimaginable discrimination |

## Improving Social Contracts with COVID-19 Technologies

We argue that a technological determinism lens is useful for thinking about the context in which people may be perceiving issues around technologies deployed by governments during a crisis. It enables a 'worst case' image for contemplation and debate. Further research can empirically test this. Such research could help us to build safeguards against not only the potential outcomes, but the fears that could limit productive debates. Further work in research and policy can also consider how to mitigate issues regarding the sensitivity of healthcare technologies by articulating and actively applying alternative perspectives of technology that highlight the malleability and co-construction by agentic humans based on their use in practice (e.g., Orlikowski, 1991, 2005). By shifting aspects of the public and policy narrative that reflect technological determinism, to technology-in-practice, a less adversarial position could be achieved. Additional research could also investigate the practices and structures at organizations working on healthcare technologies to identify or apply dimensions of responsible innovation (Metz & Rathert, 2022).

## Conclusion

In this chapter, we proposed that COVID-19 technologies deployed by governments create an unusual intersection and rearrangement of two different social contracts people typically adhere to – between citizens and the state, and between users and technology. If we consider that technologies are inscribed with political perspectives, and especially potentially authoritarian ones (Mumford, 1964; Winner, 1980), we can see how from an individual's perspective, when one is cut out from the social contract, one is forced to accept that the relationship between citizens and their states has enlarged with technology as its extension. To better interrogate COVID-19 technologies, we looked through a technological determinism lens.

Citizens, experts, and academics have expressed concerns and discomfort with COVID-19 technologies, such as issues with the data protocols of track and trace apps, or being blocked from a country by the lack of a vaccination passport. We theoretically suggest that concerns are surface tensions manifested from deeper discomfort with the idea that the state signs social contracts on citizen's behalf, which brings an implicit fear of technological determinism. In response, governments can find ways to encourage constructive iteration whereby citizens are able to negotiate these new social contracts democratically. At the same time, the notion that people are upset by this breach, brings into focus larger issues than technical concerns.

## Edits to Institutionalized Social Contracts

Overall, studying COVID-19 technologies is important. Large scale jolts, such as a pandemic, fracture and break existing norms and assumptions, clearing the way for new approaches, technologies and arrangements that may become institutionalized, or taken-for-granted, in the future (Greenwood et al., 2002). Viewing COVID-19 technologies as deterministic, we argue, can help surface hidden issues and offer clues for issue mitigation – to help manage the current and potentially future pandemics. We can be more fully aware of the normative assumptions that are perpetuated and critically assess them. We can put checks in place to ensure technologies do not develop beyond our control, and we can be aware that no matter what we try to think through, unintended consequences are bound to occur and could be negative. Ongoing debate and multi-stakeholder participation can possibly mitigate risks.

# References

Ahmed, N., Michelin, R.A., Xue, W., Ruj, S., Malaney, R., Kanhere, S. S., Seneviratne, A., Hu, W., Janicke, H., & Jha, S. (2020). A survey of COVID-19 contact tracing apps. *IEEE Access, 8,* 134577-134601.

Acquisti, A. & Grossklags, J. (2005). Privacy and rationality in individual decision making. *IEEE Security and Privacy Magazine, 3*(1), 26-33. doi:10.1109/MSP.2005.22

Adam, D. (2020). Special report: The simulations driving the world's response to COVID-19. *Nature News Feature.* https://www.nature.com/articles/d41586-020-01003-6

Barley, S. (1986). Technology as an occasion for structuring: Evidence from observations of CT scanners and the social order of radiology departments. *Administrative Science Quarterly, 31*(1), 78-108.

Berendt, B., Guenther, O., & Spiekermann, S. (2005). Privacy in e-commerce: Stated preferences vs. actual behavior, *Communications of the ACM, 48*(4), 101-106. doi:10.1145/1053291.1053295

Bimber, B. (1994). Three faces of technological determinism. In M. R. Smith & Marx, L. (Eds.), *Does technology drive history?* (pp. 79-100). MIT Press.

Chen, C., Jyan, H., & Chien, S. (2020). Containing COVID-19 among 627,386 persons in contact with the Diamond Princess Cruise Ship passengers who disembarked in Taiwan: Big data analytics. *Journal of Medical Internet Research, 22*(5), 1-9.

Chin, V., Samia, N. I., Marchant, R., Rosen, O., Ioannidis, J., Tanner, M. A., & Cripps, S. (2020). A case study in model failure? COVID-19 daily deaths and ICU bed utilisation predictions in New York state. *European Journal of Epidemiology, 35*(8), 733–742. https://doi.org/10.1007/s10654-020-00669-6

Cho, H., Ippolito, D., & Yu, Y. W. (2020). Contact tracing mobile apps for COVID-19: Privacy considerations and related trade-offs. *ArXiv, 2003*(11511). http://arxiv.org/abs/2003.11511.

Council of Europe. (2020). *Contact tracing apps.* https://www.coe.int/en/web/data-protection/contact-tracing-apps

Cudd, A., & Seena, E. (2021). Contractarianism. In E. N. Zalta (Ed.), *The Stanford Encyclopedia of Philosophy.* https://plato.stanford.edu/archives/win2021/entries/contractarianism/

Dafoe, A. 2015. On technological determinism: A typology, scope conditions, and a mechanism. *Science, Technology, & Human Values, 40*(6), 1047-1076.

Dar, A. B., Lone, A. H., Zahoor, S., Khan, A. A., & Naaz, R. (2020). Applicability of mobile contact tracing in fighting pandemic (COVID-19): Issues, challenges and solutions, *Computer Science Review, 38.* https://doi.org/10.1016/j.cosrev.2020.100307

Davidson, S. (2021). The world wants to reopen: will vaccine passes be the key? *Biometric Technology Today, 2021*(6), 5–7. https://doi.org/10.1016/S0969-4765(21)00070-9

Demeyer, T., Dobbe, R., van Eeten, M., Haan, W., Jansen-Dings, I., Leenes, R., de Raad, H., Visser, J. & de Winter, B. (2020, April 17). Reactie experts op selectieproces corona-app. https://www.veiligtegencorona.nl/reactie-experts-selectieproces.html

Doffman, Z. (2020, May 5). Why new contact tracing apps have a critical WhatsApp-sized problem. *Forbes*. https://www.forbes.com/sites/zakdoffman/2020/05/05/all-whatsapp-users-must-now-install-this-new-app-heres-why/?sh=1e53b0454221

Donaldson, T., & Dunfee, T. W. (1994). Toward a unified conception of business ethics: Integrative social contracts theory. *Academy of Management Review, 19*(2), 252–284. https://doi.org/10.2307/258705

Eker, S. (2020). Validity and usefulness of COVID-19 models. *Humanities and Social Science Communications, 7*, 54.

Ellis, J. (1975). *The social history of the machine gun*. Johns Hopkins University Press.

EU Digital, 2022. EU Digital COVID Certificate. https://ec.europa.eu/info/live-work-travel-eu/coronavirus-response/safe-covid-19-vaccines-europeans/eu-digital-covid-certificate_en. Accessed 1.5.2022

Fogel, J., & Nehmad, E. (2009). Internet social network communities: Risk taking, trust, and privacy concerns. *Computers in Human Behavior, 25*, 153–160. doi:10.1016/j.chb.2008.08.006

Friedman, J., Liu, P., Troeger, C. E., Carter, A., Reiner, R. C., Barber, R. M., Collins, J., Lim, S. S., Pigott, D. M., Vos, T., Hay, S. I., Murray, C., & Gakidou, E. (2020). Predictive performance of international COVID-19 mortality forecasting models. *MedRxiv: The preprint server for health sciences*. https://doi.org/10.1101/2020.07.13.20151233

Gauthier, D. (1986). *Morals by agreement*. Oxford University Press.

Giddens, A. (1979). *Central problems in social theory: Action, structure and contradiction in social analysis*. University of California Press.

Gioia, D. A., Corley, K. G., & Hamilton, A. L. (2013). Seeking qualitative rigor in inductive research: Notes on the Gioia methodology. *Organizational Research Methods, 16*(1), 15-31.

Glaser, B, & Strauss, A. (1967). *The discovery of grounded theory*, Aldine Publishing.

Gnanvi, J. E., Salako, K. V., Kotanmi, G. B., & Glèlè Kakaï, R. (2021). On the reliability of predictions on Covid-19 dynamics: A systematic and critical review of modelling techniques. *Infectious Disease Modelling, 6*, 258–272. https://doi.org/10.1016/j.idm.2020.12.008

Greenwood, R., Suddaby, R., & Hinings, C.R. (2002). Theorizing change: The role of professional associations in the transformation of institutionalized fields. *Academy of Management Journal*, *45*(1): 58-80.

Halasz N. A. 1959. *Biography of Alfred Nobel*. The Orion Press.

Hall, M. A., & Studdert, D. M. (June 2020). Privileges and immunity certification during the COVID-19 pandemic. *JAMA*, *323*(22), 2243–2244.

Hampton, J. (1986). *Hobbes and the social contract tradition*. Cambridge University Press.

Hansen, S., & Baroody, A.J. (2019). Electronic health records and the logics of care: Complementarity and conflict in the U.S. healthcare system. *Information Systems Research*, *31*(1) 57-75.

Herschel, R. T., & Miori, V. M. (2017). Ethics & big data. *Technology in Society*, *49*, 31-36. https://doi.org/10.1016/j.techsoc.2017.03.003

Hickson, D. J., Pugh, D. S., & Pheysey, D. C. (1969). Operations technology and organization structure: An empirical reappraisal. *Administrative Science Quarterly*, *14*, 378-397.

Holmdahl, I., & Buckee, C. (2020). Wrong but useful - What Covid-19 epidemiologic models can and cannot tell us. *The New England Journal of Medicine*, *383*(4), 303–305. https://doi.org/10.1056/NEJMp2016822

Hughes, T. P. (1987). The evolution of large technological systems. In W. E. Bijker, T. P. Hughes, & T. Pinch (Eds.), *The Social Construction of Technological Systems* (pp. 14-76). MIT Press.

Ioannidis, J., Cripps, S., & Tanner, M. A. (2020). Forecasting for COVID-19 has failed. *International Journal of Forecasting*, *38*(2), 423–438. https://doi.org/10.1016/j.ijforecast.2020.08.004

Brooks-Pollock, E., Danon, L., Jombart T., & Pellis, L. (2021). Modelling that shaped the early COVID-19 pandemic response in the UK. *Philosophical Transactions*. *376*, 20210001. https://doi.org/10.1098/rstb.2021.0001

Kruikemeier, S., Boerman, S. C., & Bol, N. (2020). Breaching the contract? Using social contract theory to explain individuals' online behavior to safeguard privacy. *Media Psychology*, *23*(2), 269-292. https://doi.org/10.1080/15213269.2019.1598434

Langley, A. (1999). Strategies for theorizing from process data. *Academy of Management Review, 24*(4), 691–710.

Lloyd, S. A., & Sreedhar, S. (2020). Hobbes's moral and political philosophy. In E. N. Zalta (Ed.), *The Stanford Encyclopedia of Philosophy.* https://plato.stanford.edu/archives/fall2020/entries/hobbes-moral/

Luciano, F. (2020). Mind the app—considerations on the ethical risks of COVID-19 apps. *Philosophy and Technology, 33*, 167–172. https://doi.org/10.1007/s13347-020-00408-5

Martin, K., & Freeman, R. E. (2004). The separation of technology and ethics in business ethics. *Journal of Business Ethics, 53*(4), 353–364.

Martin, K. E. (2012). Diminished or just different? A factorial vignette study of privacy as a social contract. *Journal of Business Ethics, 111*(4), 519–539. https://doi.org/10.1007/s10551-012-1215-8 http://www.jstor.org/stable/23324816

Martin, K. E. (2016). Understanding privacy online: Development of a social contract approach to privacy. *Journal of Business Ethics, 137*, 551–569. https://doi.org/10.1007/s10551-015-2565-9

Merrill, J. C. (2011) Overview: Theoretical foundations for media ethics. In D. Gordon, J. M. Kittross, J. C. Merrill, W. A. Babcock, & M. Dorsher (Eds.), *Controversies in media ethics* (pp. 3–32). Routledge.

Metz, A. (2022). Eindverslag COVID-19 programma: Preconditions for COVID-19 mobile apps: A feature-level investigation of user acceptance based on insights from South Korea and Canada, applied in the Netherlands. https://research.tilburguniversity.edu/en/publications/eindverslag-covid-19-programma-preconditions-for-covid-19-mobile-

Metz, A. & Rathert, N. (2022). Responsible innovation: The role of organizational practices and structures, In F. Angeli, A. Metz & J. Raab [Eds.], *Organizing for Sustainable Development: Addressing the Grand* Challenges, (pp. 31-45). Routledge.

Mumford, L. (1964). Authoritarian and democratic technics. *Technology and Culture, 5*(1), 1-8. https://doi.org/10.2307/3101118

Nageshwaran, G., Harris, R. C., & Guerche-Seblain, C. E. (2021). Review of the role of big data and digital technologies in controlling COVID-19 in Asia: Public health interest vs. privacy. *Digital Health, 7*, 20552076211002953.

Narveson, J. (1988). *The Libertarian Idea*. Temple University Press.

Orlikowski, W. J. (1991). The duality of technology: Rethinking the concept of technology in organizations. *Organization Science, 3*(3), 398-427.

Orlikowski, W. J. (2005). Material works: Exploring the situated entanglement of technological performativity and human agency. *Scandinavian Journal of Information Systems, 17*(1), 183-186.

Petrakaki, D., Klecun, E., & Cornford, T. (2016). Changes in healthcare professional work afforded bytechnology: The introduction of a national electronic patient record in an English hospital. *Organization, 23*(2), 206–226.

Shahroz, M., Ahmad, F., Younis, M. S., Ahmad, N., Kamel Boulos, M. N., Vinuesa, R., & Qadir, J. (2021). COVID-19 digital contact tracing applications and techniques: A review post initial deployments. *Transportation Engineering, 5*. https://doi.org/10.1016/j.treng.2021.100072

Plato. *Five dialogues*. (Trans. G.M.A. Grube) Hackett Publishing Company (1981).

Plato. 1968. The republic: Book I. (A. Bloom, Trans.). Basic Books.

Rodríguez, P., Graña, S., Alvarez-León, E. E., Battaglini, M., Darias, F. J., Hernan, M. A., Lopez, R., Llaneza, P., Martin, M. C., RadarCovidPilot Group, Ramiz-Rubio, O., Romani, A., Suarez-Rodriguez, B., Sanchez-Monedero, J., Arenes, A., & Lacasa, L. (2021). A population-based controlled experiment assessing the epidemiological impact of digital contact tracing. *Nature Communications 12*, 587. https://doi.org/10.1038/s41467-020-20817-6

Schultz, C. (2013). *Blame sloppy journalism for the Nobel Prizes*. Smithsonian.

Singer, N. (2020, July 8). Virus-tracing apps are rife with problems. Governments are rushing to fix them. *The New York Times*. https://www.nytimes.com/2020/07/08/technology/virus-tracing-apps-privacy.html

Snyder, J., Carpenter, D., & Slauson, G. J. (2006). MySpace.com – A social networking site and Social Contract Theory. *Proc ISECON, 23*, 1-9.

Voo, T. C., Reis, A. A., Thomé, B, Ho, C. W., Tam, C. C., Kelly-Cirino, C., Emanuel, E., Beca, J. P., Littler, K., Smith, M. J., Parker, M., Kass, N., Gobat, N., Lei, R., Upshur, R., Hurst, S., & Munsaka, S. (2021). Immunity certification for COVID-19: Ethical considerations. *Bulletin of the World Health Organization, 99*(2), 155–161. doi: 10.2471/BLT.20.280701

Waardenburg, L., Sergeeva, A., & Huysman, M. (2018) Hotspots and blind spots. In C. Østerlund, M. Mähring, U. Schultze, K. Riemer, & M. Aanestad (Eds.), *Living with monsters? Social implications of algorithmic phenomena, hybrid agency, and the performativity of technology - IFIP WG8.2 Working Conference on the Interaction of Information Systems and the Organization, IS and O 2018, Proceedings* (pp. 96-109). Springer. https://doi.org/10.1007/978-3-030-04091-8_8

Walton, S. A. (2019). Technological determinism(s) of war. *Vulcan 7*(1), 4-18.

Ward, S. (2005). Philosophical foundations for global journalism ethics. *Journal of Mass Media Ethics 20*(1), 3–21.

WHO. (2021, May 10). COVID-19 natural immunity. *Scientific Brief.* https://apps.who.int/iris/handle/10665/341241

Williams, S. N., Armitage, C.J., Tampe, T., & Dienes, K. (2020). Public attitudes towards COVID-19 contact tracing apps: A UK-based focus group study. *medRxiv*. https://doi.org/10.1101/2020.05.14.20102269.

Winner, L. (1977). *Autonomous technology-technics-out-of-control as a theme in political thought*. MIT Press.

Winner, L. (1980). Do artifacts have politics. *Daedalus, 109*(1), 121-36.

Winner, L. (1986). *The whale and the reactor – A search for limits in an age of high technology*. University of Chicago Press.

Wymant, C., Ferretti, L., Tsallis, D., Charalambides, M., Abeler-Dorner, L., Bonsall, D., Hinch, R., Kendall, M., Milsom, L., Ayres, M., Holmes, C., Briers, M., & Fraser C. (2021). The epidemiological impact of the NHS COVID-19 app. *Nature, 594,* 408-412. https://doi.org/10.1038/s41586-021-03606-z

Wynants, L., Van Calster, B., Collins, G. S., Riley, R. D., Heinze, G., Schuit, E., Bonten, M., Dahly, D. L., Damen, J., Debray, T., de Jong, V., De Vos, M., Dhiman, P., Haller, M. C., Harhay, M. O., Henckaerts, L., Heus, P., Kammer, M., Kreuzberger, N., … van Smeden, M. (2020). Prediction models for diagnosis and prognosis of Covid-19: Systematic review and critical appraisal. *BMJ, 369,* m1328. https://doi.org/10.1136/bmj.m1328

# SAME ROOTS, DIFFERENT FLOWERS: HOW ONE CATHOLIC SOCIAL TEACHING LED TO RADICALLY OPPOSED PRUDENTIAL JUDGEMENTS

**Edward Hadas**[1]

**Abstract:** Catholic Social Teaching (CST) offers a coherent and reasonably comprehensive set of ethical principles. When COVID-19 arrived, those principles were interpreted in radically different ways, as either justifying obedience to the public health decisions of legitimate governments or as questioning the wisdom of novel restrictions on social contacts. I introduce five relevant principles: the respect for both the goodness of physical life and for the fullness of life, the responsibilities of governments to support the common good, the shared responsibility of each person and group for everyone (solidarity), the preference for bottom-up over top down policy making (solidarity), and the importance of putting the good of the poor first in setting public policies (the preferential option for the poor). I explain how each of these principles can be used to support radically different judgements, relying on a dichotomy of heroic and massive misjudgement narratives of COVID-19. I argue that the disputes do not invalidate CST as a helpful analytic tool.

## Introduction

In March 2020, I obeyed and defended the newly announced anti-COVID-19 lockdowns. The endorsement should have surprised me, as my study of Catholic Social Teaching (CST) had led me to be cautious about assertive modern governments. I had even given talks and written an essay (Hadas, 2019) on the topic.[2] However, when this crisis arrived, I was no different from most of my frightened compatriots. I trusted the government.

---

[1] Research Fellow, Blackfriars Hall, Oxford University, Oxford, UK

[2] I tie this political model into the response to COVID in Hadas (2022).

The trust did not last. By June, preliminary reading had persuaded me that the principal mandated "non-pharmaceutical interventions" – lockdowns, school closures, social distancing, travel restrictions, and mandatory masking – had little or no scientific support, were contrary to the previously accepted canons of public health, and were causing significant harm. Subsequent study and events have only strengthened my convictions, while the list of public policy aberrations has lengthened to include a reckless and divisive approach to vaccines.[3] I am now a strong proponent of what I call the massive misjudgement narrative of the response to the SARS-CoV-2 virus.

I believe that CST supports my conclusion. I see in this worldview a rejection, implicit but unequivocal, of the standard heroic narrative of the anti-COVID policies. Some students of CST share my interpretation.[4] However, many others do not. Indeed, the disagreement starts at the top. Pope Francis, the leader of the Catholic Church, has steadily called for faithful obedience to all government-ordered restrictions and mandates related to COVID-19.[5] The bishops who report to him have almost all followed their boss's lead.

One exception was Daniel Fernández of Arecibo, Puerto Rico, who told his flock that "what the pharmaceutical companies or drug regulatory agencies say is in no way a dogma of faith". The Vatican hastily removed Fernández from his office (Catholic News Agency, 2022).

---

[3] For summaries, Berenson (2021) and Kheriaty (2022). On previous practices, Heriot & Jamrozik (2021) and Tognotti (2013). For a sample of previous standard guidelines, with strong bias towards minimal intervention, World Health Organisation (2019). On effectiveness of measures, Lemoine (2021). Miles et al. (2020) gives an early cost-benefit analysis, based on standard UK National Health Service measurements. For vaccines, Kostoff et al. (2021).

[4] Stefano Fontana (e.g., Fontano 2021) has been a thoughtful critic from within the CST tradition. Monsignor Charles Pope, a popular American priest-writer, was unusual in the English-speaking world. See Pope (2020) For a more recent Thomistic argument, see Farrow (2022).

[5] For a clear statement of his views aimed at a broad audience, see Francis (2020a). See also Francis (2020b, 32-34). On vaccines, Francis (2022).

That sort of treatment is likely to discourage episcopal rebellion. However, strict enforcement hardly seems necessary. There are no signs of major Catholic discontent with the Vatican line. On the contrary, the near-unanimity of the hierarchy has largely been mirrored in Catholic academic and media circles.[6] Even Catholics who are generally critical of Francis have mostly accepted this part of his teaching.

My dissent puts me in the difficult position of claiming a deeper understanding of the social teaching than most of its authoritative interpreters. Am I really more Catholic than the Pope? The current essay is an effort to answer that question.

I will proceed as follows. In the next section, I introduce some basic principles of CST. The third section discusses how the social teaching responds to modern technology and the fourth discusses how much obedience the governed owe to their governments. The fifth section goes over four divergences in Catholic responses to the anti-pandemic policies. I conclude with a brief defence of the enduring practical value of CST.

## Pandemic-relevant Catholic Social Teaching

Catholic Social Teaching is the Catholic Church's official response to the political, social, cultural, and economic innovations of the modern world.[7] Its most authoritative expression is a series of encyclicals, which are documents written by popes (or at least issued with their signatures). The first CST encyclical was Leo XIII's *Rerum Novarum*, issued in 1891, and the most recent is Francis's 2020 *Fratelli Tutti*.

A great deal has changed in the world since 1891, and the Catholic Church has learned from those developments, more or less willingly and more or

---

[6] Examples from early in the pandemic include Johnson (2020) and DeCosse (2020). McGovern et al. (2020) offers a slightly more cautious endorsement of the anti-pandemic measures. I have seen no Catholic reconsiderations of original positive judgements.

[7] In Hadas (2020) I discuss the lively debates about the contents, limits, essence, purpose, and authority (for Catholics) of the social teaching. These are irrelevant for the purposes of this article.

less completely. As should be expected from a teaching that aims to respond to current challenges, it has evolved in both emphases and practical judgements. As should be hoped for a teaching that claims to be based on the unchanging truths of human nature and God's Creation, its fundamental principles remain constant.

Before listing five of those principles, I want to mention the claimed sources of CST's authority. *Christian revelation, aided by human reason,* provides the fundamental understanding of human moral nature as all at once good, sinful, and essentially and ultimately oriented to the divine. A combination of *Christian revelation and Aristotelian philosophy* anchors the recognition that human nature is essentially social, essentially but imperfectly oriented to the common good of human communities. Finally, the understanding of individual virtues and of human flourishing in this life (as compared to eternal life) is largely *Aristotelian,* as distilled in the theological alembic of *Thomas Aquinas.*[8]

The Catholic Church teaches that there is a fundamental harmony of faith and reason, so, in that view, the social teaching's reliance on divine revelation does not make it irrelevant to non-Catholics or non-believers.[9] Many non-Catholics have in fact been inspired by the ethical and political principles that are at the core of the teaching.[10] In my judgement, CST can help all policymakers and citizens respond well to "the joys and the hopes, the griefs and the anxieties of the men of this age, especially those who are poor or in any way afflicted" (Vatican Council II, 1965, 1).

The quotation, from the Church's Second Vatican Council, is general. However, CST only deals with a collection of fairly specific joys, hopes, griefs, and anxieties. The limits are built into Aristotelian-Thomistic ethics, in which careful consideration of specific circumstances is necessary part of any effort to turn unchanging true principles into current best practices.

---

[8] Pontifical Council for Justice and Peace (2004) provides an authoritative summary with ample references.

[9] For the "unity of truth, natural and revealed" see John Paul II (1998, section 34). References to all Vatican documents are by section or paragraph number.

[10] Examples of non-Catholic appreciations of CST include Thomas (2019), Welby (2016) and Glasman (2020).

The analysis of circumstances is one part of what Thomists call the virtue of prudence, but prudence has other elements. It is dispassionate: prudential judgements avoid both foolish hopes and exaggerated fears. It is modest; the prudent observer respects the knowledge of experts but is wary of the frequent arrogance of the half-learned. And it is wise in the ways of the world; the prudent citizen respects legitimate authority but is wary of the corruption that inevitably tempts the powerful.

Prudential judgements are often morally difficult, because they can require balancing several genuine goods that cannot all be served perfectly. In a pandemic, the good of minimising the disease's toll of hospitalisations and deaths might conflict with the good of preserving the friendships, flourishing, and normal forms of everyday life. Like most conflicts of true goods, this one probably has no simple or fully satisfactory resolution.

When faced with a particular problem, CST teaches policymakers to proceed by evaluating the facts of the matter. There are several types of facts. For a pandemic, there are public health facts, including the likely effects of different measures on the severity of illnesses and the number of deaths from the disease in question. There are social facts such as the current economic and psychological state of the population and the likely overall health, social, and perhaps spiritual effects of particular collections of anti-pandemic measures. Finally, there will be ethical facts, including the nature of the possibly rival goods of the preservation of lives and the fullness of life.

As I just explained, the specificity and realism of CST counsels limit the availability of up-to-date counsels. When a new challenge arises, CST cannot offer an "off the shelf" answer. The CST method requires a gathering and analysis of whatever facts are relevant to this particular controversy.

"How should governments respond to a viral pandemic?" was one of the many questions that CST had not addressed carefully before 2020. This gap was neither surprising nor irresponsible, because there was broad agreement on the general pattern of pandemic facts and on the right basic direction of anti-pandemic policy.[11] The pandemic guidelines issued by various global and national public health authorities had three simple and ethically sound goals: the ill should be treated as much as possible, the spread of the disease should be slowed as much as is practical, and life should continue as normally as is compatible with the common good.

The goals might sometimes be in serious conflict. However, for pandemics there was a broad consensus that humans cannot do much to limit the spread of influenza and similar viruses. Under those circumstances, the guidelines all came to the prudent conclusion that the continuation of normal life was a greater good than anything that could be achieved by the imposition of disruptive antiviral measures.[12]

This prudent approach was abandoned in the response to COVID-19. In its place, governments around the world imposed severe restrictions on everyday life, including long-lasting quarantines of healthy people and restrictions on socialisation that were, arguably, more disruptive than anything previously seen in peacetime.[13] Pandemics suddenly became a pressing ethical issue. Five foundational principles of CST can help address this issue. On the truth of these principles, loyal Catholics all agree. As I said in the Introduction, there is discord on their implications for the response to COVID-19.

*1) Human life is a God-given good, but there is more to life than being alive.*

The "but" in this principle reflects the mystery of the human condition. People naturally want life, both for themselves and for others, *but* death always lurks. People naturally want to live as full and good a life as possible, *but* the fullness and goodness can sometimes bring an earlier death. And, Christians will add, people want to flourish for as long as they

---

[11] In retrospect, the political and medical response to the 2009 swine flu was a harbinger of what happened in 2020. However, only very prudent, or very suspicious observers could have anticipated the significance of this precedent.

[12] See for example World Health Organisation (2019)

[13] On quarantines, Centers for Disease Control and Prevention (2022). On social distancing Lipton and Steinhauer (2020). The novelty of the anti-COVID-19 techniques is disputed, but see Tucker (2021) with embedded article.

live, *but* they have a calling and a craving for a supernatural flourishing that somehow overcomes death.

The tension of the "but" can be seen in the social teaching about caring for *individuals*. A Vatican-approved Catholic guide to healthcare states,

> Although physical life on the one hand manifests the person and takes on his value, so that it cannot be disposed of as a thing, on the other hand it is not exhaustive of the person's whole value and does not constitute his supreme good…Bodily life is a fundamental good, the condition for all the others, but there are higher values for which it may be legitimate or even necessary to accept the danger of losing it. (Pontifical Council for Pastoral Assistance to Health Care Workers, 2017, 89)

The Social Teaching has always emphasised the *social* responsibility to go beyond keeping people alive. An official summary explains that "It is necessary to 'consider every neighbour without exception as another self, taking into account first of all his life *and* [emphasis added] the means necessary for living it with dignity'" (Pontifical Council for Justice and Peace, 2004, p. 132).

For measures against pandemics, this two-sided principle can point in two quite different directions. Because human life is a great good, it is reasonable to expect people to make some sacrifices to delay deaths. (The usual "saving lives" is misleading, since humans cannot be "saved" from bodily death. The phrase is especially misleading for COVID-19, which predominantly causes the deaths of people who are already relatively close to death, either because of age or pre-existing ill health.[14]) Alternatively, because human life should be more than simply being alive, the common good might require giving preference to the fullness of life over the delaying of deaths.

---

[14] Statista (2022) indicates that 74% of U.S. deaths attributed to COVID-19 were of people over 65. Office of National Statistics (2022) provides U.K. data, which records that 17% of people dying from the disease in the fourth quarter of 2021 had no pre-existing conditions.

*2) Governments should support the common good.*

The central responsibility of any government is to support the shared good of all the governed. This common good is inseparable from the true good of each of the governed. The *Catechism of the Catholic Church*, an official summation of the Church's teaching on faith and morals, explains what this support entails: "it is the proper *function of authority* [emphasis added] to…make accessible to each what is needed to lead a truly human life: food, clothing, health, work, education and culture, suitable information, the right to establish a family, and so on" (Catechism of the Catholic Church, 1997, 1908).

Even the best constituted political authorities often do not support the common good as they should. The causes of these failures can be seen as practical; the common good is always hard to identify and even harder to promote. More profoundly, their source is in human nature, in the sin "that clings so closely" (Hebrews 12:1) to all human endeavours.

This principle also may point in two different directions in the midst of a pandemic. One argument is that the first thing that is needed for a truly human life in a community is to be alive, so the first responsibility of political authorities in a pandemic is to protect people's physical health. An alternative argument is that the authorities should recognise that the relevant virus will successfully resist all human efforts at control. The chief political and medical task is to minimise the pandemic's damage to the communal and individual fullness of life.

*3) All people are responsible for the good of all their neighbours.*

This mutual responsibility, called solidarity in CST, is common to individuals, groups, and nations. Pope John Paul II described solidarity as "a firm and persevering determination to commit oneself to the common good…because we are all really responsible for all" (John Paul II, 1987, p. 38). Francis added that this determination should find "concrete expression in service, which can take a variety of forms in an effort to care for others" (Francis, 2020b, p. 115).

What forms of solidaristic action are called for in a pandemic? Perhaps all people should engage in painful social isolation to protect the strangers whom they might otherwise infect. Perhaps most people should avoid cancer screenings, face-to-face medical visits, and other routine healthcare to allow the medical system to deal with a pandemic-induced flood of critically ill patients. Alternatively, perhaps the most relevant form of solidarity is accepting some risks to everyone's health to ensure that education, trade, and loving attention to the ill and poor continue unabated.

*4) Public policy should build upwards, not impose downwards.*

This is the CST of subsidiarity. In concrete terms, subsidiarity calls for giving as much authority as possible to smaller organisations – from the family through local businesses and churches up to regional governments – and as little power as possible to national and international governments and organisations. In the words of John Paul II, "a community of a higher order should not interfere in the internal life of a community of a lower order, depriving the latter of its functions, but rather should support it in case of need and help to coordinate its activity with the activities of the rest of society, always with a view to the common good" (John Paul II, 1991, p. 48). The thinking behind this principle is that smaller organisations can generally make prudential judgements that are more suitable and more humane than orders dispatched from distant bureaucratic governments.

The nature of global pandemics may militate against the application of subsidiarity. Linguistically, pandemics only exist when an international organisation, the World Health Organisation, declares that they do. Practically, pandemics cannot be slowed without massive, coordinated policy responses. Alternatively, pandemics might offer especially good opportunities for subsidiarity. The common good might be well served if different communities find their own best ways to balance the various goods and evils of different anti-pandemic measures.

*5) Public policies should favour the poor over the rich.*

In CST, this principle is called the preferential option for the poor. It holds that "the poor, the marginalized and in all cases those whose living conditions interfere with their proper growth should be the focus of particular concern" (Pontifical Council for Justice and Peace, 2004, 182). For Catholics, there is little disagreement on how to apply this principle in a pandemic. Policymakers at all levels should think about how to help those least able to help themselves, whether because they lack economic resources or because they are most vulnerable to the disease. Disagreements do arise when policymakers have to balance the good of this preferential option against other social goods, most notably the delaying of deaths.

The preferential option was articulated in response to many governments' seeming indifference to poverty. That apparent indifference remains common, but pro-poor generosity sometimes flourishes in a national crisis. There are many accounts of people helping more marginalised neighbours during the time of anti-COVID-19 restrictions. However, even defenders of those restrictions generally accept that overall, they caused more pain and damage to the poor than to the rich. The sentiment that "we're all in this together", which was often expressed during the COVID-19 pandemic, did not lead to a transfer of either wealth or comforts from rich to poor, but "work from home" policies effectively transferred exposure to COVID-19 in that non-preferential direction.

## The technocratic paradigm

At least hypothetically, the five principles I just discussed are not very controversial in post-Christian and other liberal societies. I now turn to two more challenging issues. The first is the technocratic paradigm, a phrase introduced by Pope Francis in his environmental encyclical *Laudato Si'* (Francis, 2015, 106-110). By *technocratic* he means the unquestioned assumption that technologies can solve any social or individual problem. The technologies in question are not only mechanical or digital. They include the bureaucratic organisations in which people become interchangeable parts of administrative machines. By *paradigm* he means a way of thinking about the world that is comprehensive and exclusive. A paradigm guides and limits what we notice and think about, how we approach problems, and what solutions we consider acceptable.

By technocratic paradigm, Francis means a "tendency, at times unconscious, to make the *method* and *aims* of *science* and *technology* [emphasis added]an epistemological paradigm which shapes the lives of individuals and the workings of society" (Francis, 2015, 107).

The COVID-19 pandemic can help clarify that somewhat murky description. People who are stuck inside the technocratic paradigm trust numbers, so their pandemic thoughts are likely to start with statistical calculations, for example of death rates and life expectancies. When they measure a surprising increase of deaths, they do not look to God or philosophy for comfort or explanation. Rather, they instinctively use even more of the *method* of *science*. They map genetic sequences and measure viral concentrations. They create mathematical models of contagion. Equally instinctively, they turn to the *aims* of *technology*. They demand human mastery over this phenomenon of nature.

In other words, inside the paradigm, there is no reason to be fatalistic about a fatal disease. Technocratic thinking is the only thinking available within the paradigm, and it can only see disease as a problem to be solved. This thinking cannot easily – or perhaps at all – blend the desire for better physical health with the recognition that illnesses and death are conjoined, continuing, and unavoidably spiritual challenges of the human condition.

Today's Christians are not immune from the paradigm's seductive logic. In a pandemic, they may struggle to remember their faith's teaching about the redemptive value of suffering for both sufferers and those who accompany them.[15] Instead, they will be tempted to join in with the technocratic chorus: "Something must be done to stop this. Science, technology, and modern governments should overpower the virus."

In *Laudato Si'*, Francis does not discuss pandemics, but he writes eloquently about the distortions and damage that the technocratic paradigm has brought to modern societies. He starts with the physical environment and moves on to decry the effects of the paradigm's de-spiritualisation on many aspects of personal and social relations. In my judgement, though, Francis has not been prudent in his judgements of the technocratic policy responses to COVID-19. He has totally ignored the possibility that some of these

---

[15] For an explanation of this Christian teaching, see John Paul II (1984).

policies might exemplify the paradigm's fundamental weaknesses.[16] Obviously, the pope and most thoughtful Catholics see something quite different: technical thinking used to support the common good.

## Obedience and justice

The anti-COVID policies were designed by public health specialists, but they were imposed by governments. How closely and critically should the governed question the wisdom and justice of these or any other dictates of their governments? When one person or a group of people decide that some laws or rules are unwise or unjust, under what circumstances do they have the privilege, right, or obligation to disobey?

Such philosophical and practical questions concerning governments, justice, and obedience have been posed for millennia. They have become much more pressing in recent decades, as the number and intrusiveness of governmental rules and regulations increased. The strict anti-pandemic limits on healthy people's normal activities can be seen as the latest deepening of that governmental expansion.

CST has three quite different approaches to what might be called the government obedience challenge. Each might be relevant to anti-COVID policies. The first approach is to assume that governments should be obeyed. In the Bible, the apostle Paul tells the Christians in Rome, "Let every person be subject to the governing authorities. For there is no authority except from God…Therefore he who resists the authorities resists what God has appointed, and those who resist will incur judgement" (Revised Standard Version, Rom. 13.1-2).

This principle clearly points to accepting without question all government decrees. If anything, obedience should be especially fervent to pandemic-related decrees, because so many lives are at stake.

---

[16] I have written in somewhat more detail about this in Hadas (2021). Hanby (2015) provides a philosophical introduction to the paradigm's reshaping of our understanding of nature and science. Cayley (2020) and Cayley (2021) bring the related approach of Ivan Illich to the particular circumstances of Covid-19.

The second approach starts with the universal obligation – to God, conscience, and the common good – to act justly. This higher duty points towards just disobedience of human injustice. In the Bible, the apostle Peter, whom Catholics consider to be the first pope, refused to obey the commands of the Jewish religious leaders. He explained that "We must obey God rather than men" (Acts 5:29, Revised Standard Version). Thomas Aquinas drew out the legal implications of this principle: "if in any point [a human law] deflects from the law of nature, it is no longer a law but a perversion of law.... Wherefore such laws do not bind in conscience, except perhaps in order to avoid scandal or disturbance..." (Aquinas, 1920, II.I.95.2 corpus and II.I.96.4 corpus).[17]

This approach points to serious questioning of anti-pandemic restrictions. Do they support the common good? If not, do they create significant and unjust harm? Is disobedience prudent or a cause of unnecessary scandal or disturbance? Is some disobedience an ethical necessity?

The third approach starts with a critical suspicion of the goodness of the distinctly modern "all-encompassing welfare state" (Benedict XVI, 2009, 57). As Pope Benedict XVI explained, "The State which would provide everything, absorbing everything into itself, would ultimately become a mere bureaucracy incapable of guaranteeing the very thing which the suffering person—every person—needs: namely, loving personal concern. We do not need a State which regulates and controls everything..." (Benedict XVI, 2005, 27).

The anti-pandemic regulations and controls that various states imposed did not extend to "everything". However, some people might conclude that they have smothered society under a totalising and love-denying administrative blanket – a plethora of rules of how far you can travel, how many people you can see, how close to them you can get, and under what circumstances you can attend school. If that image is accurate, then the anti-Covid policies deserve especially critical moral scrutiny.

---

[17] See also Wyma (2014).

## Four axes of diverging judgement

I hope that the discussion so far has made clear in a general way how loyal and prudent Catholics could strongly disagree about what responses to COVID-19 were best aligned with CST. In this section, I describe four specific divergences in the interpretation of the Covid-relevant circumstances.

*1) The choice of narratives.*

Earlier in this essay, I suggested that there were basically two opposing narratives of COVID-19 and the governmental and social response to it. One is the hard but inspiring tale of heroism in a great global crisis. The other is a recounting of a long series of massive misjudgements.

My duality of narratives is undoubtedly an oversimplification. There are also many centrist narratives, substituting, for example, caution and confusion for heroism or mild misjudgements for massive ones. However, focusing on the extreme narratives helps clarify what is at stake in fitting the pandemic response into the moral framework of CST.

A Catholic heroic telling of the Covid story might go something like this: "Governments demanded great and virtuous sacrifices from citizens for the sake of the common good. The authorities acted as governments are supposed to act in a crisis equivalent to a war.[18] Yes, the choice to follow the best available scientific and public health advice undoubtedly led to suffering among the governed, but any other response would have been irresponsible. Even if the chosen measures were not very effective in reducing mortality, indeed even if they did more harm than good, they were adopted for good reasons and the popular response to them was, for the most part, morally exemplary."

The massive misjudgement narrative sounds very different. A Catholic-tinged version might be: "The choice of anti-COVID-19 policies was imprudent in many ways, starting with the unjustified abandonment of

[18] Castro Seixas (2021) surveys war imagery from politicians in early 2020.

standard anti-pandemic polices. The authorities' understanding and analysis of the common good was deficient, as it basically ignored the social, medical, psychological, and economic effects of the various anti-Covid measures. The stoking of exaggerated health fears was a dereliction of governments' responsibility to serve the governed, as was the governmental indifference to the preferential option for the rich that their anti-pandemic policies created."

*2) The value of life.*

I have already alluded to the inevitable ethical tensions between the good of delaying deaths and the good of promoting the fullness of lives. Prudential judgements about which good to favour in a particular situation will always depend on circumstances. However, there is often a fundamental preference in favour of one or the other: life itself or the fullness of lives.

The heroic narrative of the COVID-19 pandemic focuses first and foremost on the first, the good of life itself. More specifically, it barely recognises any good other than delaying as many deaths as possible for as long as possible. That judgement was encapsulated in the often repeated slogan, "If we save one life, it was worth it".

The respect for the value of life led to such antisocial anti-pandemic policies as isolating very old people from their families and keeping children from attending schools or seeing friends. Ironically, those two policies so distressed the people affected that they might have accelerated more deaths than they delayed. Still, the principle that misery should sometimes be accepted in exchange for extra time alive is defensible, even if earthly life itself is not considered to be the greatest human good, and even if physical death is not thought to be the greatest evil.

The other approach, to focus more on promoting good lives, necessarily leads to a lesser focus on warding off deaths. Arguably, this second approach is more congruent than the first one to the Catholic understanding of the human condition. Because humans naturally desire to be good and because bodily death is inevitable, the common good includes the nurturing of good lives, which must include good deaths.[19] Because humans are naturally social creatures, the common good is harmed when lives are not lived and ended in communal love.

It is not necessary to endorse the "good lives" approach to the common good to conclude that the massive misjudgement narrative is right. The anti-pandemic measures may have been wrong simply because it was imprudent to believe that they would on balance delay deaths. However, in my judgement, anyone who does endorse this second understanding of the good of human life would be at least tempted by the misjudgement narrative.

The temptation need not lead to full adoption. A temporary suspension of normal arrangements during a pandemic might promote good lives exactly *by* delaying more deaths. However, in the "good lives" approach to the common good, any fullness-denying measures should be undertaken with deep regret and should be questioned constantly. Were the anti-COVID-19 antisocial policies accompanied by sufficient hesitation, doubts, reconsiderations, and regrets?

*3) The need for strong controls.*

Governments responded to the pandemic in line with the militaristic framing of the heroic narrative. Normal democratic processes of law-making were suspended in almost all countries and the defence of such traditional civil liberties as the freedoms of speech, assembly, and worship was often treated as a near-treasonous support of the viral enemy. Such "treason" was rare. The restrictions were mostly accepted willingly and obeyed carefully.

In the heroic narrative, the controls and the obedience amount to a good example of how the Catholic call to respect legitimate political authority should work. This narrator might say something like, "Yes, the chosen measures caused some harm and injustice. But harsh and imperfect rules

---

[19] Not all Christians actually use this broader understanding of life in their ethical analyses. Illich (1977, 209 fn. 62) condemns a "practical convergence of Christian and medical practice [that] is in stark opposition to the attitude to death in Christian theology."

are necessary to deal with crises. The authorities were heroic in creating them, as were the people who suffered in obeying them."

The massive misjudgement narrator would give a quite different speech: "The pandemic was not an emergency that required the suspension of normal political practices. The laws and regulations that took minute control of everyday life were unjust in concept and execution. The use of dishonest propaganda was a further abuse of power. The anti-Covid measures amount to a clear example of the unjust dictates that the Catholic tradition holds to be violence rather than law."

If the critical narrator is wary of intrusive governments, she might continue, "The depredations are also a clear example of the bureaucratic smothering that Benedict XVI warned against. Many parts of governments' extensive welfare and regulatory apparatus were turned against the users whom they are supposed to help and protect. The use of a culture of expertise to do such damage demonstrates the moral weakness of today's almost omnipotent bureaucratic governments."

*4) The possible religion of science.*

One of the proudest boasts of the heroic COVID-19 narrative is that governments followed "the Science". In the massive misjudgement narrative, this boast is frustrating, irritating, and, at least for Christians, frightening.

The claim of scientific backing is *frustrating* because, in this narrative, the approach was largely untouched by the critical objectivity of genuine science. Having cast aside the prior consensus of public health scientists about pandemics and vaccines, the politicians and their chosen experts engaged in "policy-based evidence-making". They found or created dubious scientific studies to support their essentially unscientific fears and hopes.[20]

Public health was not only pandemic-relevant scientific discipline that was ignored. From the perspective of CST, the most frustrating anti-scientific

---

[20] Prasad (2022) discusses the U.S. Centers for Disease Control and Ioannidis (2020) discusses epidemiological forecasting.

decision was the refusal to heed the warnings from the scientific experts in the fullness of life. Psychologists, sociologists, and a slew of other specialists warned that the suspension of normal social interactions would seriously damage the common good. These scientists of the heart and of humanity were ignored – in the name of "the Science".

From both a Catholic and a secular liberal perspective, the reliance on "the Science" is *irritating* because it shows political leaders abdicating their essential responsibility to judge and promote the common good. Instead, the legitimate authorities outsourced decisions to a group of people with no political legitimacy and often with only dubious competence in genuine science. These self-declared experts told politicians what to do, claiming the authority of a technocratic "Science".

Finally, Christians, who condemn all types of idolatry, are *frightened* when science, or something given that name, is treated as a higher-than-human authority. In the misjudgement narrative, that is exactly what happened in the response to COVID-19. Political leaders proffered blind obedience to the cruel commands of the unquestionable deity whom they called "the Science". The worldly discourse of democratic politics was replaced with a quasi-religious frenzy, including a sort of Holy War against anyone who showed signs of scepticism about the oracular teachings on masks, lockdowns, social distancing, and vaccines. These heretics were judged to threaten not only the civil order but the cosmic one. It would be their fault if the Science did not work.

## Conclusion

The analyses provided by the two CST-based narratives are almost diametrically opposed to each other, as are their judgements of the wisdom of the anti-pandemic policies. However, they are not radically different, in the etymological sense of "radical". On the contrary, they are both growths out of the same intellectual-moral-theological root: the human, humane, and divine principles of CST.

In a pragmatic age, the contradictions of interpretation and judgement might seem to invalidate the method, as if all that emerged from this promising root were useless weeds. Such a dark conclusion is far too hasty.

On one side, the CST reading of the heroic narrative effectively brings out what is best in that understanding of reality. The pope is certainly right to draw attention to the virtues brought out by measures that "momentarily revived the sense that we are a global community, all in the same boat, where one person's problems are the problems of all" (Francis, 2020, 32). The spiritual lesson he draws from the pandemic may be timeless, but it could still be apt. "The pain, uncertainty and fear, and the realization of our own limitations, brought on by the pandemic have only made it all the more urgent that we rethink our styles of life, our relationships, the organization of our societies and, above all, the meaning of our existence" (Francis, 2020, 33)

On the other side, the CST reading of the misjudgement narrative expresses the ethical core of that understanding. What was most wrong with these measures was their disregard for the true good of human life and human communities, along with their abuse of the legitimate authority of governments.

The CST versions readings of both narratives point to two common conclusions, the need for societies that are better prepared for pandemics and the need for anti-pandemic policies that are both virtuous and prudent.

The simplest way to understanding disagreement within CST about COVID-19 is as one version of the broader disagreement between the heroic and misjudgement narratives. However, the CST debate is particularly illuminating, for non-Catholics as well as Catholics, because it never loses its focus on what is truly most important, the common good.

Finally, to answer my initial question: I am certainly not more Catholic than the Holy Father. In our disagreement over this pandemic, we are both doing what Catholics, and others, should always do – apply the Church's great wisdom to the troubles of the world.

## References

Benedict XVI (2005). *Deus caritas est: Encyclical letter on Christian love*. Libreria Editrice Vaticana. https://www.vatican.va/content/benedict-xvi/en/encyclicals/documents/hf_ben-xvi_enc_20051225_deus-caritas-est.html

Benedict XVI (2009). *Caritas in Veritate: Encyclical letter on integral human development in charity and truth*. Libreria Editrice Vaticana. https://www.vatican.va/content/benedict-xvi/en/encyclicals/documents/hf_ben-xvi_enc_20090629_caritas-in-veritate.html

Berenson, A. (2021). *Pandemia: How Coronavirus hysteria took over our government, rights, and lives*. Regency.

Catechism of the Catholic Church. (1997). (2nd ed.) Libreria Editrice Vaticana http://www.scborromeo.org/ccc/p3s1c2a2.htm#II

Catholic News Agency (2022, March 10). Pope sacks bishop who claimed it was 'legitimate' for Catholics to question safety of Covid vaccines. *Catholic Herald*. https://catholicherald.co.uk/pope-sacks-bishop-who-claimed-it-was-legitimate-for-catholics-to-question-safety-of-covid-vaccines/

Castro Seixas E. (2021). War metaphors in political communication on Covid-19. *Frontiers in Sociology, 5*,583680. https://doi.org/10.3389/fsoc.2020.583680

Cayley, D. (2020). *Pandemic revelations*. davidcayley.com. https://www.davidcayley.com/blog/category/Pandemic+2

Cayley, D. (2021). *Concerning life*. davidcayley.com. https://www.david cayley.com/blog/2021/6/11/concerning-life-1

Centers for Disease Control and Prevention (2022). *History of quarantine*. https://www.cdc.gov/quarantine/historyquarantine.html

DeCosse, D. (2020, March 20). *Five ethical basics in the face of the coronavirus pandemic*. Markkula Center for Applied Ethics, Santa Clara University. https://www.scu.edu/ethics-spotlight/covid-19/five-ethical-basics-in-the-face-of-the-coronavirus-pandemic/

Farrow, D. (2022, January 27). *Whether there is a moral obligation to disobey the coercive mandates*. Theopolis. https://theopolisinstitute.com/conversations/whether-there-is-a-moral-obligation-to-disobey-the-coercive-mandates/

Fontana, S (2021, December 20). *Emergenza perenne: I motivi sono politici non sanitari. Andrea Gagliarducci intervista Stefano Fontana.* Osservatorio Internazionale Cardinale Van Thuân sulla dottrina sociale della chiesa. https://www.vanthuanobservatory.org/emergenza-perenne-i-motivisono-politici-non-sanitari-andrea-gagliarducci-aci-cna-intervista-stefano-fontana/

Francis (2015). *Laudato Si': Encyclical letter on care for our common home.* Dicastero per la Comunicazione – Libreria Editrice Vaticana https://www.vatican.va/content/francesco/en/encyclicals/documents/papa-francesco_20150524_enciclica-laudato-si.html

Francis (2020a, November 26). Pope Francis: A crisis reveals what is in our hearts. *New York Times.* https://www.nytimes.com/2020/11/26/opinion/pope-francis-covid.html

Francis (2020b). *Fratelli Tutti: Encyclical letter on fraternity and social friendship.* Dicastero per la Comunicazione – Libreria Editrice Vaticana. https://www.vatican.va/content/francesco/en/encyclicals/documents/papa-francesco_20201003_enciclica-fratelli-tutti.html

Francis (2022, January 10). *Address to the members of the diplomatic corps.* Dicastero per la Comunicazione – Libreria Editrice Vaticana. https://www.vatican.va/content/francesco/en/speeches/2022/january/documents/20220110-corpo-diplomatico.html

Glasman, M. (2020, June 12). How Catholic Social Teaching rescued me from an academic crisis. *Catholic Herald.* https://catholicherald.co.uk/lord-glasman-how-catholic-social-teaching-rescued-me-from-an-academic-crisis/

Hadas, E. (2019, September 24). *Individualism, statism and the common good.* Together for the Common Good. https://togetherforthecommon good. co.uk/leading-thinkers/individualism-statism-and-the-common-good

Hadas, E. (2020). *Counsels of imperfection: Thinking through Catholic Social Teaching.* Catholic University of America Press.

Hadas, E. (2021, November 18). *Covid and the technocratic paradigm.* Together for the Common Good. https://togetherforthecommongood.co.uk/leading-thinkers/covid-and-the-technocratic-paradigm

Hadas, E. (2022, March 16). Locke, Hegel, and Covid-19. *Humanum Review.* https://humanumreview.com/articles/lock-hegel-and-covid-19

Hanby, M. (2015). The gospel of creation and the technocratic paradigm: Reflections on a central teaching of Laudato Si'. *Communio: International Catholic Review, 42*(Winter 2015), 724-727. https://www.communio-icr.com/files/42.4_Hanby_website.pdf

Heriot, G.S. & Jamrozik, E. (2021). Imagination and remembrance: What role should historical epidemiology play in a world bewitched by mathematical modelling of COVID-19 and other epidemics? *History and Philosophy of the Life Sciences 43*(81). https://doi.org/10.1007/s40656-021-00422-6

Illich I. (1977). *Limits to medicine: Medical nemesis: The expropriation of health*. Penguin.

Ioannidis, J., Cripps, S., & Tannerc, M. (2022, August 25). Forecasting for COVID-19 has failed. *International Journal of Forecasting, 38*(2), 423-438. https://doi.org/10.1016/j.ijforecast.2020.08.004

John XXIII (1963). *Pacem in terris: Encyclical on establishing universal peace in truth, justice, charity, and liberty*. Libreria Editrice Vaticana. https://www.vatican.va/content/john-xxiii/en/encyclicals/documents/hf_j-xxiii_enc_11041963_pacem.html

John Paul II (1984). *Salvifici doloris Apostolic letter on the Christian meaning of human suffering*. Dicastero per la Comunicazione – Libreria Editrice Vaticana. https://www.vatican.va/content/john-paul-ii/en/apost_letters/1984/documents/hf_jp-ii_apl_11021984_salvifici-doloris.html

John Paul II (1987). *Sollicitudo rei socialis: Encyclical letter for the twentieth anniversary of* Populorum progressio. Dicastero per la Comunicazione – Libreria Editrice Vaticana. https://www.vatican.va/content/john-paul-ii/en/encyclicals/documents/hf_jp-ii_enc_30121987_sollicitudo-rei-socialis.html

John Paul II (1991). *Centesimus annus: on the hundredth anniversary of* Rerum novarum. Dicastero per la Comunicazione – Libreria Editrice Vaticana. https://www.vatican.va/content/john-paul-ii/en/encyclicals/documents/hf_jp-ii_enc_01051991_centesimus-annus.html#-2S

John Paul II (1998). *Fides et ratio: Encyclical letter on the relationship between faith and reason*. Dicastero per la Comunicazione – Libreria Editrice Vaticana. https://www.vatican.va/content/john-paul-ii/en/encyclicals/documents/hf_jp-ii_enc_14091998_fides-et-ratio.html

Johnson, K. (2020, March 17). *Pandemic and the common good*. Catholic Moral Theology. https://catholicmoraltheology.com/pandemic-and-the-common-good/

Kheriaty, A. (2022, April 5). *This is not normal, and no one should accept it.* Brownstone Institute. https://brownstone.org/articles/this-is-not-normal-and-no-one-should-accept-it/

Kostoff, R., Calina, d., Kanduc, D., Briggs, M., Vlachoyiannopoulos, P., Svistunov, A., & Tsatsakis, A. (2021, September 14). Why are we vaccinating children against COVID-19? *Toxicology Reports, 8,* 1665-1684. https://doi.org/10.1016/j.toxrep.2021.08.010

Lemoine, P. (2021, March 24). *The case against lockdowns*. CSPI. https://cspicenter.org/blog/waronscience/the-case-against-lockdowns/

Lipton, E., & Steinhauer, J. (2020, April 26). The untold story of the birth of social distancing. *The New York Times.* A1.

McGovern, T., Flood, A., Carson, P. (2020, August 10). COVID-19 policy-making in a country divided: Catholic Social Teaching as a path to unity. *The Linacre Quarterly, 87*(4). https://doi.org/10.1177/0024363920942431

Miles, D., Stedman, M., & Heald, A. (2020, July). Living with Covid-19: Balancing costs against benefits in the face of the virus. *National Institute Economic Review.* https://doi.org/10.1017/nie.2020.30

*Number of coronavirus disease 2019 (COVID-19) deaths in the U.S. as of March 30, 2022, by age* Statista (2022. April 4) Retrieved April 5, 2022. https://www.statista.com/statistics/1191568/reported-deaths-from-covid-by-age-us/

Office of National Statistics (2022, January 21). Monthly mortality analysis, England and Wales. https://www.ons.gov.uk/peoplepopulationandcommunity/birthsdeathsandmarriages/deaths/bulletins/monthlymortalityanalysisenglandandwales/december2021#pre-existing-conditions-of-people-whose-death-was-due-to-covid-19-deaths-registered-in-october-to-december-2021

Pontifical Council for Pastoral Assistance to Health Care Workers (2017). *New charter for health care workers* (The National Catholic Bioethics Center, trans.). The National Catholic Bioethics Center. (Original work published 2016 by Libreria Editrice Vatican) https://www.ncbcenter. org/free-scribd-texts/new-charter-for-health-care-workers

Pontifical Council for Justice and Peace (2004). *Compendium of the social doctrine of the church.* Libreria Editrice Vaticana. https://www.vatican.va/roman_curia/pontifical_councils/justpeace/documents/rc_pc_justpeace_doc_20060526_compendio-dott-soc_en.html#

Pope, C. (2020, May 6). *'Coronavirus,* "Where is thy sting?' — Why this gripping fear is useless. *National Catholic Register.* https://www.ncregister.com/blog/coronavirus-where-is-thy-sting-why-this-gripping-fear-is-useless

Prasad, V. (2022, February 15). How the CDC abandoned science. *Tablet.* https://www.tabletmag.com/sections/science/articles/how-the-cdc-abandoned-science

Thomas Aquinas (1920). *Summa theologiciae.* (Fathers of the English Dominican Province, Trans., online edition, 2017) https://www.newadvent.org/summa/

Thomas, J. (2019, October 18). *Catholic Social Teaching and the non-Catholic writers who advocate it.* The Wanna Bee. https://medium.com/soli-deo-gloria/catholic-social-teaching-and-the-non-catholic-writers-who-advocate-it-b17f063bfb69

Tognotti, E. (2013). Lessons from the history of quarantine, from plague to influenza A. *Emerging Infectious Diseases 19*(2), 254–259. https://doi.org/10.3201/eid1902.120312

Tucker, J. (2021, January 12). *In the Asian flu of 1957-58, they rejected lockdowns.* AIER. https://www.aier.org/article/in-the-asian-flu-of-1957-58-they-rejected-lockdowns/

Vatican Council II (1965). *Pastoral constitution on the church in the modern world, Gaudium et spes.* The Holy See. https://www.vatican.va/archive/hist_councils/ii_vatican_council/documents/vat-ii_const_19651207_gaudium-et-spes_en.html

Welby, J (2016, November 17). *Archbishop Justin Welby on 'the common good and a shared vision for the next century'.* Archbishop of Canterbury. https://www.archbishopofcanterbury.org/speaking-writing/speeches/archbishop-justin-welby-common-good-and-shared-vision-next-century

World Health Organisation (2019). *Non-pharmaceutical public health measures for mitigating the risk and impact of epidemic and pandemic influenza.* https://apps.who.int/iris/bitstream/handle/10665/329438/9789241516839-eng.pdf?ua=1

Wyma, D. (2014). When and how should we respond to unjust laws? A Thomistic analysis of civil disobedience. *Christian Scholar's Review, 43*(2), 157-170. https://christianscholars.com/when-and-how-should-we-respond-to-unjust-laws-a-thomistic-analysis-of-civil-disobedience/

# PART THREE
# Lived experiences

# HEALTHCARE WORKERS' LIVED EXPERIENCES AT THE PEAK OF COVID-19 OUTBREAK IN NEW YORK HOSPITALS

**Cheryl Patton**[1]

**Abstract:** The first recorded case of COVID-19 in the U.S. state of New York during the pandemic occurred in early March 2020. The greater New York Metropolitan area soon became an epicenter of the pandemic. Hospitalizations soared during this time, overwhelming healthcare workers as they struggled to treat the sudden onslaught of patients. Four nurse practitioners and four registered nurses who were employed in greater New York Metropolitan hospitals were interviewed between May and July of 2020 for a phenomenological study conducted to determine healthcare workers' lived experiences when caring for patients hospitalized with COVID-19. It was evident from the data that the pandemic introduced unprecedented ethical challenges within the healthcare systems, many of which stemmed from the scarcity of resources, both equipment resources and human resources. This chapter details some of those ethical challenges, while concomitantly integrating other studies and healthcare workers' experiences that dealt with hospitals' ethical, moral and practical lessons from the COVID 19 pandemic.

In spring of 2020, I conducted a qualitative study on healthcare workers' lived experiences when caring for patients hospitalized with COVID-19 in greater New York Metropolitan hospitals. Specifically, I interviewed four registered nurses and four nurse practitioners, none of whom worked at the same hospital as the other participants. The greater New York metropolitan area comprises New York City, New York Metro – Long Island, and northern New Jersey; this region contains approximately 100 hospitals (NYS Health Profiles, n.d.). This geographic area was chosen for the study because, at the time, it was considered the "heart of the [COVID-19] outbreak in the United States" (Warren, 2020, para. 1). Furthermore, according to Mogul (2020), "no U.S. city suffered

---

[1] Adjunct Professor, Eastern University, St. Davids, Pennsylvania, USA

more in the first wave of the coronavirus pandemic than New York City, where more than 24,000 people died, mainly in the spring" (para. 1). The purpose of my study was to explore impacts to the nursing personnel's wellbeing, and throughout the interview process, the nursing personnel revealed various ethical dilemmas that arose due to the crisis. In basic terms, health care ethics involves the sense of right and wrong as well as beliefs about personal rights and duties owed to others. The most common ethical concerns were associated with the allocation of scarce resources at a time when COVID-19 patients overwhelmed the healthcare workplaces in the greater New York Metropolitan area. The scarcity of personal protective equipment (PPE) issues and human resources arose most frequently in the data analysis. According to Gaudine et al. (2011), "the distribution of limited health care resources can be a major source of ethical conflict" (p. 756). These conflicts exist in routine healthcare contexts; in times of a major pandemic, when resources are significantly scarce, exacerbated conflicts arise. This chapter will tie the study participants' concerns regarding the lack of personal protective equipment (PPE) and human resources to the existing literature on these ethical conundrums.

## Personal Protective Equipment Scarcity

Masks, gowns, goggles, face shields, hairnets, shoe coverings, germicidal wipes, and body bags were specific items that my study participants mentioned were in short supply within their hospital workplaces at the height of the pandemic (Patton, 2020). Of these, a shortage of protective facemasks was by far the most concerning to the study participants, primarily because COVID-19 was a respiratory disease. While most of the participants bemoaned the mask shortage, three of the eight mentioned that their supervisors admonished staff members early on during the pandemic for wearing any type of facemask (either medical or N95 masks[2]) unless

---

[2] Medical masks are also referred to as surgical masks. Particulate respirators include National Institute for Occupational Safety and Health-certified N95, N99, U.S. Food and Drug Administration surgical N95, and European Union standard FFP2 or FFP3.

they had not received the flu vaccine[3] (Patton, 2021). This reprimand even took place when the hospital employee personally supplied the mask, as opposed to wearing hospital-provided masks. Other nurses in direct contact with patients with COVID-19 who were offered a medical mask wanted a better-filtering particulate respirator, an N95 mask, for higher protection. One participant voiced concerns to her supervisors regarding the safety and ethical consequences of withholding this type of PPE from direct contact patient care workers, inquiring, "How are you asking our frontline staff-- both nurses and providers that are actually seeing patients, some of them are positive COVID, and you are not giving them an N95? You're giving them a [medical] facemask. That's not acceptable." Other participants noted that when in training, they had been instructed that N95 masks were disposable after one use and had used N95 masks as such prior to the pandemic. Yet, now they were required to use the same N95 mask "indefinitely," according to one participant or until they were no longer functional, according to another, or for a "whole week," according to a third participant.

The eight participants in the study were not alone in their concerns about the PPE shortage. The literature is rife with ethical considerations regarding masks for healthcare workers during the COVID-19 pandemic. Griffith (2020) relayed the cases of two U.S. nurses who felt that they were persecuted for trying to protect their health during the early stages of the pandemic. One of the nurses worked in California and was sent home after refusing to wear a medical mask instead of an N95 mask when caring for COVID-19 patients. The second, a Kentucky nurse, received an insubordination reprimand and reassignment for refusing to treat COVID-19 patients when her hospital workplace would not provide her with an N95 mask. Similar to my participants' experiences, providing one's own N95 was unacceptable as well in many hospitals. Across the country, U.S. nurses were told that they were not allowed to wear their personal N95 masks at work, with consequences that included termination (Davis, 2020; Firth, 2020; Lacy, 2020). In one case, the nurse was fired shortly after she

[3] In 2013, New York State mandated that all healthcare workers with direct patient contact wear a mask if they have not received a flu vaccine to avoid potentially infecting patients (Caplan, 2013).

was told to clock out and go home when she insisted that she would wear her own mask and gloves during her work on a floor with COVID-19 patients. She then was told that she had the choice of resignation or termination. Within a day of the nurse going public with her experience, in her attempt to do "what was right in the midst of this pandemic," the hospital changed its policy to allow nurses to wear personally acquired masks (Broadt, 2020, para. 19). Griffith (2020) quoted Arthur Caplan, head of the division of medical ethics at the New York University Grossman School of Medicine, who stated "it's important to speak up if you see inadequate conditions for patients or yourself." The medical ethicist believed that those who do speak up should be protected rather than punished. Frontline healthcare workers across the globe complained of the lack of PPE as they felt pulled between choosing their health or their livelihood. For example, Shaibu et al. (2021) explained how nurses in Kenya threatened to go on strike during March and April of 2020, while public hospital nurses in Zimbabwe did strike due to the lack of PPE. Nurses in Botswana sued the government over the issue, while dozens of nurses and doctors from two hospitals in Bulgaria's capital resigned due to inadequate supply of PPE (Schuklenk, 2021; Shaibu et al., 2021).

The aforementioned U.S. nurses' employers cited the Centers for Disease Control and Prevention (CDC) mask recommendations when justifying the use of medical masks and their responses to the nurses' complaints. At the time of the nurse complaints, the CDC recommended that healthcare professionals use N95 respirators during aerosol-generating procedures (e.g., intubation, tracheotomy, and bronchoscopy) on patients with possible severe acute respiratory syndrome coronavirus 2 (SARS-CoV-2) infection. In essence, the CDC and other public health agencies such as the World Health Organization (WHO) recommended that healthcare professionals reserve the scarce, more protective respirators for procedures that they perceived posed a greater risk of transmission. However, subsequent studies showed that some aerosol-generating procedures actually generate less infectious aerosol than a coughing patient with acute COVID-19 (Hamilton et al., 2021; Klompas et al., 2021). Public health agency guidelines (e.g., CDC and World Health Organization) changed repeatedly throughout the pandemic due to changes in supply as well as in response to improved research on issues surrounding the novel coronavirus.

For example, during the time of their interviews, the participants in my study were required to wear the same N95 respirator for long periods of time. This variation from the norm was due to capacity problems. The CDC has created capacity strategies for optimizing the supply of N95 respirators. As many participants noted during interviews, N95 respirators are to be disposed of after each use, in conventional, everyday practice. When supplies diminish, contingency strategies are put into effect. Contingency strategies include the use of respirators beyond manufacturer shelf life for fit test and training and may be used for an extended time, with multiple patients. In times of extreme crisis, the crisis capacity strategies are enacted, which include the use of respirators beyond manufacturer shelf life for healthcare delivery, allowance for limited reuse, and prioritized use dependent on healthcare activity type. Crisis capacity strategies are not compatible with U.S. standards of care; they are only used when there are recognized shortages of N95 respirators, and the previous two strategies were already implemented. These strategies were an attempt at distributive justice, which involves the use of ethics concepts and criteria to determine how scarce resources should be divided among people, groups, organizations, and communities" (Reamer, 2015, para. 1).

## Scarcity of Healthcare Staff

Allocation of scarce resources occurred beyond PPE. My study's participants explained that the influx of COVID-19 patients overwhelmed their hospitals in a short period of time. Shortly thereafter, due to the lack of adequate protection, many nurses fell ill and some, many participants speculated, stayed home due to fears of infection. This combination of factors created a massive staffing shortage. In order to meet the demands, scope of practice expansions were made and healthcare personnel from other areas of the hospital, as well as nationwide, were deployed to COVID-19 units (NYSED, 2020). Prior to receiving help from traveling nurses, the hospitals mitigated the problem by shifting workers from their typical area of expertise to the COVID-19 units. One participant, who typically worked in a clinic caring for patients with chronic diseases, was pulled in to work in the inpatient unit. She stated that she just did what she was able, since she did not have access to the inpatient electronic records.

That participant shared that she told the nurses on the inpatient unit, "I can give patients their trays, I can feed them, I can make sure they are on oxygen. I can clean their bed. I can put them on stretchers. I can do all that…and that's exactly what I did." She expressed that the help she offered was highly appreciated and she received feedback such as "Please tell me when you're coming again." She assured them that she would return the next day and perform the same duties. Not every participant relayed a similar story, however.

Another nurse I will refer to as Mary[4], revealed, "Our entire hospital became a COVID-19 hospital." Furthermore, she explained, "All of our nurses in our hospital were redeployed doing things that they were not used to doing." Mary typically worked in an area where she did not have prolonged contact with patients. She relayed that this type of short-term care suited her since it prevented her from becoming too emotionally close to the patients. Due to her redeployment to COVID-19 units, the personalization was difficult on her. She divulged:

> When you are doing the intimate kind of care that you need to do for an [intensive care unit] ICU patient, you're doing bed baths, you're turning them, you're doing oral care, you know, you're telling them what you're doing because you're moving them. And they now have a name and a face, and you talk to the family. And they know your voice when you pick up the phone, you know. And it's a very different experience than what I'm used to. Um, I- I'm experiencing- honestly PTSD, um, which I recognize now because I'm having panic attacks just out in the grocery store…I can't go out.

One critical care nurse practitioner participant stated that she was "forced to work to the extent of [her] license" due to the high volume of patients. She recalled, "If things needed to be done, you couldn't necessarily reach out to an attending physician for every decision. We didn't have time for that, or they could die if you don't make that decision in the next 10 seconds." Fortunately, due to her typical role as a critical nurse practitioner, she was already accustomed to caring for critically ill patients. Others were not, acknowledging that they assumed responsibilities of patient care that were atypical due to staffing issues. This caused frustration and fears of

---

[4] All participant names have been changed for confidentiality purposes.

patient safety. One nurse, relaying her fear for the physical safety of patients, stated that nurses were redeployed with "no training, no nothing, just thrown in there." Another nurse, Ann, also revealed that being pulled into a new role could have an impact on patients. Ann disclosed that she typically did not offer critical care to acute patients:

> We normally have a rapid response team, and we have rapids [response team members] that are ICU nurses. But they were all sick. So, we would have rapids, and no one would come. Or we would have a stat intubation patient, and no one would come. So, then we became the people who were giving Levophed and pushing fentanyl. But we don't normally have meds on our floor, we don't normally do that.

Ann went on to explain that the unfamiliarity with procedures and medications typically handled by a specialized team created dilemmas for the nurses. She recalled conversations with physicians:

> The doctor's like, "Here, hang this Levophed," and I'm like, "Can this go in the peripheral line or does this have to go in a central line?" And they're like, "The nurses do it." And I'm like, "I don't know." Or they would be like, "Oh, nobody did this tie out for the central line." And I was like, "I don't know what I'm doing, guys. You tell me. I'm not an ICU nurse, you have to prompt me to do things." People would [say], "Where is your OT tube?" I'm like, "I don't even know what that is. You tell me. Where is it normally? This isn't an ICU floor." They were like, "Can you get me Versed?" And I'm like, "It has to come from pharmacy, we don't keep that here." So, then I'm running down to pharmacy to try and get Versed. It's just stuff like that. Yeah. Which I think would've been fine if we had more staffing.

Nurses were not the only healthcare professionals to get redeployed. Multiple participants stated that physician specialists from other fields disassociated from ICU care (e.g., gynecology and psychiatry) were pulled to work in the COVID units. One participant felt that her job as a nurse was to be "responsible" for the patients throughout this time. She added, "I felt that my job meant so much at that time because we were the advocates for the patients. We were fighting with the physicians" to try to provide the best care. Sometimes that ideal of offering the patients high quality, "best care" was out of the hands of both physicians and nursing staff, however. A few participants discussed the changes in emergency resuscitation practices in their hospital workplaces. One participant shared that at her hospital, many units within the hospital were not calling codes[5] on futile patient cases since the risk of spreading COVID-19 during chest compressions was considered a great risk to the healthcare staff and the chances of the patients' successful return to health was considered minimal. Another nurse shared that his hospital "did have criteria on who's eligible for code" and thus, there were a "high number of patients that became DNR [do not resuscitate]." A third nurse disclosed, "We weren't coding any patients." The nurse continued, "Chest compressions weren't a thing [at that time] because they were concerned for…aerosolizing" that would place the limited healthcare staff at risk of transmission. Yet, the nurse recalled that one patient received a full code, complete with chest compressions. The resuscitation attempt was in vain, however, as the patient, a long-time employee of the same hospital, expired despite the efforts.

The aforementioned participant experiences raise a number of ethical questions. Can a healthcare professional ethically treat a patient without proper training or experience? What role do nurses play when involved in ethical conflicts with physicians? When is it ethical to withhold life saving measures? The following paragraphs illuminate the unfortunate typicality of the nurses' experiences at the height of the early pandemic in hotspot[6] areas.

Jia et al.'s (2020) qualitative study involved 18 Chinese nurses who provided care to COVID-19 patients in China. The research specifically sought to explore the ethical challenges nurses encountered while caring for the

---

[5] Code status can be defined as the emergency response treatment patients would or would not receive if their heart or breathing were to stop. Codes are called in a hospital if the patient does not have "do not resuscitate" code status.

[6] To be considered a COVID-19 hotspot county on a particular date, as defined by the Centers of Disease Control the county must meet the following four criteria: 1) >100 new COVID-19 cases within the past 7 days, 2) an increase in the most recent 7-day COVID-19 incidence over the preceding 7-day incidence, 3) a decrease of <60% or an increase in the most recent 3-day COVID-19 incidence over the preceding 3-day incidence, and 4) the ratio of 7-day incidence/30-day incidence exceeds 0.31. Also, hotspots must have met one or both of the following criteria: 1) >60% change in the most recent 3-day COVID-19 incidence, or 2) >60% change in the most recent 7-day incidence (CDC, 2020).

patients. The study was conducted quite early in the pandemic, with participant interviews taking place in February and March 2020. Upon analysis of the data, the ethical challenges identified involved: 1.) Patients' neglected rights and emotional support, where the lack of medical support and patients' inability to communicate led to patients not choosing their medical plans as well as lack of family hospital visitation, 2.) Inequality, where nurses spent far more time in patients' rooms compared to physicians and some physicians expected the nurses to perform their duties for them in order to avoid patient contact, 3.) Professional ethics, which involved nurses' slow response time to patients caused by donning of protective equipment or the purposeful delayed responses to avoid compromising their health, and 4.) Job competency, where one participant stated, "I used to do surgical nursing, but now internal medicine knowledge is needed for nursing COVID-19 patients, and I am not familiar with that" (p. 39). The authors also included the feeling of powerlessness and the worry of nurses' inability to treat patients adequately within the realm of job competency.

Job competency issues were echoed in Panda et al.'s (2021) qualitative study. The authors interviewed nine hospital leaders from nine hospitals in the United States, United Kingdom, New Zealand, Singapore and South Korea. Seven hospitals redeployed their healthcare staff during peak surges of critically ill COVID-19 patients. Their findings showed that one of the top three concerns for the redeployed involved their skills and patient safety. Moyal-Smith et al. (2020) address these concerns upon analyzing the interviews from a data set of nine physicians and another of 12 clinicians who were rapidly redeployed during the pandemic in peak admission times. The authors advised that having a structured framework for rapid training would be useful in the onboarding process. Nearly all the interviewees stated that shadowing another provider is essential during onboarding. One interviewee posited that if they knew they would be paired with another provider, they would have entered the redeployment role with much less anxiety, adding, "I was nervous that I would be a fish out of water. We are perfectionists and are used to doing things really well. Fear of making mistakes is extremely anxiety-producing" (p. 4). Many interviewees also noted that they "depended on the 'elbow support' (i.e., real-time answers) that they received from core teams of physicians and advanced practice providers who were familiar with the clinical care and the unit" (p. 4).

Redeployment of healthcare workers was essential when patient volume quickly increased. This occurred at varying times across the globe. Louisiana surpassed its record for the number of COVID-19 patients in August 2021. At that time, the state's public health officer lamented, "There's just not enough qualified staff in the state right now to care for all these patients" (Chavez, 2021, para. 3). As such, hospitals redeployed many team members. Ochsner Health redeployed 800 team members from across its system. Dr. Robert Hart, Ochsner's chief medical officer and executive vice president, relayed that "We've shut down a lot of our procedure areas and moved those staff members into bedside care areas to help out on the floor or in the intensive care unit" (Chavez, 2021, para. 12).

Redeployment led to some healthcare professionals lacking the knowledge to properly care for patients. However, the crisis of an overburdened health system due to an overabundance of positive COVID-19 cases led to extreme measures. Healthcare staffing shortages were already problematic pre-pandemic; once the onslaught of COVID-19 patients began, the lack of personnel rose significantly (Parrott, 2022). The atypical influx of inpatients required hospital administrators to rapidly redeploy workers and sometimes seek outside help from traveling healthcare professionals. These times of crisis serve as a reminder to healthcare professionals of the ethical responsibility of teamwork and interprofessional collaboration. Though physicians traditionally regarded nurses as subordinates, with the former giving orders and the latter implementing them, this can create an unethical environment. Unfortunately, according to Elsous et al. (2017), these traditional understandings of the physician-nurse relationship can adversely affect healthcare professionals' attitudes toward collaboration. Thus, a more collaborative relationship is often needed. The authors posit that with effective collaboration, problem solving involves a mutual effort with no hierarchical physician-nurse relationship. With this approach, there would be less "fighting with physicians" as one of my study participants had experienced, and more cooperation as the team works toward the common goal of caring for the patients. Regardless, nurses must act on behalf of the patient in cases where they believe that the physician's actions or orders are not in the best interest of the patient. They are morally obligated to do so (Kroeger Mappes, 1989).

Interprofessional collaboration can certainly help in the training of those onboarding in the hospital setting. As Moyal-Smith et al. (2020) recommended, rapid training upon onboarding must be a prime consideration, as is the potential of pairing the redeployed with a more seasoned healthcare professional when possible. This seasoned professional might be an employee who is typically considered lower in hierarchy than the novice. For example, a critical care nurse can help onboard a physician who has been redeployed from an area that typically does not treat critically ill patients in times of crisis in a strained healthcare system.

The withholding of life support during the height of the crisis created much debate among medical ethicists. Western nations with outstanding healthcare systems rarely face the concerns of how to best allocate standard life-saving medical resources when demand exceeds supply. Unfortunately, these challenges are not unfamiliar to those working in resource-poor countries (Chan et al., 2020). Yet, when patients inundated hospitals during peak times of COVID-19 in certain geographical areas, decisions about what patients to save had to be made. Chan et al. explained that deontological ethics, where "each person is valuable and should have an equal chance of receiving life-saving care (i.e., first-come, first-served)" was threatened in some areas, replaced by utilitarian ethics, where clinicians were forced to face the possibility of prioritizing "saving the most lives in settings with extremely limited resources" (para. 2). They explained that until the COVID-19 pandemic, U.S. physicians generally practiced medicine via an individual, versus a societal lens. The pandemic challenged that. Some healthcare professionals were put in a situation that caused them "imminent moral distress," deciding "which patient receives life-saving care when the alternative outcome is certain death" (para. 3). This was the case in hospitals within the greater New York Metropolitan Area during the spring of 2020, according to some of my participants' accounts. Voytko (2020) reported that while the greater New York City area was considered the "epicenter of the nation's coronavirus crisis" (para. 10), some of the hospitals had not instated hospital-wide policies on resuscitation efforts, one hospital was reported to have stopped "performing chest compressions on COVID-19 patients, due to the risk of exposure and the amount of protective gear needed" (para. 4), another hospital's leader "advised doctors to 'think more critically' about which patients should receive one of their limited number of ventilators, and that the institution would support doctors who 'withhold futile intubations'" (para. 6), while yet another hospital reportedly bullied "older COVID-19 patients into signing DNR and 'do not intubate' orders" (para. 5). Other areas of the United States were not spared of these discussions, either. Cha (2020) reported that a Seattle hospital "severely" limited "the number of responders to a contagious patient in cardiac or respiratory arrest" while the city was considered a COVID-19 hotspot (para. 6) and a hospital in the District of Columbia utilized "modified procedures" during resuscitation, such as "putting plastic sheeting over the patient to create a barrier" (para. 6). Cha (2020) cited some bioethicists' views, including those of R. Alta Charo, from the University of Wisconsin – Madison. Charo opined that it is pragmatic to withhold treatment during these critical times of scarcity, despite how unsettling it is in a country that is not used to facing these difficult decisions on a regular basis. Charo continued, "It doesn't help anybody if our doctors and nurses are felled by this virus and not able to care for us...The code process is one that puts them at an enhanced risk" (para. 11). University of Pennsylvania bioethicist, Scott Halpern was also quoted, stating that stopping all resuscitation efforts for all COVID-19 patients is too "draconian" but the problem of infecting healthcare workers and the scarcity of staff and PPE is a major consideration when making such decisions. He added, "If we risk their well-being in service of one patient, we detract from the care of future patients, which is unfair" (para. 31). Bruno Petinaux, the chief medical officer at George Washington University Hospital, stated that the decisions are ultimately dependent upon the individual hospital's resources at the time (Cha, 2020). When a hospital is fortunate enough to have sufficient equipment and manpower, these decisions are not commonplace. Yet, the COVID-19 pandemic clearly illustrated that scarcity can become problematic, even in countries unaccustomed to such crises.

## Post-Pandemic Staffing Impact

The COVID-19 pandemic placed extreme stress on the healthcare workforce in the United States, leading to hospital shortages and an increase in healthcare employee burnout, exhaustion, and trauma (ASPE,

2022). These issues added to the U.S. "workforce shortages and maldistribution, as well as in a workforce where burnout, stress, and mental health problems" that pre-existed the pandemic (p. 1). Pre-pandemic data on 116 New York hospitals' nurse-patient staffing ratios found great variation across the New York hospitals. ICU ratios ranged from 1.8 to 4.3, with an average of 2.5 patients per nurse; medical-surgical units ranged from 4.3 to 10.5 patients per nurse and an average of 6.3 patients per nurse (Lasater et al., 2021). The optimal nurse-patient ratio is 1:2 for ICUs and 1:5 for medical-surgical units (Sharma & Rani, 2020). Thus, there were staffing issues already at play in New York prior to the onslaught of COVID-19 patients. Afterward, the situation worsened considerably. According to an analysis by Epic Health Research Network, U.S. hospital staffing demands increased 245% from September 2020 to December 2020 (Teriakidis et al., 2021). Yet, after a year of the pandemic, three out of 10 healthcare workers are considering leaving the profession (Wan, 2021). Mercer (2021) predicted that "demand for nurses will grow by at least 5% over the next five years" and during that time period, the profession is projected to lose 900,000 nurses (p. 6). That creates a need to hire over 1.1 million nurses by 2026. Mercer predicts that 29 U.S. states will be unable to keep up with the demand, "coming up almost 100,000 nurses short in the next five years" (p. 6). Of the 29 U.S. states set to experience significant demand, "the largest projected shortages of nursing talent will be in Pennsylvania, North Carolina, Colorado, Illinois, and Massachusetts" (p. 6). To keep up with demand today, hospitals have been increasingly depending on travel nurses. U.S. hospitals' use of contract temporary labor has risen over 130% (AHA, 2022). A Kaufman Hall analysis determined that the use of contracting work has contributed to increased hospital expenses of 17% over pre-pandemic levels (AHA, 2022). Immediate attention to the healthcare worker crisis is essential for the ethical treatment of patients and healthcare workers alike.

## Conclusion

This chapter identified significant ethical challenges faced by healthcare professionals, administrators, and patients during the COVID-19 pandemic, particularly during a time when the SARS-CoV-2 virus swept through areas, infecting masses with COVID-19. Scarcity of equipment and staff caused havoc as hospital stakeholders faced issues most had never before experienced in their entire careers. Though the ethical boundaries of right versus wrong were blurred during these perilous times, the courses of action employed were decided upon after as much deliberation as time would allow and changed as fast and furious as the prevalence of COVID-19 itself, within specific geographic areas. Since it is now well recognized that healthcare resources are impermanent, greater preparedness may improve patient outcomes and healthcare professionals' wellbeing in the future. The time to act is now, as it is predicted that the demand for healthcare workers will increase and exacerbate the current crisis, with insufficient number of professionals able to meet the healthcare needs of our patients.

## References

AHA. (2022). Data brief: Health care workforce challenges threaten hospitals' ability to care for patients. American Hospital Association. https://www.aha.org/fact-sheets/2021-11-01-data-brief-health-care-workforce-challenges-threaten-hospitals-ability-care

ASPE. (2022). Impact of the COVID-19 pandemic on the hospital and outpatient clinician workforce. Assistant Secretary for Planning and Evaluation: Office of Health Policy. https://aspe.hhs.gov/sites/default/files/documents/9cc72124abd9ea25d58a22c7692dccb6/aspe-covid-workforce-report.pdf.

Ault, A. (2020). *Amid PPE shortage, clinicians face harassment, firing for self-care.* MedScape Medical News. https://www.medscape.com/viewarticle/927590#vp_2

Broadt, L. (2020). Virtua okays masks brought from home; nurse who raised concerns fired. *Burlington County Times.* https://www.burlingtoncountytimes.com/news/20200411/virtua-oks-masks-brought-from-home-nurse-who-raised-concerns-fired

Caplan, A. L. (2013). The law! Get a flu shot or wear a mask, healthcare workers! *MedScape.* https://www.medscape.com/viewarticle/812959

CDC (2020). Trends in number of distribution of COVID-19 hotspot counties – United States, March 8 – July 15, 2020. *Weekly, 69*(33), 1127–1132. https://www.cdc.gov/mmwr/volumes/69/wr/mm6933e2.htm

Cha, A. E. (2020, March 25). Hospitals consider universal do-not-resuscitate orders for coronavirus patients. *The Washington Post.* https://www.washingtonpost.com/health/2020/03/25/coronavirus-patients-do-not-resuscitate/

Chan, P. S. Berg, R. A., Nadkarni, V. M. (2020). Code blue during the COVID-19 pandemic. *Circulation: Cardiovascular Quality and Outcomes, 13*(5). https://doi.org/10.1161/CIRCOUTCOMES.120.006779

Chavez, R. (2021). *Surgery by day, bedpans at night: Staffing shortages in Louisiana hospitals mean some workers pull double duties.* PBS News Hour. https://www.pbs.org/newshour/health/surgery-by-day-bedpans-at-night-staffing-shortages-in-louisiana-hospitals-mean-some-workers-pull-double-duties

Davis, K. (2020). *Coronavirus latest: South Jersey nurse says she was fired from hospital for wearing own PPE.* CBS Philly. https://philadelphia. cbslocal.com/2020/04/17/coronavirus-latest-south-jersey-nurse-says-she-was-fired-from-hospital-for-wearing-own-ppe

Elsous, A., Radwan, M., & Mohsen, S. (2017). Nurses and physicians' attitudes toward nurse-physician collaboration: A survey from Gaza Strip, Palestine. *Nursing Research and Practice, 2017,* 7406278. https://doi.org/10.1155/2017/7406278

Firth, S. (2020). Told she can't wear her own mask, nurse walks off job. *MedPage Today.* https://www.medpagetoday.com/infectiousdisease/covid19/85760

Gaudine, A., LeFort, S. M., Lamb, M., & Thorne, L. (2011). Ethical conflicts with hospitals: The perspective of nurses and physicians. *Nursing Ethics, 18*(6), 756-766. doi: 10.1177/0969733011401121.

Griffith, J. (2020). *Nurses are protesting working conditions under coronavirus — and say hospitals aren't protecting them.* NBC News. https://www.nbcnews.com/news/us-news/nurses-are-protesting-working-conditions-under-coronavirus-say-hospitals-aren-n1181321

Grimaldi, M. E. (2007). Ethical decisions in times of disaster: choices healthcare workers must make. *Journal of Trauma Nursing, 14*(3): 163–164.

Hamilton, F., Arnold, D., Bzdek, B. R., Dodd, J., AERATOR group, Reid, J., & Maskell, N. (2021). Aerosol generating procedures: are they of relevance for transmission of SARS-CoV-2? *Lancet Respiratory Medicine, 9*(7), 687-689. doi: 10.1016/S2213-2600(21)00216-2

Jia, Y., Chen, O., Xiao, Z., Xiao, J., Bian, J., & Jia, H. (2021). Nurses' ethical challenges caring for people with COVID-19: A qualitative study. *Nursing Ethics, 28*(1), 33–45. https://doi.org/10.1177/0969733020944453

Klompas, M., Baker, M., & Rhee, C. (2021). What is an aerosol-generating procedure? *JAMA Surgery, 156*(2), 113-114. doi:10.1001/jamasurg. 2020.6643

Kroeger Mappes, E. J. (1989). Ethical dilemmas for nurses: Physicians' orders versus patients' rights. In J. Arras & N. Rhodes (Eds.), *Ethical issues in modern medicine* (pp. 110-117). Mayfield Publishing.

Lacy, A. (2020). Kaiser threatens to fire nurses treating COVID-19 patients for wearing their own masks, unions say. *The Intercept.* https://theintercept.com/2020/03/24/kaiser-permanente-nurses-coronavirus/

Lasater, K. B., Aiken, L. H., Sloane, D. M., French, R., Anusiewicz, C. V., Martin, B., Reneau, K., Alexander, M., & McHugh, M. D. (2021). Is hospital nurse staffing legislation in the public's interest?: An observational study in New York State. *Medical Care, 59*(5), 444–450. doi: 10.1097/MLR.0000000000001519

Mercer (2021). U.S. healthcare labor market. https://www.mercer.us/content/dam/mercer/assets/content-images/north-america/united-states/us-healthcare-news/us-2021-healthcare-labor-market-whitepaper.pdf

Mogul, F. (2020, December). *Battle-weary nurses wonder if New York hospitals can handle another coronavirus surge.* NPR. https://khn.org/news/nyc-hospital-workers-knowing-how-bad-it-can-get-brace-for-covid-2nd-wave/

Moyal-Smith, R., Sinyard, R. D., Goodwin, C., Henrich, N., Molina, G., & Haas, S. (2020). *New England Journal of Medicine.* doi: 10.1056/CAT.20.0570

NYSED. (2020). *COVID-19 pandemic and professional practice.* http://www.op.nysed.gov/COVID-19_EO.html

NYS Health Profiles. (n.d.) Hospitals by region/county and service. *New York State Department of Health.* https://profiles.health.ny.gov/hospital/county_or_region/region:new+york+metro+-+new+york+city

Panda, N., Sinyard, R. D., Henrich, N., Cauley, C. E., Hannenberg, A. A., Sonnay, Y., Bitton, A., Brindle, M., & Molina, G. (2021). Redeployment of health care workers in the COVID-19 pandemic: A qualitative study of health system leaders' strategies. *Journal of Patient Safety, 17*(4), 256–263. https://doi.org/10.1097/PTS.0000000000000847

Parrott, M. (2022). *Why isn't New York enforcing its staffing law?* New York Focus. https://www.nysfocus.com/2022/02/15/why-isnt-new-york-enforcing-its-nurse-staffing-law/

Patton, C. M. (2020). Caring for COVID-19 patients: Nurses' mental and emotional impact and management. *The Internet Journal of Healthcare Administration. 12*(1).

Patton, C. (2021). A phenomenological study of COVID-19's impact on US nursing personnel. *Workplace Health and Safety.* Sage. https://doi.org/10.1177/21650799211030294

Reamer, F. G. (2015). Eye on ethics. *Social Work Today.* https://www.socialworktoday.com/news/eoe_011515.shtml

Schuklenk, U. (2020). What healthcare professionals owe us: Why their duty to treat during a pandemic is contingent on personal protective equipment (PPE). *Journal of Medical Ethics, 46*, 432–435. doi:10.1136/medethics-2020-106278

Shaibu, S., Kimani, R. W., Shumba, C., Maina, R., Ndirangu, E., & Kambo, I. (2021). Duty versus distributive justice during the COVID-19 pandemic. *Nursing Ethics, 28*(6), 1073–1080. https://doi.org/10.1177/ 0969733021996038

Sharma, S. K., & Rani, R. (2020). Nurse-to-patient ratio and nurse staffing norms for hospitals in India: A critical analysis of national benchmarks. *Journal of Family Medicine and Primary Care, 9*(6), 2631–2637. https://doi.org/10.4103/jfmpc.jfmpc_248_20

Teriakidis, A., McNitt, J., McAllister, M., Sizemore, O., & Lindemann, P. (2021). *COVID-19 impact on nurse staffing and ICU beds.* Epic Research. https://epicresearch.org/articles/covid-19-impact-on-nurse-staffing-and-icu-beds

Voytko, L. (2020, April 1). Overwhelmed NYC hospitals reportedly implementing 'do not resuscitate' policies for coronavirus patients. *Forbes.* https://www.forbes.com/sites/lisettevoytko/2020/04/01/overwhelmed-nyc-hospitals-reportedly-implementing-do-not-resuscitate-policies-for-coronavirus-patients/?sh=6d9aa5733146

Wan, W. (2021). Burned out by the pandemic, 3 in 10 health-care workers consider leaving the profession. *The Washington Post.* https://www.washingtonpost.com/health/2021/04/22/health-workers-covid-quit/

Warren, M. S. (2020). *Here's why New Jersey and New York are the epicenter of the coronavirus pandemic. NJ.com.* https://www.nj.com/news/2020/03/heres-why-new-jersey-and-new-york-are-the-epicenter-of-the-coronavirus-pandemic.html

# EMERGENCY TIMES' KINDNESS IN COVID-19 TIMES

## The Community Action Network and Finding Ethical Languages

**Agnese Roda**[1]

**Abstract:** This case study considers conversations about COVID-19 pandemic support undertaken by members of Citizen Action Networks or CANs during the initial stages of lockdown in Cape Town, South Africa. I analyse the voices of volunteers and coordinators from two very different sides of the city providing assistance in the emergency. This illuminates how language and self- and social awareness in the time of pandemic emergency became significant elements for affecting social change. Cape Town is still shaped by spatial apartheid; 28 years after apartheid's end, Black people living in impoverished communities still struggle for recognition, access to basic rights and human dignity. In contrast, White people can choose to live disconnected from the pain of these communities or act to alleviate some of their hardship in an attempt to change the continuing historical narratives of race-based inequality and privilege. The conversations reveal the emergence of a new language of kindness during pandemic/emergency time based on citizen dialogue, space, community, and shared norms and values. The time of pandemic is seen to hold possibilities for people in vastly unequal social circumstances to create new ways to effect and sustain change via finding new ethical grammars and conditions for social collaboration and care.

Post-apartheid South Africa is one of the most unequal countries on the planet, with approximately 60% households dependent on social grants rather than earned income for a living. Strong patterns of racial and gender inequalities persist (StatsSA, 2015). This inequality, birthed by apartheid segregation laws, is still reflected in the social order and uneven access to rights in the city despite the end of legislated apartheid in 1994.

---

[1] Independent Social Anthropologist, University of Cape Town, South Africa

On 31 December 2019, the World Health Organization (WHO) reported a cluster of pneumonia cases in Wuhan City, China, confirming SARS-CoV-2 as the causative agent of the "Coronavirus Disease 2019" or COVID-19. National lockdown began in South Africa on 27 March 2020 while the infection rate was still low. All work and travel ceased, except for some essential activities. The lockdown was one of the most severe globally, and reinforced the inequalities experienced by the majority Black population, in particular Black Africans, the most disenfranchised group under apartheid. Working class and poor Black households suffered major loss of income and ability to access food. Within two weeks communities began experiencing extreme hunger which lasted for at least five months until lockdown restriction eased.

Foreseeing this scenario, Community Action Networks (CANs) were established by citizens on 23 March 2020 to operate as compensational providers of necessary items to poor communities. Food, PPE, sanitation support such as water, cooking fuel and data, amongst others, were distributed to households in Black townships, the homeless, non-locals/foreign nationals from the continent and other vulnerable groups such as the elderly and those living with disabilities. Civil society successfully lobbied government to address food access via allocation of a special COVID-19 relief grant for those impacted. However, corruption and government mismanagement still saw many vulnerable people falling through the gaps.

The CANs self-organized localized assistance networks for the vulnerable. CAN networks formed rapidly around the city with no specific structure. The historically apartheid shaped city produced the dynamic of wealthy and impoverished neighbourhoods pairing up to undertake such assistance. This strategy for providing social assistance via the CANs quickly took root during the initial stages of lockdown. Both CAN organizers and recipients appeared keenly aware that more than twenty years post–apartheid, segregated and racialized realities would need to be negotiated between communities on different sides of the city.

Once established, the CANs began collaborating with existing structures such as NGOs, community activists and citizen volunteers. They organised locally and digitally, using social media platforms such as WhatsApp and

Facebook. Dialogues began about where to access resources and how to improve the logistics of assistance such as organizing soup kitchens and delivering blankets, food, PPE, and basic toiletries as well as connecting people to data and airtime for communication beyond their homes. CAN volunteers and community activists began to engage about reworking or dispensing with ideas about charity, turning co-dependency into sustainability and locating volunteer efforts more visibly as social justice activism by directly confronting their respective positionalities.

Thus emerged an engaged ethical and moral dialogue about kindness, giving and receiving among individuals and communities involved in the Cape Town CANs. It enabled reflection on the extent of the "emergency" in the current system, that is, acknowledging past and continued social failures on both sides of the city. Those new to "community emergency" work became more aware of the existence of a grossly unequal globalized world in which the majority of people are abandoned to deal with life at the margins. The issue of governmental corruption and mishandling of grants, the pandemic and support for vulnerable communities became urgent foci and goal to tackle for both sides.

Focus on kindness helped to create a new behavioral lens and ethics relating to social assistance. Questions emerged about what previous help initiatives undertaken as charity and philanthropy failed to take into account. For example, on the receiving side of assistance, the dynamics of giving were interrogated, with "White saviour" behavior in receiving communities criticized as enhancing division and a dependency system. The persistent divide between classes and races prompted the challenging of ideas about help and assistance based on the Western notion of charity. Failure of social justice and difficulty accessing fundamental rights for the majority, highlighted by the COVID-19 emergency, dispelled once and for all the myth of a rainbow nation constitution in which all are equal, and reinforced ideas about a new struggle for equality.

The CAN partnership between Sea Point, a wealthy White neighbourhood on the Atlantic seaboard, and Gugulethu, a Black township on the city outskirts, is instructive as a case study. Apartheid Segregation laws from 1948 to 1994 shaped Cape Town into a geography of racial classification with the key aim of socio-spatial control (Christopher, 2000). Post-apartheid, most neighbourhoods have experienced very little change. Sea Point remains predominantly mute about confronting its past and is a cultural-racial exemplar of Cape Town as a "city of exclusions" (Lemanski, 2004). Teppo (2009, p. 367) describes Sea Point as a "space of White behaviour", a proper behaviour, where "loudness is frowned upon, and White aesthetic ideals are presented in every shop window." This language of architectural and social division based on race has severe repercussions on community identity and formation, especially Black communities at the city's margins.

The conversations about assistance among members in the CAN network created a platform for reconsidering and reshaping narratives about identity in some communities. To me, kindness is a useful concept to understand the language in these conversations in order to ascertain and understand ethical shifts of awareness in words and actions in vastly unequal communities spotlighted by the pandemic. Ethics usually speaks to a broad morality rooted in religion, upbringing, and privilege. However, in ethics, there is seldom only one way or right or wrong; instead, it is possible that differences can prompt reconsideration to shape a new, ethical language and collaboration for a common good in a vastly unequal space.

The pandemic time was a very particular moment for reconsidering philanthropic and care acts performed by individuals involved in the Seaboard and Gugulethu CANs. The assistance helped to fill gaps of unawareness with new knowledge and challenge assumptions held by these vastly different communities in the city space. The break produced by the halting of usual activities during the lockdown prompted reimagining, challenging and attempting transforming of charity actions into a new social way of uniting and relating in communities. Here, the receivers of assistance/care and ability to give back and sustain efforts became important.

For example, donations were often replaced by skills building, with Sea Point CAN members assisting Gugulethu CAN members to identify and develop their talents to break dependency on donations. This enabled the Gugulethu CAN members to design and expand a future vision for their community amongst themselves. The township community confronted its own identity and power in its undertaking of community help actions and systems of care as well as challenging exclusions and urban life dynamics.

Castaneda (2006) defines ethics as performance in society of rules and behaviors as well as its use as a reflective tool to understand the politics behind actions. In care relationships, related political, economic and moral dimensions intersect with one another (Mc Kearney & Armith, 2021). Kindness is a behaviour marked by ethical characteristics, concern for and consideration of others. Kindness is an embodiment of compassion and care in relation to our behaviour in society. But in an emergency situation, what does kindness reflect about ethics, about the way we relate to each other? Does kindness lead us to reflexivity? If so, how does reflexivity unfold in the present moment and in comparison to marginalization in our historical past?

My questions about kindness are theoretically situated at the threshold of Anthropology studies on affect and ethics that connect our ordinary, private actions and beliefs to our social actions when we perform our habitual practices. Our feelings, beliefs and ideas reverberate at the intersection of the actions we perform in society as well as their repercussions. Sentiment and intimacies in our daily life can tell us a lot about the social realm, mirrored through us (Ahmed, 2004; Massumi, 2015). By abstracting affect, we attempt to find a bridge between ourselves and the cultural and political systems in which our lives are embedded. Understanding the language emerging through our actions is thus critical, as is understanding that our actions and language are connected with the morality structure from which they emerge or that they want to affect (Das, 2012). These processes significantly informed interactions between members of the Sea Point and Gugulethu CANs, which I explore in this study.

The motto of the Seaboard CAN is: "Our response is not to wait, but to do what we can." Its members, from suburbs of the "Atlantic Seaboard"--Sea Point, Green Point, and Mouille Point--form a network of individuals with different expertise and work backgrounds. The CAN constitutes in a 130 member WhatsApp group, and is part of the larger Cape Town Together movement of 13.000 Capetonians self-organized into 150 autonomous CANs. I joined the Seaboard CAN a few days after lockdown began, and my activities there mainly comprised participating via social media to organize food assistance in the city through WhatsApp and Facebook.

This was where I first met one of the group coordinators, Lisa (pseudonym), whom I interviewed via Zoom after having met her once in person to introduce her to my research project. The story Lisa told me about starting the Sea Point CAN has to do with vulnerability and being practical about it. Lisa shared her definition of kindness with me: "The more people have been taken away from you, the more you can understand what it means to give. That, I think, is kindness." After many years of involvement in social justice circles in South Africa, Lisa had pulled the strings and connected the dots of a big circle of contacts to form a support structure--a network of assistance called the Seaboard CAN.

Despite her attempt to offer people the opportunity to get involved during the COVID-19 emergency, Lisa was angry at the reactionary behaviour of some community members towards the homeless in the Seaboard area. In May 2020, a car belonging to neighbours assisting homeless people with food was set on fire one night, a clear warning to those assisting the homeless. The violence horrified CAN members but only reinforced Lisa's need to take action.

Lisa identifies responsibility and reflexivity about personal pain against collective pain as critical in volunteer work. She sees the potential of personal pain to transform into concern and care for others and a collective good: "I think it is a choice… For me it is all about them …the homeless people. The ... group against them … [h]ow can these people think they can do that?"

The Pentecostal Church in Sea Point and the CAN run a soup kitchen, with morning preaching as mainly homeless people line up on the pavements to be fed, which some residents resent. For Lisa, it is important to look at why people object to this: "I really blame the government for why people are against each other." But Lisa also finds people's ethics challenging, which in this context is recognizing the historical privileging of Whites, their sense of entitlement and focus only on personal responsibility as well as the country's long history of racialisation. According to Lisa, "The way that Whiteness works here in this country is that we are extremely well resourced and connected... I might not have loads of money, but I have been to universities, I have friends overseas, I have travelled overseas. I have access to a network that people in the township do not have. And that is social capital and very powerful with loads of money in the end, and potential."

In my understanding, social capital is the effective functioning of social groups through interpersonal relationships, a shared sense of identity and of norms and values as well as mutual trust, cooperation and reciprocity. In the case of Sea Point, the White minority retains many resources that the Black majority lacks. Opposition to the CAN's assisting the homeless reflects the lack of engagement of a section of the community not only with the idea of social capital but also the stories and needs of homeless people living in the community. They thus fail to recognize the notion of social responsibility and the political and historical dynamics of the space in which they live.

Lisa explained: "A friend of mine challenged me the other day. What point has doing things based on guilt? she asked. I do not think it is about guilt. I think it is about... a sense of responsibility to others and that needs to be coupled with kindness... ." Lisa recognizes the possibility for engagement with a new alphabet of potential focused on reconsidering the narrative of inherited history. Stewart (2007) observes responsibility of emotions geared towards public and intimate feelings as offering possibilities for change. In the above conversation, the feelings of guilt and responsibility provide possibilities to shift towards influencing the affective dimensions of daily life in order to form a new norm and new ethical ground. The new ground is not only composed of words and actions but also objects--the soup bowl, a warm blanket, a new document obtained, a seed planted. These objects transform assistance into a space of new dignity for ourselves and others as a collective (Berlant, 2000).

Lisa explains how her positionality leads to a specific type of affective self-making: "Certainly a person like me [is] privileged and Black people [are] oppressed and that makes me feel particularly responsible for what happens in this country and a huge need to give back." Here, the idea of Black and White as stereotypes translates as stereotypes of the self, affecting ethics. I observed palpable feelings of personal discomfort when speaking to White CAN members about White culture; there is always sharing of feelings about self. They express particular discomfort at differences in people's access to society as a result of capitalism and racism. Hence the CAN members' need to offer assistance is based not only money but sharing of emotional support and participation.

Working with discomfort induces people to reach out to diverse peoples and intellectual traditions in an attempt to understand how to fill the gaps (Salo, 2013). Thus lockdown presented a possible way out of predetermined narratives, compelling historically privileged people to consider the idea of collective good, in the process offering White communities the possibility of becoming more inclusive. It also gave Whites an opportunity to become more visible to Black people as engaging in privilege reconsideration.

Another activist in a psycho-social support group from a Muslim background, I spoke with offered another view. She stressed that assisting Black people is not only about working with but empowering communities by rejecting Western colonial, racist and capitalist ideas about charity, monetary donations and volunteerism. She observed: "Communities in a non-Judeo-Christian environment are raised to consider others, no matter what. For instance, when you cook dinner, you will cook a bit more, to give to others. No matter what you get back from it. You just know that whenever there is enough for you, there is enough for others." She observed that unless those in privileged spaces understand this intrinsic system of assistance as gifting undertaken within poor communities and work within that dynamic, they will fail to understand and respect the power and agency of their volunteer counterparts there. This closes the space for equal partnering and relationships of true care and kindness in the giver-recipient exchange.

In response to the above, a White Jewish Seaboard CAN member stated: "About money and the narrative of we have enough to feed… South African society is the way it is, because of centuries of… explicit dispossession. For a community to have enough to care for themselves but be cut out and for us to sit here in Sea Point and the main concern during lockdown – it was that we could not have champagne... I do not think it is fair! Those people with so many limited resources are expected to solve their own problems or do everything for themselves, while others have been let off the hook... at the end of the day, you… need shelter, food and healthcare. Sure you could survive, but what does that survival look like? I am not saying it is impossible, but maybe it is something we have not found our way through."

Here, the words are not nearly enough in the conversation; they reveal an unspoken problem and question. The language of both sides possess infinite forms and registers with potential to reveal the complex and uncertain terrain of shifting the word and its meaning from the past to a new present. But the problem is they appear still as parallel rather than intersecting languages. The question then is: What is still needed to effect intersections in which emerge the mutual needs of each side for reconsidered identity and position in relationships of assistance/care? Lisa concluded our Zoom with a wish for a new way that embraces ongoing thinking about new forms of living that can include everyone's differences, be performed socially, and resonate collectively in everyone's lives. She repeated that kindness finds a space to flourish in vulnerability, in the opening up of the wounds of the past, in trying to find ways to heal and change despite such limits as government inaction, "politics", and regular lack of funds in assistance/care work.

Lisa's story in Sea Point intersects with the Seaboard CAN's area of assistance that is far from the White coastal neighbourhoods and located at the city's margins. Gugulethu, a historically Black African township, is approximately 20 km from Sea Point. The township, its name in isiXhosa means "Our Pride" was established in the 1960s after the Group Areas Act (1950) which dispossessed Black people of land and segregated the areas in which the different races lived and conducted their social and economic activities. Thus Black African, coloured, and Indian people from areas inside the city were relocated to new suburbs, often far from their places of work. Gugulethu was established to accommodate migrant workers from the rural Eastern Cape.

The young woman Belinda, who runs the Gugulethu CAN shared she started it with skills gained from volunteering for an NGO at the beginning of lockdown. The government failing her community, she, with the help of her family, began assisting the vulnerable, the elderly, women and children in partnership with the Seaboard CAN. She tells me over the phone: "I recently lost my brother, so my family and I needed some way to give back and do something that matters because life is short and we need to do something. We thought about what people need the most. Food. Without food in your stomach, there is nothing people are going to obey."

Access to food is difficult in many poor Black communities, even before COVID-19, and needed urgent tackling during lockdown. The first place I visited in Gugulethu was the CAN's soup kitchen. Well organised, it served a disciplined group of people, mainly children. The closure of schools during lockdown meant many learners lost their only solid meal for the day, provided by the public education system. A group of volunteers assisted with food preparation. The woman who cooked the food shared she finds strength in God to serve the community and that her food is delicious, which the community appreciates. Her eyes shine when she tells me she has realized a dream: "Before the CAN started, I was a volunteer and unemployed [working] in an organisation called OFW, which means organising for work…helping unemployed people. As I [am] also unemployed I tend to volunteer a lot as I think if I am not getting experience, I will not have skills. When the lockdown came I found myself …unemployed, with no source of income and the government was telling me to lock myself inside the house and not go anywhere. So when I heard about Cape Town Together, I said to myself this [is] the opportunity to help my community."

On both sides of the network, the presence of women is remarkable, yet there are differences between them. White women from Sea Point could choose to be volunteers; the Black women from Gugulethu had no real choice other than to undertake the care work at the battle front of exclusion the majority of the population experiences. Gender representation post-apartheid is still below the 50% mark for women in influential roles, with women more likely than men to be involved in unpaid work (Gini coefficient, 2011). Amy Nelson (2020) estimates of approximately 13.000 members on the CAN's Facebook page, 72% are women, 24% men and 4% unspecified. This clearly shows women constitute the main workforce in assistance/care work; yet Black women undertaking this work experience some of the greatest vulnerability in the extremely unequal post-apartheid society that is specifically designed for their exclusion.

The Gugulethu-Seaboard CANs' partnership is based on interdependence. Without each other, they would struggle to exist, but together they make a difference in people's lives. What makes them work well together is a common language with the main aim to serve the community. They also trust each other by working collaboratively to identify needs and growth possibilities via a chat group and regular administrative meetings to advance their work and goals. They share good practices; giving and receiving occur via support of and listening to the community's needs and sharing skills. Thus assistance is not just about providing funds for the community's basic needs. The chat also acts as a sort of emotional support structure for sharing photos of the community receiving goods, distributing vouchers, sending letters to the media about their care work and personal views about the CAN collaboration.

These are examples of collaborative behaviour negotiated through work involving virtue ethics and a common intention. "Central to this ethic is the set of dispositions to behave systematically in one way rather than the other, in order for someone to lead a particular kind of life" (MacIntyre, 2007, p. 38). Such norms help at the collaborative level, the most important of which is what Merritt (2000, p. 374) calls "the sustaining social contribution to the character", that is, in particularly challenging social relationships and settings. Thus, even individuals not wholly endowed with 'internal' stability are supported by consistent 'external' frames of reference such as etiquette or routines. In the case of the Gugulethu-Seaboard CANs partnership, collaborative language speaks consistently of a shared set of norms.

In April 2020 the Gugulethu CAN launched their own project, community gardening in people's backyards and establishing a large soup kitchen. "I realized that CAN thing, I thought WOW, this is an opportunity," one of Gugulethu's oldest farmers shared. The community united to create a Green Gugulethu to sustain itself, its practice of assistance and its CAN to benefit everyone via a common goal and permaculture teaching and practices.

The above initiatives and conversations show two critical things emerging from assistance collaborations during the COVID-19 pandemic. One is the realisation that some narratives about collaboration can be challenged in urban and community spaces. Another is different sides of the city uniting during an emergency to create a common good for the community. Via saving schemes and soup kitchens, the emergency moment was transcended, leading to better understanding about access to rights and working as a collective to find new ways to care.

The emergency moment enabled new dynamics to take shape. For one side, this became a time for reflection and reconsideration due to the lockdown silence and break from normal life routines. Volunteers and coordinators tackled local narratives of daily living by working together to understand the daily struggles of those still disenfranchised, by participating in community life outside their neighbourhoods, and assisting marginalized communities to engage in restructuring their internal collaboration efforts for greater sustainability to claim their rights. For the other side, the emergency time accelerated decision making, focused on new organisational systems and more efficient ways to organize socially to serve and provide the community and its needs, all crucially informed by its own members and not outsiders. These disrupted previous and pre-conceived charity and philanthropy notions that even if well-meant maintain a disconnection and separation between communities made unequal by historical legacies. This process was enabled by and operated primarily around a new language and its performativity in actions.

Kindness is seen to have transformed into a shared concept that enabled the givers to listen to the receivers and the receivers to give back in their own way care work from within their own community. These relationships went beyond apartheid stereotypes and pre-pandemic city dynamics. Kindness became the main parameter in collaboration to sustain lives. In this way, during the time of emergency, a new ontology of ethics emerged and began to take shape in the city of Cape Town.

## References

Ahmed, S. (2004). Affective economies. *Social Text, 22*(2), 117–139. https://doi.org/10.1215/01642472-22-2_79-117

Berlant, L. (2007). Cruel optimism: On Marx, loss and the senses. *New Formations, 63*, 33-51.

Castañeda, Q. E. (2006). Ethnography in the forest: An analysis of ethics in the morals of anthropology. *Cultural Anthropology, 21*(1), 121-145.

Christopher, A. J. (2002). *Atlas of changing South Africa*. Routledge.

Das, V. (2015). What does ordinary ethics look like? In G. deCol (Ed.), *Four lectures on ethics. Anthropological Perspectives* (pp. 53-125). Hau Books.

*Gini coefficient on South Africa inequality*. (2011). World Bank Atlas 2011. The World Bank.

Lemanski, C. (2004). A new apartheid? The spatial implications of fear of crime in Cape Town, South Africa. *Environment and Urbanization, 16*(2), 101-112.

MacIntyre, A. C. (2007). *After virtue* (3rd ed.). University of Notre Dame Press.

Massumi, B. (2015). *Politics of affect*. John Wiley & Sons.

McKearney, P., & Amrith, M. (2021). *Care. Cambridge Encyclopedia of Anthropology*. https://www.anthroencyclopedia.com/entry/care

Merritt, M. (2000). Virtue ethics and situationist personality psychology. *Ethical theory and moral practice, 3*(4), 365-383.

Nelson, A. (2020). In the communities, the SA Covid-19 ground response is mostly female. *The Daily Maverick*. https://www.dailymaverick.co.za/opinionista/2020-05-21-in-the-communities-the-sa-covid-19-ground-response-is-mostly-female/

Salo, E. (2013). *Lessons in race and African feminism*. Independent Online. https://www.iol.co.za/sundayindependent/lessons-in-race-and-african-feminism-1574641

Stats SA. (2015). Statistics South Africa. https://www.statssa.gov.za/

Stewart, K. (2007). *Ordinary affects*. Duke University Press.

Teppo, A. (2009). My house is protected by a dragon: White South Africans, magic and sacred spaces in post-Apartheid Cape Town. Suomen Antropologi.

# COVID-19 AND THE FRAIL RIGHTS OF THE 'ORDINARY MAN' IN NIGERIA

**O. Sherina Okoye**[1]

**Abstract:** This chapter will consider the implications of COVID-19 from inception to the 'post-lockdown' era, from a legal standpoint vis-a-vis its effect on the common man particularly in Nigeria. In Nigeria, it has long been established that sometimes laws are observed in breach and the rights of the indigent are sometimes trampled upon with impunity by persons in authority or persons with access to those in authority. This article will explore and attempt to depict the lasting effects of this global epidemic on the already poorly-protected rights of the average Nigerian. Has it improved or worsened the narrative? Can government actors and stakeholders find middle ground against a common enemy? Will the ordinary man remain the grass that suffers in this battle or is there more the justice system of this developing nation can do to help stem the worst of the tide? This work will attempt to bring to the fore, the unheard voices of citizens.

## Introduction

Nigeria watched in stark horror and helpless fascination as COVID-19 cut a morbid swath through the rest of the world in late 2019. Finally, it majestically rested its unwelcome oars on the shores of Nigeria in the first few weeks of 2020.

Prior to the invasion by COVID-19, there were already frissons of alarm about the potential catastrophe the notorious virus could unleash on a country with a burgeoning population crisis and a scant ability to contain it. Melinda Gates led the way with a 'crystal-ball' prediction that dead bodies would be littered all over the streets of Africa from COVID-19 (Nwachukwu, 2020).

[1] Executive Director, African Kids and Women Rights Empowerment Initiative

In a country that still vividly remembers its unique Ebola scare of the year 2014, and how it barely escaped mass depopulation, those words were like the proverbial death knell, fuelling internal fears, tension, and worries. In homes and on street corners, Nigerians could be seen murmuring about the virus and exchanging worried looks. In offices, and in large organizations, the use of masks was already being insisted upon even though the official figures were still minimal at the time.

As soon as COVID-19 began to gain ground, Nigeria joined the rest of the world in adopting full lockdown measures on March 30, 2020 (Eagle Online, 2020) and therein began the woes of the common man in the territory.

## COVID-19 in Full Bloom: The Nigerian Narrative

### The effect of the pandemic on abuse by security operatives, crimes and impunity, discrimination

Halima Sambo[2], a small road-side shop owner in Gwagwalada, Abuja-Nigeria, locked up her shop on the first night of the ordered lockdown and returned a scant few weeks later to a wide-open shop with its doors standing on drunken hinges. Halima had at first frozen in disbelief, convinced she was seeing things. But then a wail from a similarly-affected neighbor jerked her back to awareness of reality. The shop *had* been broken into and looted! It wasn't just a bad dream. She had stocked the space full of beverages, bread, and the usual everyday household requirements her customers required. Every food item was gone, leaving in its place just a few brooms and buckets and notebooks (H. Sambo, Personal Communication, January 15, 2022).

Mercy Friday[3], another small shop owner had an even more disastrous tale. Whoever had broken into her shop had not been satisfied with just looting what they could carry. They had also helped themselves to the items a friend had stored in her shop and had also emptied packs of sachet water all over the floor of the shop, effectively damaging what was left. Then they

---

[2] Halima was personally interviewed by the writer at the time of researching this article; but the name used herein is an alias.

[3] Mercy was personally interviewed by the writer at the time of researching this article; but the name used herein is an alias.

had gone ahead with acts of vandalism gouging holes in the walls and breaking windows and ceilings (M. Friday, Personal Communication, December 15, 2021).

Security agents killed and maimed several innocent Nigerians in a bid to enforce the lockdown, adopting excessive force with impunity and drawing international attention (Azu, 2020). In the first few weeks of lockdown, one of the several victims was a medical doctor who was accosted on his way to work. His protestations that he was essential personnel fell on deaf ears and his hands were irreversibly damaged in the scuffle that followed— he was a surgeon (B. Abraham, Personal Communications, June 12, 2020).

Nigerian women were also specially victimized during the pandemic. The lockdown saw an astronomical increase in an already boggling and disheartening volume of sexual abuse cases and domestic violence cases (Umokoro, 2020). One woman, Halima Bulama, actually had her hand hacked off by her husband during the lockdown thus emphasizing the fact that most victims were now on lockdown with their abusers (Umokoro).

When persons who had taken ill (even post lockdown), were diagnosed with any semblance of a cough, they were confined in Holding Areas in hospitals against their will, to check if they had the virus. No one cared about their rights to liberty. We were after the 'greater good' and it did not seem to matter if non-infected persons could effectively get the virus from infected persons in the Holding Area since everyone was lumped together while the test results were being awaited (personal experience). Interestingly, when you tried to buy drugs for those persons in the hospital and mentioned that your relation was in the "Holding Area," you were immediately given a wide berth by the hospital staff, met with stiff silence, and treated as if you had the very plague. Sometimes patients' relations had to practically *beg* to get doctors to come check on their relations in such Holding Areas. It didn't matter what the Constitution said; discrimination was pretty much par for the course during and after COVID-19 in Nigeria (personal experience).

Through all of this, COVID-19 served to emphasize social stratification with most of the human rights abuses being meted out to the common man on the streets of Nigeria.

## The effect of the pandemic on the pace of justice delivery and access to courts by the common man

Pre-COVID, the Nigerian justice sector was already bedeviled by persistent delay in the dispensation of justice hence resulting in crippling clogs in the already-wobbly wheels of justice. These delays were due to the deluge of cases relative to the small number of judges; infrastructural inadequacies like lack of constant electricity to enable the court staff carry out their duties; judges being relegated to ancient practices of long-hand jotting during sessions rather than use of court stenographers and of course, budgetary shortcomings.

Several experts have long decried the Nigerian tradition of delayed litigation. In the now famous words of the Vice-President of Nigeria, Prof. Yemi Osinbanjo SAN, the problem of the common man in Nigeria now "is not access to justice but *exit* from justice" (NBA Pushes Justice, 2022, sec. 7).

Extra-judicial killings were common in Nigeria even before COVID-19, with several tales of killing with impunity dating as far back as Nigeria's early post-independence days and running into thousands of lives lost (Ejikwonyilo, 2021). These killings were often committed by government actors and even ordinary citizens for all manner of reasons; some of them trivial in the extreme. The message was received long ago that in the wrong situation, the difference between life and death could be one misplaced mob action or an accidental discharge from a trigger-happy fellow in uniform.

During the initial stage of the pandemic, CLEEN Foundation[4] reported a total of at least 23 documented incidents of extra-judicial killing in enforcement of the lockdown (Eagle Online, 2020). But what was more worrisome was that almost none of those cases showed a conclusive crime and punishment ending. Of course, the courts were shut down too and the security agencies who should have protected the common man were the culprits.

---

[4] CLEEN Foundation (formerly known as Centre for Law Enforcement Education) is a non-governmental organization with a bias for access to justice and justice sector reforms.

The banking sector was sadly not left out of the quagmire. There was an increase in internet fraud with some people receiving alarming bank alerts indicating that their monies had been swiped. This fact was corroborated by Nigeria's Director of Corporate Communications in the Central Bank, Isaac Okoroafor (Agbedo, 2021) Even when the lockdown was partially lifted, there were massive hordes in front of the various banks, due to the efforts to prevent over-crowding in the banking halls. This meant that the victims of internet fraud could scarcely access their bankers in good time to make reports and try to stem the theft of their hard-earned resources. Nor could they access the courts either, due to the same virus.

After the lockdown, the number of cases in courts increased astronomically, with the Country's Chief Justice admitting that the virus and the subsequent nationwide strike by the Judiciary Staff Union of Nigeria (JUSUN) had served the country's justice sector with its worst crises yet, in recent history (Ejekwonyilo, 2022). As a result, the access of citizens to justice were further hampered with people being forced to wait in long queues outside in the sweltering heat. Some cases were for enforcement of contracts frustrated by the lockdown, some were for recovery of premises from defaulting tenants. But there were very few cases indeed for enforcement of fundamental human rights breached during the lockdown. It would seem that the concept of breach of rights during the lockdown had been largely swept under the carpet.

## The effect of the pandemic on finances of the poor

When the pandemic officially hit Nigeria in March 2020, like the rest of the world, the entire country went on lockdown. However, due to the economic realities and prevailing hardship, as well as the relatively lesser impact of the disease in terms of lesser spread of contagion in the tropics, the lockdown was partially lifted in May 2020. Within the span of less than three months, many had lost their businesses, their homes, and some even their loved ones (Omogbolagun, 2020).

Several people were rendered homeless, several had to return to rural areas, and several others lost their jobs as businesses went under after the pandemic. Of course, most small and medium enterprises in Nigeria as well as a couple of banks and larger companies adopted the no-work-no-pay approach and stopped paying salaries entirely during the pandemic (Adigin et al., 2020).

Like the rest of the world, many educated Nigerians converged on the internet scene in 2020 seeking remote work. However, their chances were hampered in some instances because several high-paying remote jobs require PayPal as means of payment whereas, PayPal still does not allow Nigerians receive payments on their platform. Although recent reports in 2021 indicate that a new partnership has emerged between Flutterwave and PayPal to allow Nigerian businesses (but not Nigerian individuals) receive money on PayPal (Paul, 2021).

As at 2020, only 49.14% of the Nigerian population had access to the internet (Statista, n.d.). The concept of remote work or indeed any form of work at all, was thus inaccessible to more than 50% of the population. In several localities, many families could be seen selling off their cars, their lands, and in some cases even their clothes to try to have money for feeding. The rate of local begging increased as some families in desperation went door to door seeking assistance with feeding.

In a bid to stem the rising hunger, palliatives began to come into the country some by foreign donors and some from wealthy Nigerians. But rather than disperse them among the poor and needy, the food items were mostly stored in warehouses while cash palliatives were dispersed in a way that remains largely a mystery as to how the "beneficiaries" were chosen. As hunger and frustration increased, Nigerians began to raid those warehouses where the palliative items were stored in a show of self-help (Orjinmo, 2020). Some of the palliative food items were found in the homes of politicians and some in government warehouses (Orjinmo, 2020). The looters were uncontrollable and violent, and their actions resulted in several stampedes that left many people dead.

## The Fallout Between Vaccines and Human Rights

In trying to stem the virus, Nigeria joined the rest of the world in insisting on vaccination of its citizens. The vaccines were largely inaccessible to common citizens at government facilities forcing people to try to get them from private hospitals (Okunola, 2021). In Nigeria, government hospitals are state-owned and run by the government whereas private hospitals are often owned and run by individuals, groups of persons, or even non-profit organizations. However, the masses often prefer to visit government hospitals because of the over 300% price difference in addition to which the government hospitals tend to have more doctors and nurses on staff as well as better experienced consultants. In private hospitals, the astronomical cost of the vaccine in a country where most people live on less than a dollar a day is laughable. The Nigerian current minimum wage is N30,000 per month, (approximately $53 USD) and so much of the population earns far *less* than that minimum wage. Whereas the COVID-19 vaccine was being administered in some private centers for as much as N50,000 (approximately $89.3) per dose. The cost sent a clear signal that the vaccine was for the elite and thus enforced social stratification and discrimination even more.

Assuming, but without conceding, that the vaccines were the only guarantee of surviving the virus, would preventing access to the vaccines not amount to an attempted violation of the right to life?

In Nigeria, the vaccines met with stiff resistance and suspicion, especially since the bulk of the populace seemed to be "just fine" without it. And most of those who wanted it, could not access or afford it.

In a survey of 440 persons in Ibadan-Nigeria, 359 persons expressed an unwillingness to take the vaccines due to the cost (Ilesanmi et al., 2021).

Chapter IV of the 1999 Constitution of Nigeria insists that the citizens are, amongst other things, entitled to freedom of thought, conscience, private and family life. However, the Nigerian government shocked everyone post-COVID when it passed what could only be termed a "decree" that all civil servants were expected to be vaccinated and to present their vaccine cards before being allowed into their work premises (Owolabi, 2021). The requirement was later relaxed but the harm had already been done; a clear message had already been passed that in this battle against COVID-19, the common man was the grass to be trampled upon.

Sadly, the government was not alone in its draconian tactics. Some workers in private sector and non-governmental organizations in the country have reported being forced to take the vaccines at the threat of losing their jobs (Ekwowusi, 2022). Sadly, this development met with approval in some quarters (Odiegwu 2022)

In the Nigerian case of ***Medical and Dental Practitioners Disciplinary Tribunal v Dr. John Emewulu Nicholas Okonkwo***[5] their Lordships of the Supreme Court held conclusively that the failure to extract a patient's informed consent before administering a blood transfusion on him constituted an infraction of his fundamental human rights to privacy (section 37) and right to freedom of religion and conscience (section 38). It further held that the right to object to any form of medical treatment is constitutionally protected by the mentioned sections.

Global experts have incessantly lent their voices to the cry for mass vaccination as a prerequisite to stem the tide of the virus. But the question continued to be whether the vaccines were indeed helpful in stemming the tide especially since some reports indicated that some persons who were vaccinated still fell casualty to the virus like the late Chief Ladi Williams SAN (Ojerinde, 2021). Local suspicion towards the vaccine remained very high.

The suspicion and distrust of the vaccine and the motivations behind it, was further worsened when newspaper headlines asserted that Prof. Mojisola Adeyeye, Director-General of the National Agency for Food and Drug Administration and Control (NAFDAC) had indicated that Nigerians would *"no longer"* take expired vaccines (NAN, 2021). The common man took that to mean that many Nigerians had been jabbed with expired vaccines already and even though there were strenuous denials by the incumbent government, the jury's still out on that in the eyes of average Nigerians.

## Conclusion

In the wake of the pandemic, the world has been as one coming out of a slumber to witness the explosion of change around it. Most communities

---

[5] LOR (2/3/2001) SC

seem to only just be coming to a full realization of the extent of the damage that humans wrought on each other using the pandemic as an excuse. In the words of the Secretary General of the UN, Antonio Guterres (2021), "One year on, another stark fact is tragically evident: our world is facing a pandemic of human rights abuses."

It is easy to see that most of the reactions trailing the scourge of the virus were borne out of fear; and understandably so. But if global experts are to be believed, COVID-19 may not be the last pandemic the world will ever see (Are, 2021). Perhaps we can all collectively return to the drawing board; reassess and standardize towards a uniform approach in the event of crisis such as this in the future. Perhaps then, such incidences of gross violations would be minimized if not totally stemmed.

International treaties *simpliciter* may not be very effective. In war-torn nations, there have been post-war trials for war crimes which has effectively served as a measure of deterrence. A global or even national consensus on institution of post-pandemic trials for gross acts of human rights violations during pandemics should be as a matter of course. Governments must be more dogged about data collection and follow through with appropriate punitive actions especially for government actors who violate human rights during health crises.

COVID-19 drives home the need to install an absolute and unbending respect for the Rule of Law rather than subjecting it to the whims and caprices of those in power. If human rights are truly recognized for what they are, vaccines would not be forced on persons who are unwilling to take them especially when available evidence suggests that those vaccines, while perhaps helpful, are not necessarily a guarantee for the vaccinated.

Nations, especially those in the developing world, must be encouraged to strengthen their mode of emergency response, which includes coordination, surveillance and epidemiology, case management, lab facilities, points of entry (PoE), infection prevention and control (IPC), risk communication, logistics, and research and even contact tracing and surveillance. The Nigerian narrative saw a backlash of citizens blaming the government for not doing enough, and government not catering to the basic needs of citizens whilst accusing the citizens of not cooperating enough. The end result was an unwieldy dance, with everyone effectively burying their heads and waiting for the scourge to pass.

It is trite that global action on strengthening response to such crisis is important as COVID-19 drives home the fact that we are all connected and a health crisis in a little town in China could literally affect the entire world.

The trust of citizens is very important in any crisis, and it is apparent that when state actors resort to *ultra vires* modes of law enforcement like bullying or beating up citizens, then that trust would be next to impossible. Many may never recover from the injuries the pandemic brought into their lives and it is hypocritical indeed for any responsible government to expect loyalty when it reacts unpredictably in times of crisis.

Governments at all levels must entrench accountability and basic compassion in dispensing their duties. They must also learn to work *with* the people in the face of a pandemic rather than adopting a divergent approach that seems to create an "us-against-them" scenario in the minds of the citizens.

No Government can effectively govern if it has the mandate alone without the trust and confidence of the people.

Global action towards pandemics must be expressly defined and respected with a clear understanding that fundamental human rights are inalienable; and even when exceptions exist, such exceptions must be clearly within the ambit of exceptions recognized by law.

## References

Adigun, O., Oyesole, B., Agbota, S., & Obiernyi, C. (2020, May 18). COVID-19: Bleak future for workers as employers cut jobs, salaries - experts urge FG to restart economy with stimulus. *The SUN*. https://www.sunnewsonline.com/covid-19-bleak-future-for-workers-as-employers-cut-jobs-salaries-experts-urge-fg-to-restart-economy-with-stimulus/

Agbedo, O. (2021, September 4). How banks are grappling to safeguard funds against e-fraud. *The Guardian.* https://guardian.ng/business-services/how-banks-are-grappling-to-safeguard-customers-funds-against-e-fraud/

Are, J. (2021, December 28). UNL COVID won't be the last pandemic: We need to prepare for the next. *The Cable.* https://www.thecable.ng/un-covid-wont-be-the-last-pandemic-we-need-to-prepare-for-the-next

Azu, J. C. (2020, May 19). Nigeria: How COVID-19 affects human rights. *Daily Trust.* https://allafrica.com/stories/202005190061.html

Eagle Online. (2020, April 21). *COVID-19: 23 killed, many maimed by security agents enforcing lockdown- report.* https://theeagleonline.com.ng/covid-19-23-killed-many-maimed-by-security-agents-enforcing-lockdown-report/

Ejekwonyilo, A. (2021, December 6). How Nigerian security operatives extra-judicially killed 13,241 in 10 years-CDD. *Premium Times.* https://www.premiumtimesng.com/news/499472-how-nigerian-security-operatives-extra-judicially-killed-13241-in-10-years-cdd.html

Ejekwonyilo, A. (2022, January 1). COVID-19, JUSUN strike add to Nigeria's justice sector woes. *Premium Times.* https://www.premiumtimesng.com/news/more-news/503319-2021-covid-19-jusun-strike-add-to-justice-sectors-woes-other-highlights.html

Ekwowusi, S. (2022, January 25). The illegality of COVID mandates. *The Guardian.* https://guardian.ng/opinion/the-illegality-of-covid-mandates/

Guterres, A. (2021, February 22). The pandemic faces a pandemic of human rights abuses in the wake of COVID-19. *The Guardian.* https://www.theguardian.com/global-development/2021/feb/22/world-faces-pandemic-human-rights-abuses-covid-19-antonio-guterres

Ilesanmi, O., Afolabi, A., & Uchendu, O. (2021, March 26). The prospective COVID-19 vaccine: Willingness to pay and perception of community members in Ibadan, Nigeria. *PeerJ, 9,* e11153. https://doi.org/10.7717/peerj.11153

NAN. (2021, December 29). Nigeria won't take expired vaccines again- NAFDAC DG. *The Guardian.* https://guardian.ng/news/nigeria-wont-take-expired-vaccines-again-nafdac-d-g/

NBA pushes justice sector reform to the front burner (2022). *This Day*. https://www.thisdaylive.com/index.php/2022/02/01/nba-pushes-justice-sector-reform-to-the-front-burner/

Nwachukwu, J. O. (2020, April 13). COVID-19: I see dead bodies littered all over Africa- Melinda Gates warns. *Daily Post*. https://dailypost.ng/2020/04/13/covid-19-i-see-dead-bodies-littered-all-over-africa-melinda-gates-warns/

Odiegwu, M. (2022, February 22). *Compulsory vaccination helps conquer fears in Nigeria*. Gavi.org. https://www.gavi.org/vaccineswork/compulsory-vaccination-helps-conquer-fears-nigeria

Ojerinde, D. (2021, 4 October). Fully vaccinated 74-year old SAN, Williams, dies of COVID-19. *Punch*. https://punchng.com/fully-vaccinated-74-year-old-san-williams-dies-of-covid-19/

Okunola, A. (2021, May 11). I tried to get a COVID-19 vaccine in Lagos, Nigeria. Here's what happened. *Global Citizen*. https://www.globalcitizen.org/en/content/i-tried-to-get-the-covid-19-vaccine-in-nigeria/

Omogbolagun, T. (2020, May 30). How we lost our loved ones rejected by hospitals amid COVID-19 pandemic bereaved families. *Punch*. https://punchng.com/how-we-lost-our-loved-ones-rejected-by-hospitals-amid-covid-19-pandemic-bereaved-families/

Orjinmo, N. (2020, October 26). Why Nigerian looters are targeting COVID-19 aid. *BBC News*. https://www.bbc.com/news/world-africa-54695568

Owolabi, F. (2021, October 13). FG makes COVID-19 vaccination compulsory for civil servants. *The Cable*. https://www.thecable.ng/just-in-fg-makes-covid-19-vaccination-compulsory-for-civil-servants

Paul, E. (2021, March 16). Nigerians, other African merchants can now accept PayPal via Flutterwave partnership. *TechPoint, Africa*. https://techpoint.africa/2021/03/16/africa-accept-paypal-via-flutterwave

Statista. (n.d.). Internet user penetration in Nigeria from 2016 to 2026. https://www.statista.com/statistics/484918/internet-user-reach-nigeria/

Umokoro, E. (2020, May 30). Amidst COVID-19 lockdown Nigeria sees increased sexual and gender violence. *Premium Times*. https://pulitzercenter.org/stories/amidst-covid-19-lockdown-nigeria-sees-increased-sexual-and-gender-violence

# PART FOUR
# Healthcare personnel: Fighting in the frontline

# BURNOUT AND BOUNDARIES: ETHICAL CONSIDERATIONS FOR ESSENTIAL WORKERS DURING CRISES

**Devin J. Rapp**[1]

**Abstract**: For many workforces, the pandemic's onset and nature dramatically changed how their workers experienced pre-existing work-nonwork boundaries. However, for so-called "essential workers," like healthcare workers, there were added burdens and changes that blurred boundaries in ways that increased job demands, decreased job resources, and exacerbated burnout. Utilizing research from a recent grounded theory study of 93 healthcare workers (Rapp et al., 2021), I highlight a number of physical and cognitive boundary violations—unwanted disruptions between work and personal life—which, if not adequately addressed, were associated with specific dimensions of burnout (i.e., emotional exhaustion, detachment, and sense of incompetence). I also describe specific physical and cognitive boundary work tactics utilized by some of these same workers to effectively manage boundary violations. I offer several practical and ethical implications for decision-makers and educators moving forward to plan for and protect essential workers who can be especially vulnerable during times of crisis.

## Burnout and Boundaries: Ethical Considerations for Essential Workers During Crises

The COVID-19 pandemic dramatically changed the way workers experienced pre-existing work-nonwork boundaries across the planet (Vaziri et al., 2020). However, for so-called "essential workers," there were often added levels of demands that blurred their existing boundaries between work and nonwork domains. **Essential workers** *perform operations and services that are critical to the continuity of needed functions in society* (CISA, 2020). Essential workers, such as healthcare workers, are critical for the well-being of communities in both times of stability and times of crisis.

---

[1] Ph.D. researcher, University of Utah, Utah, USA

While pandemics have been (and hopefully will continue to be) infrequent, large **contextual shocks** (Crawford et al., 2019), which *disrupt how workers manage work and nonwork boundaries*, are more common and generally impact essential workers first and foremost (e.g., September 11th, 2001 terrorist attacks heavily impacted firefighters). This chapter aims to share grounded theoretical findings generated from a grounded theory analysis of what 93 healthcare workers experienced during COVID-19 (Rapp et al., 2021) in order to raise ethical considerations for essential workers, organizations, educators, and society going forward.

Throughout this chapter, and especially at its conclusion, ethical questions and implications are identified that concern stakeholders at all levels. Given the novelty of the pandemic, it is understandable that many of these issues arose in real-time and were not adequately dealt with by healthcare leaders and organizations. However, with the benefit of hindsight, scholars and practitioners are responsible for identifying ethical issues and considering solutions for future events. We can determine what happened during the pandemic and the crucial lessons learned by highlighting these quotes and the grounded theory that emerged. This chapter includes examples of how some essential workers effectively managed the interruptions of the pandemic by responding with specific tactics that allowed them to renegotiate their work-nonwork boundaries. Armed with this knowledge, workers, decision-makers, and organizations can help facilitate boundary management tactics tailored to specific dimensions of burnout that we explain below.

## Burnout and Boundary Theory

Along with two colleagues, I set out to understand how healthcare workers were experiencing work during the pandemic (see Rapp et al., 2021). Our sample included 93 healthcare workers from a variety of low and high-status workers such as housekeepers, doctors, nurses, physician assistants, physical therapists, and more from the United States (87) and South America (6). We quickly found that their work had been highly disrupted and many of our participants complained of worsening burnout. Our 93 grounded theory interviews (Corbin & Strauss, 2008; Glaser & Strauss, 1967) revealed that the COVID-19 pandemic had adversely impacted many boundary violations for healthcare workers. The rest of this chapter will discuss the findings of this study and the healthcare workers we interviewed.

**Boundary violations** are *undesired disruptions between work and other important life domains such as personal and family life* (Kreiner et al., 2009; Rapp et al., 2021). These boundary violations are classified as either physical or cognitive in nature. **Boundary theory** concerns *how people classify and perceive the world around them with socially constructed boundary domains*, such as those between "home" and "work" (Ashforth et al., 2000, Rapp et al., 2021). These boundaries may vary in thickness and permeability (Ashforth et al., 2000). Individuals also vary in their preferences toward integrating or segmenting different domains, such as life domains and facets of their workplace (Kreiner et al., 2006; Kossek et al., 2012). Boundary violations are categorized as either an intrusion or distancing event. **Intrusion events** are *boundary violations that disrupt boundaries like those between the worker and elements of their work* (e.g., an outsider's ignorant beliefs of the virus, an element of healthcare workers' jobs). **Distancing events** consisted of *aspects of work that were perceived as overly or newly segmented between the worker and the work domain* (e.g., social distancing policies that required workers to eat meals apart; Kreiner et al., 2009).

## Boundary Violations and Burnout During the Pandemic

**Burnout** is defined by three dimensions (Maslach, 1982; Maslach & Jackson, 1981). First, *emotional exhaustion results from being "drained" from excessive job demands* (Demerouti et al., 2001). Second, *detachment and cynicism represent disengagement from work and relevant actors at work*. Last, *inefficacy consists of a lack of accomplishment and sense of incompetence*. Our study (Rapp et al., 2021) and other empirical research during the pandemic (Jalili et al., 2020; Khasne et al., 2020) confirmed what newspapers, anecdotes, and common sense suspected; the pandemic was exacerbating and increasing burnout for healthcare workers. In fact, the very first of the 93 participants interviewed for our grounded theory study was an experienced nursing home administrator in San Diego, CA. The interview occurred a few weeks after he had experienced 53 of his 59 nursing home residents catch COVID-19 in the span of two weeks. In his words, the "hardest and heaviest" part of so many

COVID-19 cases was "dealing with the burnout of so many employees who were ready to quit." Supervisors like this one had to deal with the challenges of taking care of both employees and vulnerable patients. An intensive care unit nurse described the impact of such burdensome boundary violations on the widespread worker burnout as follows:

> Most everybody that I work with has experienced a level of burnout that we didn't really anticipate... Honestly, this year is the first time in my six years of working in healthcare that I have not been able to leave work at work... all of [it] comes home with healthcare workers... Nurses during this pandemic have had their personal and professional boundaries tested like never before. All of that has caused the burnout and exhaustion level of nurses to increase exponentially.

Many healthcare workers reported experiencing the most demanding working conditions of their life while, at the same time, a pandemic was impacting their home life too. The cumulative results were often burnout and cumbersome spillover that they could not easily abandon because of their moral and ethical commitments to their patients, coworkers, and employers. A nursing home administrator in Pennsylvania summarized her experience succinctly: "My work-life encroached on home life. There was little separation between work and home [and] this led to exhaustion." Meanwhile, other pandemic forces pushed workers away from coping resources they had long relied upon, such as coworker social support and meaningful connections with their patients. The result was exacerbated detachment from work. The same intensive care unit nurse from above, who described exponential increases in burnout, explained how the reduction of job resources was contributing to burnout:

> Now reduce the trained staff, reduce the resources, add in false and empty praise from management, take away lunch and bathroom breaks, don't provide any compensation for the change in workload, and take away important benefits, and you have a frustrated, overworked, underpaid, and under-appreciated staff that quite literally can't continue to show up to work and feel like they are worth anything.

In summary, the boundary violations of the pandemic disrupted work and nonwork life for healthcare workers in ways that increased job demands and decreased job resources, resulting in new or worsening outcomes of burnout.

## Physical Boundary Violations

While the rest of society was socially distancing and making changes to the work interface, quite simply, healthcare workers had to go to work. Furthermore, work was a place that seemed to be growing more and more physically dangerous every day. While healthcare workers might appear an extreme example of physical work for essential workers, the nature of essential work often includes close proximity to other people like patients, customers, and other workers. Such work is inherently less flexible and difficult to control. Research during the pandemic highlighted the chaotic and unfortunate conditions that often limited personal protective equipment (PPE) and other legally required safety protections, especially at the pandemic's beginning (Gaitens et al., 2021; Gershon, 2020; Gould & Barone, 2020; Redman, 2020). This inability to protect healthcare workers and the increasing prevalence of the virus, put healthcare workers and their loved ones at higher risk of infection (Baker et al., 2020). A hospital nurse in Missouri spoke to us of the anxieties and fears of those she worked with regarding PPE and the virus: "Am I going to get exposed [or] have the right equipment? All that [was] weighing on you and then coming home, you were still anxious... There'd be nurses throwing up before their shifts; they were so worried." The ethical implications of inadequate PPE were that healthcare workers were often forced to decide between their personal safety and their duty to care for their patients and perform their job roles as clinicians. Going forward, it is paramount that adequate personal protective equipment is available for essential workers for future crises.

The healthcare workers in our study also reported fearing that they could infect their family members. An experienced housekeeping supervisor explained why he and his wife, a dietary manager at a different nursing home, slept apart since the pandemic: "We work in separate facilities, so we sleep in separate bedrooms." Many of our participants disrupted their family or nonwork domains to avoid physical spillover effects of either bringing the virus into work by infecting their patients or residents and from the work domain into the home domain by infecting their loved ones. These spillover stressors induce questions on ethical considerations for whether or not essential workers like healthcare workers should be entitled to external assistance when contextual shocks disrupt their work and nonwork lives.

While some workers had the means and the willingness to avoid risk by not entering public places or sleeping in separate bedrooms from their spouses, many did not. Should workers be expected to sacrifice their personal lives to benefit patients and the broader society? Perhaps. Nevertheless, given the personal risk, perhaps they should also be helped with the financial and other costs incurred by their sacrifices to remain ethically correct and provide the necessary resources to engage in such challenging work.

Another source of boundary violations originating from PPE protocols was the cumbersome nature of wearing it for long periods of time. An early career stage nurse spoke about the physical toll of PPE and how it contributed to burnout:

> My burnout mainly comes from the PPE. I don't want to wear a mask all day, every day. It's honestly really hard for me. It gets really hot, and my skin feels irritated, and I just feel like I can't breathe appropriately.

This nurse was not alone, as time wearing PPE is associated with increased stress (Hoedl et al., 2020), in part due to the increased incidence of headaches and other pains. A different nurse complained about the burden of so much extra work wearing PPE: "You get minimal breaks because of the severity of how sick these patients are, carrying around a PAPR unit for twelve hours or wearing an N95 mask for twelve hours a shift, minimal water breaks, minimal bathroom breaks."

Conversely, some policies meant to limit co-contamination unwittingly increased social distance between coworkers, reducing social support, a vital job resource for buffering burnout (Halbesleben, 2006). An intensive care unit nurse in Southern California said: "You can't even have a human connection with your coworkers that are going through the same thing you are." This insight that healthcare workers were facing unique challenges is important because it provides a reminder that when essential workers are most needed for work, these are the times when resources like social support might be most under threat. Therefore, the instinct managers might have to make quick changes to protocols around eating meals or taking breaks must also be challenged. Such protocols that increase the distance between workers seemed to diminish resources and foster burnout as workers felt more isolated and less supported.

Therefore, practical solutions in such cases must balance preserving physical safety while also avoiding isolation protocols. Where possible, outside spaces or transparent semi-barriers (e.g., glass or plastic divides) could strike such a balance.

## Cognitive Boundary Violations

Many healthcare workers dealt with a spillover of work into time off. Examples included higher quantities and quality of workload, exhaustion spilling over, and an inability to escape from ignorant outsiders. Since the pandemic worsened existing healthcare staffing shortages (Yang et al., 2021), patient loads often increased, adversely impacting time off and spillover. A Physician Assistant in a small town said, "That's where you get more burnout, because I'm taking 16 notes home that I still have to finish, so I'm at home now doing two to three hours' worth of work, whereas, before the pandemic, it wasn't as bad." Unfortunately, it was not only the quantity of workload that weighed on healthcare workers; they were not immune to the effects of witnessing such intense sickness and isolation as they cared for patients with COVID-19 while juggling the distancing protocols and heavy PPE. A medical doctor described the emotional spillover experienced during his time-off:

> You come home emotionally, mentally drained... I'm so fried by the time I get home that I become a zombie... I want my mind and my heart to be at home as much as at work, and it's gone by the time I get home. And my kids are excited to see me... but, you know, it's tough.

Another stressor frequently cited was frustration with the ignorance of outsiders from the media, government leaders, strangers, friends, and even close family members. These conversations or discussions became annoying intrusions that gave workers the sense they could not get away from work-related matters. Additionally, healthcare workers, already depleted of emotional resources from work, lost patience with ignorant outsiders who questioned their competence and expertise with talking points they adopted from social media or other questionable sources. An intensive care unit articulated the interaction of excessive job demands with ignorant outsiders taking shots at them:

> Now we are all exhausted from hundreds of hours of mandatory overtime or the dozens of people I have watched die alone, while the general population began to condemn us for taking things seriously. People told me, "We all have bad days at work. You signed up for this." People accused us of making the pandemic out to be worse than it really was. People called us sheep for wanting [or] taking vaccines. When really, we were desperate for help.

Even when outsiders were not spouting conspiracy theories, constant talk of work was still intrusive. An experienced intensive care unit nurse in California complained about the disruption of suddenly having a job that is an active topic of conversation:

> I feel like that part has been more frustrating, you know, turning it off when you go home. Now, all of a sudden, it's like your career choice is now in the news. Like we were never, as nurses, that, like, frontline in news stories every single day.

During contextual shocks like the pandemic, non-essential workers must better broadcast and understand that sensitivity is necessary with workers on the frontlines. Media outlets and public educators can help report on the conditions of essential workers based on empirical and verified observations. In crises, essential workers are likely to be incredibly busy and exhausted; we should not expect them to tell their own stories and educate others. These healthcare workers provide a powerful example for how essential workers experienced the many disruptions of the COVID-19 pandemic and how such boundary violations often led to or exacerbated worker burnout. In addition to the several practical and ethical implications already given, the following sections provide boundary tactics that were reported as having best buffered burnout during the COVID-19 pandemic.

## Boundary Work Tactics: What Buffered Burnout During the Pandemic

In response to boundary violations, workers reported the best results when they employed **boundary work tactics**, *effortful attempts to increase or decrease the distance (or boundaries) between domains, such as work and nonwork (e.g., personal or family lives)*. Boundary work tactics can be categorized as

**segmentation tactics**—when the worker seeks greater separation—usually employed after an intrusion event or **integration tactics**—*when the actor intended to create greater self and work immersion*—generally in response to distancing events.

## Physical Boundary Work Tactics

When the physical boundary violations disrupted work life, we found that healthcare workers best-buffered burnout when they thickened and segmented their boundaries between work and home. Such segmentation tactics included habits and physical routines to transition back safely and purposely work less overtime. An intensive care unit (ICU) physician spoke of his transition between work and home: "I have to stand outside of my door and take off all of my scrubs down into my underwear, take everything off. Leave them outside. Sneak into my side door, go wash my hands, and then I'm fine. That's become a ritual." Such routines and rituals were typical to reduce physical contamination risks during the pandemic.

Another segmentation tool was taking on less overtime. Staffing shortages often provided the need and opportunity for lucrative overtime work. However, several healthcare workers spoke about the need to manage boundaries on how often and how much they worked, often for the first time in their careers. Such renegotiations of boundaries demonstrated powerful examples of burnout risk providing a sense of empowerment and leading to healthier boundary management. A physician assistant in New York City who had regularly sought out overtime pay explained how she changed during the pandemic: "We have three shifts a week, and usually I will work extra, but during COVID, I [didn't] because I was so exhausted, but it was good for me to prevent being burned out." Participants also shared newly focused boundaries around attending the many off-day meetings about COVID-related protocols to segment their time further. Often this meant spending the time while at work to learn about new protocols or attending meetings on working days instead of off-days as they may have before the pandemic.

Given the tremendous increases in workload, we were surprised but inspired to hear several stories where healthcare workers seemed to be "diving deeper" into work despite all of the novel demands. As previously mentioned, healthcare workers observed a lot of suffering and loneliness in their patients during the pandemic. Well-meaning distancing protocols often exacerbated isolation. There are a number of inspiring accounts of frontline workers sacrificing time, attention, and personal safety as they compensated for the physical barriers and protocols brought on by the pandemic. While such profoundly personal and physically close engagement with patients carried extra physical contamination risks, not to mention emotional resources, these efforts often paid off by paradoxically increasing emotional resources as workers found meaning at work. A medical doctor located in a small town in Utah reported one of these examples:

> I was in the room for almost 40 minutes. I tried to console her, to hold her hand, and being in a room for 40 minutes; obviously, everyone is thinking about [potential contamination]. Ultimately, we were able, she was unconscious, but we were able to finally make an exception and get her husband in to be with her at the end of life; and she died within 15 minutes of him getting there, and I got just the sweetest letter, just about the hospital making that happen and having him be able to be there and say goodbye to her for the last 15 minutes. So that's how the pandemic started for me.

As interviewers, we were surprised but impressed to hear such examples of healthcare workers choosing to dive deeper into work when they were already doing and giving so much. In Santiago, Chile, an emergency room physician provided another example of great attention: "The worst thing was attending patients with [heavy PPE] because they didn't see you. They were [scared]... alone... and we were the last people they'd see." To compensate for these barriers, this doctor had photos added to worker name tags in order to humanize these otherwise scary and problematic interactions. There was pride and excitement in his voice when he talked about how much this small intervention had helped and how he had shared the best practice with other departments and healthcare workers through word of mouth and social media. While potentially increasing job demands, such engaging acts also paradoxically increased job resources as they crafted their jobs (Wrzesniewski & Dutton, 2001). Such efforts could then restore their emotional reserves and increase their sense of commitment to the job and their patients.

## Cognitive Boundary Work Tactics

Cognitively, segmentation tactics also aided healthcare workers who had to deal with the annoying intrusions between themselves and non-healthcare workers who would make ignorant comments. Some people used the tactic of simply ignoring hurtful or judgmental comments in order to reduce existing or avoid potentially added emotional exhaustion. Whereas some healthcare workers sought to advocate for themselves and their occupation, ignoring outsiders in-person, on social media, or at the dinner table simplified interactions. An experienced physician spoke about the political or conspiracy theories that would arise in conversations with friends and strangers: "I don't get into it too much with these people... getting into that type of debate or trying to persuade or change their mind, it's never that productive, and it usually ends badly."

Other means of cognitively segmenting work came by leveraging technology. For example, due to the constant changes of the novel environment of the pandemic, emails on changing protocols and staffing needs came several times a day, in some cases, and some workers segmented domains by turning off email, text, and other notifications that intruded on time off. Because of the charged nature of the pandemic and related conspiracies and ranging opinions, social media was deliberately ignored or turned off. As a result, healthcare workers were rewarded with greater peace of mind and fewer intrusions of work and nonwork. Cognitively, healthcare workers faced similar dilemmas for managing their various domains. As mentioned, a frequent scenario occurred when non-healthcare workers wanted to discuss the pandemic. Such discussions carried a potential threat of frustration as ignorant beliefs were rampant and annoying to answer (Rapp et al., 2021). Nevertheless, some chose to advocate for the pandemic's veracity and public health initiatives by citing science and expert opinions. A special COVID ICU unit nurse saw advocating on social media in this way as a responsibility or duty of his role as a clinician:

> And so, we take it upon ourselves to combat pseudoscience... Being in the realm that I was, being in the COVID ICU unit, seeing it first-hand, having that unique perspective, I did feel early on a very strong responsibility to just put things out there.

An assisted living administrator said, "I educate. If I hear someone say they won't wear a mask or social distance, I just say I work with a vulnerable population... I think it's important to educate and lead by example." A physician assistant in New York City who witnessed first-hand the early days of the pandemic in New York City reported her efforts to educate loved ones through weekly emails. Ultimately, this means of communicating the stories she was witnessing provided her a way to cope with all of the burnout and suffering she experienced:

> I would write this weekly email and send it out to family and friends because I was just like, "You can't even believe it. I could never even believe how crazy it was unless I went through it myself." And the amount of people dying and everything and it was just, at the time, in April or March, you heard on the news, people like: "This is not really going on, this is a political thing." [Of my patients,] ten people died this week from COVID. One of them was 32 years old. One of them was a couple that was 60. Just like nightmare after nightmare story... It was therapeutic to sit down and write the email… about the stories of people. I felt like I was getting… them the attention and respect that they needed from people who wouldn't otherwise be taking it seriously.

As discussed, social distancing protocols at work made it increasingly difficult to make and maintain meaningful connections at work. However, some participants would take time outside of work to integrate work and nonwork time. A hospice and home health nurse spoke of her late-night calls with a fellow hospice nurse that helped increase coping resources that distancing protocols had depleted:

> It's really easy to bounce things off her… because one of us has been there usually, and so it's healthy... She can relate and tell me a story... I just really appreciate my team and being able to talk through it… I don't think I could have gotten through some of those hard, dark days.

In summary, there is much to learn from courageous healthcare workers about how essential workers and others can manage boundary violations effectively, against all odds.

## Ethical Implications for Essential Workers

There are many ethical implications to draw from practical and theoretical findings of healthcare workers during the COVID-19 pandemic. Perhaps most importantly is knowledge and awareness that essential workers are among those most likely to experience boundary violations and burnout when contextual shocks happen. Knowledge of boundary violations and their effects on burnout can underscore the need for empathy and action (Kanov, 2021). Such action should be especially sensitive to the marginalized and underprivileged groups who are more likely to belong to essential worker occupations (Gaitens et al., 2021).

Boundary violations can come in the form of intrusion and distancing events. Intrusion events cause workers to experience more job demands and are thus more likely to suffer emotional exhaustion. Workers can thus seek segmentation of such intrusive events to reduce job demands. From distancing events, the greater isolation can result in reduced job resources and increasing detachment and cynicism. In response, workers can be helped and encouraged to bring themselves deeper into work domains where they can involve their identity, interests, etc. Such integration may develop greater job resources and thus lower their potential for detachment at work. For example, having outlets for coping at work and away from work is incredibly important to cope with the results of contextual shocks. Healthcare workers observed increased death, sickness, and loneliness in their patients. Simultaneously, they were less able to be physically and cognitively close with their patients and less able to be similarly close with coworkers who were uniquely able to understand, empathize, and encourage one another. This simultaneous thickening and thinning of boundaries exacerbated burnout.

Workforces and leaders would be wise to consider such costs to distancing protocols or other well-meaning interventions to contextual shocks. Instead, systemic nudges that safely facilitate social support will likely reduce adverse outcomes and increase morale and other emotional resources. Given the cumbersome and cumulative impacts of existing PPE, organizations and other stakeholders should consider innovations that address safety, comfort, and the ability to communicate with patients and coworkers while it is worn.

The other major ethical and moral dilemma for civic and organizational leaders is the responsibility to better support essential workers during crises. For many of our participants, wages were not increased, and some lost supplementary benefits like 401K matches because many healthcare organizations and systems lost large amounts of revenue when highly paid services like elective surgeries were suspended or limited due to the virus. Health systems and healthcare policy will vary by country and region, but decision-makers must ask difficult relevant questions. Should financial and health assistance be provided when needs arise directly because of a contextual shock? For example, many healthcare workers contracted the COVID-19 virus from work and then passed this risk on to their children or spouses. There were then implications for childcare, healthcare expenses, and even lodging implications to avoid or treat the effects of contamination (Kreiner et al., 2021) that would not be covered under traditional workers' compensation protocols. Who, then, should be responsible for such additional costs resulting from essential work? The Essential Workers Project, a collaboration between the Johns Hopkins Berman Institute of Bioethics and the University of Colorado Boulder's Masters of the Environment program, has advocated for adequate PPE, safe locations for their dependents while they are at work, as well as transportation and other considerations (Johns Hopkins Berman Institute of Bioethics, 2020).

The healthcare workers we interviewed during the COVID-19 pandemic provide a powerful example of how holistically, life can be interrupted for essential workers during a crisis and how such changes can exacerbate burnout. However, healthcare workers also demonstrated a number of tactics that helped manage the disruptions they experienced. Scholars, organizations, and civic leaders are responsible for learning from the COVID-19 pandemic and preparing for future contextual shocks (Hertelendy et al., 2021; Sriharan et al., 2021). Just as burnout may provide opportunities and empowerment for workers to reconsider and more purposefully address their boundaries, so too can the pandemic provide opportunities and empowerment for decision-makers and organizations to reconsider how we take care of our essential workers.

## References

Ashforth, B. E., Kreiner, G. E., & Fugate, M. (2000). All in a day's work: Boundaries and micro role transitions. *Academy of Management Review, 25*(3), 472–491. https://doi.org/10.2307/259305

Baker, J. M., Nelson, K. N., Overton, E., Lopman, B. A., Lash, T. L., Photakis, M., Jacob, J. T., Roback, J. D., Fridkin, S. K., & Steinberg, J. P. (2021). Quantification of occupational and community risk factors for SARS-CoV-2 seropositivity among health Care workers in a large US health care system. *Annals of Internal Medicine, 174*(5). https://doi.org/10.7326/M20-7145

CISA (2020). Identifying critical infrastructure during COVID-19. https://www.cisa.gov/identifying-critical-infrastructure-during-covid-19.

Corbin, J., & Strauss, A. (2008). *Basics of qualitative research: Techniques and procedures for developing grounded theory*. Sage Publications. https://dx.doi.org/10.4135/9781452230153

Crawford, W. S., Thompson, M. J., & Ashforth, B. E. (2019). Work-life events theory: Making sense of shock events in dual-earner couples. *The Academy of Management Review, 44*(1), 194–212. https://doi.org/10.5465/amr.2016.0432

Demerouti, E., Bakker, A. B., Nachreiner, F., & Schaufeli, W. B. (2001). The job demands-resources model of burnout. *Journal of Applied Psychology, 86*(3), 499–512. https://doi.org/10.1037/0021-9010.86.3.499

Gaitens, J., Condon, M., Fernandes, E., & McDiarmid, M. (2021). COVID-19 and essential workers: A narrative review of health outcomes and moral injury. *International Journal of Environmental Research and Public Health, 18*(4), 1446. doi: 10.3390/ijerph18041446

Gershon, R. (2020). Impact of COVID-19 pandemic on NYC transit workers: Pilot study findings. https://www.nyu.edu/content/dam/nyu/publicAffairs/documents/PDF/GershonTransitWorkerPilotStudy

Glaser, B. G., & Strauss, A. (1967). *The discovery of grounded theory: Strategies for qualitative research*. Aldine-Athestor.

Gould, J. & Barone, V. (2020). 45 NYC doormen and janitors dead from coronavirus, union says. *New York Post*. https://nypost.com/2020/04/16/45-nyc-doormen-and-janitors-dead-from-coronavirus-union-says/

Halbesleben, J. R. B. (2006). Sources of social support and burnout: A meta-analytic test of the conservation of resources model. *Journal of Applied Psychology, 91*(5), 1134–1145. https://doi.org/10.1037/0021-9010.91.5.1134

Hertelendy, A. J., McNulty, E., Mitchell, C., Gutberg, J., Lassar, W., Durneva, P., & Rapp, D. J. (2021). Crisis leadership: The new imperative for MBA curricula. *The International Journal of Management Education, 19*(3), 100534. https://doi.org/10.1016/j.ijme.2021.100534

Hoedl, M., Eglseer, D., & Bauer, S. (2020). Associations between personal protective equipment and nursing staff stress during the COVID-19 pandemic. *Journal of Nursing Management. 29*(8), 2374-2382. https://doi.org/10.1111/jonm.13400

Jalili, M., Niroomand, M., Hadavand, F., Zeinali, K., & Fotouhi, A. (2020). Burnout among healthcare professionals during COVID-19 pandemic: A cross-sectional study. *International Archives of Occupational and Environmental Health, 94*(6), 1345-1352. https://doi.org/10.1007/s00420-021-01695-x

Johns Hopkins Berman Institute of Bioethics (2020). The essential workers project. https://bioethics.jhu.edu/research-and-outreach/covid-19-bioethics-expert-insights/essential-workers-project/

Kanov, J. (2021). Why suffering matters! *Journal of Management Inquiry, 30*(1), 85-90. https://doi.org/10.1177/1056492620929766

Khasne, R. W., Dhakulkar, B. S., Mahajan, H. C., & Kulkarni, A. P. (2020). Burnout among healthcare workers during COVID-19 pandemic in India: Results of a questionnaire-based survey. *Indian Journal of Critical Care Medicine, 24*(8), 664. https://doi.org/10.5005/jp-journals-10071-23518

Kossek, E. E., Ruderman, M. N., Braddy, P. W., & Hannum, K. M. (2012). Work–nonwork boundary management profiles: A person-centered approach. *Journal of Vocational Behavior, 81*(1), 112-128. https://doi.org/10.1016/j.jvb.2012.04.003

Kreiner, G. E., Hollensbe, E. C., & Sheep, M. L. (2006). On the edge of identity: Boundary dynamics at the interface of individual and organizational identities. *Human Relations, 59*(10), 1315-1341. https://doi.org/10.1177/0018726706071525

Kreiner, G. E., Hollensbe, E. C., & Sheep, M. L. (2009). Balancing borders and bridges: Negotiating the work-home interface via boundary work tactics. *Academy of Management Journal, 52*(4), 704–730. https://doi.org/10.5465/AMJ.2009.43669916

Kreiner, G. E., Mihelcic, C. A., Mishina, Y., Dinhof, K., Hughey, J., Kleber, J., Mikolon, S., Rapp, D. J., Ruebottom, T., & Toubiana, M. (2021). Stigma as a double-edged sword: Exploring both the positive and negative effects of stigma at work. In *Academy of Management Proceedings, 1,* 11048. https://doi.org/10.5465/AMBPP.2021.11048symposium

Maslach, C. (1982). Understanding burnout: Definitional issues in analyzing a complex phenomenon. In W. S. Paine (Ed.), *Job stress and burnout* (pp. 29-40). SAGE.

Maslach, C., & Jackson, S. E. (1981). The measurement of experienced burnout. *Journal of Organizational Behavior,* 2(2), 99-113. https://doi.org/10.1002/job. 4030020205

Rapp, D. J., Hughey, J. M., & Kreiner, G. E. (2021). Boundary work as a buffer against burnout: Evidence from healthcare workers during the COVID-19 pandemic. *Journal of Applied Psychology, 106*(8), 1169-1187. http://dx.doi.org/10.1037/apl0000951

Redman, R. (2020). UFCW: Over 11,500 grocery workers affected in first 100 days of pandemic. https://www.supermarketnews.com/issues-trends/ufcw-over-11500-grocery-workers-affected-first-100-days-pandemic

Sriharan, A., Hertelendy, A. J., Banaszak-Holl, J., Fleig-Palmer, M. M., Mitchell, C., Nigam, A., Gutberg, J., Rapp, D. J., & Singer, S. J. (2021). Public health and health sector crisis leadership during pandemics: A review of the medical and business literature. *Medical Care Research and Review,* Advance online publication. https://doi.org/10.1177/10775587211039201.

Vaziri, H., Casper, W. J., Wayne, J. H., & Matthews, R. A. (2020). Changes to the work–family interface during the COVID-19 pandemic: Examining predictors and implications using latent transition analysis. *Journal of Applied Psychology, 105*(10), 1073-1087. http://dx.doi.org/10.1037/apl0000819

Wrzesniewski, A., & Dutton, J. E. (2001). Crafting a job: Revisioning employees as active crafters of their work. *The Academy of Management Review, 26*(2), 179-201. https://doi.org/10.5465/amr.2001.4378011

Yang, B. K., Carter, M. W., & Nelson, H. W. (2021). Trends in COVID-19 cases, deaths, and staffing shortages in US nursing homes by rural and urban status. *Geriatric Nursing, 42*(6), 1356-1361. https://doi.org/10.1016/j.gerinurse.2021.08.016

# ESSENTIAL WORKERS AND ETHICAL CONSIDERATIONS: ETHICAL CHALLENGES FOR HEALTHCARE PROFESSIONALS IN THE ERA OF COVID-19 PANDEMIC

**Alim Monir**[1]

**Abstract:** Since the beginning of COVID-19 pandemic healthcare workers have conquered ethical challenges in providing standards of care in the health systems. At the first wave of the pandemic, shortages of skillful professional, personal protective equipment (PPE), and ventilator supplies inflicted tremendous strain among healthcare workers. Hospital administrators had to prioritize treatment of patients who were most likely to survive, as well as make life or death decisions such as who would be admitted to the intensive care unit and when to withdraw life support. A quantitative data collection was carried out by using purposive survey questions. Frontline healthcare workers (n=564) in the New York City hospitals responded to the online Qualtrics survey. The IBM SPSS 26 data analysis was conducted to identify the significant relationship of Pearson's *r* correlation coefficient to enhance the depth of the study. During pandemic 96.7% of the healthcare workers were greatly concerned about workplace safety (p=0.032); 66.3% were working extra or long hours mandated by their employer which caused moral distress (p=0.040); and almost 90.5% felt that COVID-19 caused great stress at work. About 77.3% respondents identified issues that led to worsening psychological wellbeing. The study findings supported four ethical implications of healthcare workers with regards to work related stress, psychological wellbeing, moral distress, and workplace safety. During the COVID-19 pandemic, healthcare workers' additional stress levels at work led to wrongdoing, psychological exhaustion, and unsafe work environment among healthcare professionals. Lack of protection of healthcare workers and increase in morally distressing situations are associated with ethical challenges across the world.

---

[1] Administrator of Clinical Pathology & Laboratory Services, Bellevue Hospital, New York, New York, USA

## Introduction

The global spread of the novel coronavirus has dramatically changed the image of the U.S. healthcare delivery system. As of April 9th, 2022, over 497,923,672 civilians across the globe have been infected with COVID-19, resulting in 6,175,735 deaths. The United States has the topmost deaths of 985,296 lives that accounted for 16% of all confirmed fatalities across the globe (John Hopkins University Coronavirus Resource Center, April 9th, 2022). The frontline healthcare workers are actively involved in taking care of COVID-19 patients who are facing a lot of difficulties and ethical challenges in providing the best health care. Since the breakout of COVID-19, discrimination and inequalities on allocating resources, disparity on clinical judgement based on survival, analogous practices on healthcare policies have raised questions among healthcare professionals (McGuire et al., 2020).

Ethics is an imminent and inextricable part of clinical medicine. The healthcare professionals have an ethical obligation to obey the law to prevent or minimize harm during patient care. To date, non-maleficence, autonomy, beneficence, and justice are four main constituents of bioethical principles (Varkey, 2020). The principle of non-maleficence refers to doing no harm to the patient, especially in end-of-life care decisions regarding withholding or withdrawing life-support. Autonomy is the obligation of a healthcare provider to disclose treatment options. Beneficence emphasizes the benefits to the patient, and justice obliges fair, equitable, and appropriate treatment of the patient. The clinician has an impartial moral viewpoint on patient care and the decision-making process. Violating or ignoring any of those four foremost ethical requirements may be considered unethical behaviors. While the COVID-19 pandemic continues to be dominant, there are likely to be persistent challenges within the near future; therefore, the frontline healthcare workers are gaining legitimate attention across the world (Lai et al., 2020). Due to high levels of patient deaths, long working hours in an unsafe environment, contradicted resource allocation, lack of full protection and moral distress have raised various ethical questions throughout the healthcare industry (Gebreheat & Teame, 2021; Turale et al., 2020).

Since March 2020, the novel coronavirus disease has created extensive moral agony towards healthcare workers behavior especially in the emergency and intensive care unit. When it comes to essential workers' physical and psychological wellbeing, various ethical issues could arise that include employee work-related stress, psychological exhaustion, unethical practices, and workplace safety. Violating ethical regulations is an unethical behavior and healthcare professionals had difficulties finding ethical differences between withholding or withdrawing treatment for patient care (Boyd, 2020). The ongoing work-related stress among healthcare workers, psychological wellbeing, unethical practice due to moral distress, and workplace safety are the major ethical concerns. In this editorial, I will address these four ethical challenges of healthcare professionals, who find themselves in an unpleasant situation and adopt a strategy to reduce COVID-19 disease spread.

## Literature Review

A significant number of articles have been published on the complexity of ethical issues during COVID-19 pandemic. In an integrative literature review, Gebreheat and Teame (2021) reported that healthcare worker safety, moral distress, resource allocation, and patient-caregiver relationship are major ethical concerns across the healthcare system. Lack of PPE, prolonged pressure in maintaining resources, and prioritizing or refusing to provide patient care brings burning ethical concerns among healthcare professionals. In a descriptive correlational study among hospital registered nurses, Zho et al. (2020) stated that COVID-19 added tension, ethical dilemmas, perceived risk, and negative impact to provide care. About 81% believed that patients have the right to optimal and equal treatment, hospital management should be prioritizing allocation of respirators for older patients, and some of them believed that they have a right to refuse certain treatment of patients with COVID-19 victims (Zho et al., 2020).

The COVID-19 pandemic dramatically affects the healthcare system and compounded more issues among healthcare professionals. Normal work routines abruptly overturned into online or virtual environments. The social-distancing and stay-at-home guidelines became the new standard and mostly affected all normal activities (Ford, 2020). Due to the shortages of PPE, many healthcare professionals stopped showing up at work throughout the initial stage of the novel coronavirus. The major operational changes in the work practices among essential and non-essential employees work practices. The essential workers were required to be on site care with the patients who had underlying medical complications from COVID-19. The non-essential workers were allowed to work remotely, patient visits were handled over the phone and a video consultation. Hospital management quickly modified and deployed existing disaster plans into high-level medical care units whether things can wait until the risk for COVID-19 diminishes (Bowden et al., 2020). Temporary holds on all ambulatory surgery allowed healthcare professionals to put more focus on COVID-19 patients. Determine the urgency and balance the pros and cons regarding the in-person examination or testing versus risk of exposure to COVID-19. Daily communications increased to ensure adequate supplies of medications, ventilators, and pumps.

In a cross-sectional study, Labrague and Santos (2020) reported that the COVID-19 pandemic's changes to healthcare professionals' work outcomes, increases psychological disturbances, job dissatisfaction and turnover intentions. Hospital nurses in the United States and Australia posed an unpalatable ethical challenge in ensuring equity and fairness in patient care (Turale et al., 2020). The high levels of patient deaths, long working hours, and increased acuity were identified as ethical conflicts and moral dilemmas during the COVID-19 pandemic. Jia et al. (2020) revealed that healthcare professionals encountered ethical challenges in caring for patients that include neglecting patient rights, unequal exposure to the infectious environment, role of ambiguity, inadequate response to urgency, lack of responsibility, and lack of knowledge or skills to provide care. In a phenomenological study of New York City hospital nursing personnel, Patton (2021) identified that COVID-19 impacted on healthcare workers physical safety, psychological exhaustion, and sleep deprivation. The healthcare workers felt that they were understaffed, lacked knowledge sharing capabilities, and suffered increased anxiety when caring for COVID-19 patients. However, the COVID-19 pandemic braces hospital management to develop a series of policies, education, contingency plans, and operating procedures in response to the disaster plan.

## Materials and Methods

### Study Design and Sampling

The study involved the use of qualitative correlational data collection to explore the ethical dilemmas during the COVID-19 pandemic. After receiving the Institutional Review Board approval, participant recruitment was undertaken by the researcher via LinkedIn social media requests. The survey was hosted in Qualtrics and administered through the LinkedIn platform. All the participants completed the informed consent, and no identifiable information was collected from the participants that could potentially cause a confidentiality problem. The study population considered clinical and nonclinical healthcare employees in the New York City hospitals. A convenience sampling method with a minimum of 89 participants came from the recruitment process. The statistical G* Power software determined the minimum sampling sizes to conduct data analysis. The survey was available for 96 hours, during May 8th through May 11th, 2021, and the researcher did not limit the respondent to answer all survey questions. The response rate was higher and significantly greater than the projected sample size of 89 as a priori estimated, based on a mathematical assumption of the population. The sample size was large enough to achieve statistically significant data for both the Pearson *r* correlation coefficient and Chi Square test.

### Instrumentation

The Qualtrics survey was conducted via basic demographic and ethical factors questions. The demographic part of the survey was assessed from respondent information about gender, age, employment status, and work schedule. The ethical factors survey questions were concentrated on healthcare workers' work-related stress, psychological wellbeing, moral distress, and workplace safety issues. Three ethical factors survey questions were related to Likert scale of 1 to 2, 1 to 4, and 1 to 5. Workplace safety question has been asked on "how often you have had trouble going to sleep." Work-related stress ethical question is composed of "how often do you find your work stressful, and COVID-19 put me in great stress at work." Two of the ethical challenge questions were assessed by using direct "yes/no" responses regarding workers' moral distress issues. A numeric fill-in question was asked with "the number of days employees have been affected on doing usual activities due to COVID-19 fear" such as failure of self-care and/or recreational activities. In this study, research used bias-corrected bivariate bootstrapping procedure for each question set to eliminate possible Type I error rates. The Person's $r$ correlation coefficient test was appropriate to examine the viability and reliability of the instruments.

## Statistical Analysis

The IBM Statistical Package for Social Science (SPSS 26) data analysis was conducted to identify the significant relationship of Pearson's $r$ correlation coefficient and Chi Squared tests. All data analyses were two-tailed with an alpha of 5% for the SPSS 26 premium software for Windows. The Chi-Square analysis identified the relationships between clinical and nonclinical hospital employee positions. The statistically significant level achieved when $p$-value $\leq 0.05$.

## Ethical Statement

The study was conducted by following the official protocols of Northcentral University Institutional Review Board. Before and during the data collection procedure, the researcher adhered to the regulation of local, state, and federal government agencies on researching human subjects regarding confidentiality, anonymity, privacy, minimizes risks, deception, and informed consent. The participants were members of the LinkedIn social network. A risk was mitigated, while participation was voluntary, self-reported, and provided without any intimidation or fear of recrimination. The participants were allowed to leave at any time without completing the Qualtrics survey. About 54 respondents stopped taking the survey prior to completion; the incomplete responses were not included in the data analysis.

## Results

The goal of this study was to explore ethical factors associated with healthcare workers during COVID-19 pandemic. The study participants included 564 healthcare workers (54% male and 43% female) at New York City hospitals. Of the respondents, 63% were clinical workers who directly dealt with patient care. Table 1 represents survey demographic information where 97% of the participants were between 21 to 54 years of age. About 92% respondents were full-time clinical and nonclinical healthcare employees. The sample consisted of 354 employees who were from clinical, and 210 employees who were from nonclinical groups. The classification for this study were 24% physician, 16 % nursing practitioner, 11% physician assistant, 9% pharmacist, 6% registered nurse, 5% counselor, and remainder were from executive leadership, therapist, psychologist, management, technicians, human resource, maintenance engineer, secretary, cafeteria staff, janitor/housekeeping, social worker, IT/telecommunication, supervisor, and business developer.

**Table 1 .** *Survey Demographics*

| Variable | Category | N | % |
|---|---|---|---|
| Gender[a] | Male<br>Female<br>Unknown | 245<br>303<br>16 | 43%<br>54%<br>3% |
| Age[b] | Under 21<br>21-54<br>55 or older | 9<br>548<br>7 | 2%<br>97%<br>1% |
| Employment Status[c] | Full-time<br>Part-time | 516<br>48 | 92%<br>8% |
| Work Schedule[d] | Day shift<br>Evening Shift<br>Night Shift<br>Others | 234<br>74<br>39<br>217 | 42%<br>13%<br>7%<br>38% |

**Note:** Total Participant, N = 564; [a] Gender: Mean = 1.47, SD = 0.55, Variance = 0.30; [b] Age: Mean = 2.66, SD = 0.68, Variance = 0.47; [c] Employment Status: Mean =1.09, SD =0.28, Variance = 0.08; [d] Work Schedule: Mean =74.80, SD =1.95, Variance = 3.81

Table 2 represented the SPSS 26 data analysis and findings of two-tailed Pearson's Chi Square test values. The study was classified into four ethical factors to healthcare workers: work-related stress, psychological wellbeing, moral distress, and workplace safety (see Table 2).

**Table 2.** *Statistical Summary for Ethical Challenge Questions*

| Ethical Factors | Survey Questions | Total Participant (clinical/non-clinical) | *P-value** |
|---|---|---|---|
| Work related stress | How often do you find your work stressful? | 546 (348/198) | 0.217 |
| | *Always* | 47 (8.6%) | |
| | *Sometimes* | 241 (44.1%) | |
| | *Often* | 205 (37.6%) | |
| | *Hardly ever* | 47 (8.6%) | |
| | *Never* | 6 (1.1%) | |
| | COVID-19 put me in great stress at work | 545 (349/196) | 0.329 |
| | *Strongly disagree* | 5 (0.9%) | |
| | *Disagree* | 47 (8.6%) | |
| | *Agree* | 333 (61.1%) | |
| | *Strongly agree* | 160 (29.4%) | |
| Psychological wellbeing | Number of days effect on doing usual activities due to COVID-19 fear (e.g., self-care or recreational activities) | 554 (361/193) | - |
| | *0 day* | 126 (22.7%) | |
| | *1-5 days* | 394 (71.2%) | |
| | *6-10 days* | 26 (4.7%) | |
| | *11-30 days* | 8 (1.4%) | |
| Moral distress | Access to reduce stress management program at current workplace | 542 (344/198) | 0.001 |
| | *Yes* | 101 (18.6%) | |
| | *No* | 441 (81.4% | |
| | Working extra hours is mandated/required by employer | 552 (353/199) | 0.040 |
| | | | |
| | *Yes* | 366 (66.3%) | |
| | *No* | 186 (33.7%) | |
| Workplace safety | How often have you had trouble going to sleep? | 546 (348/198) | 0.032 |
| | *Often* | 69 (12.6%) | |
| | *Sometimes* | 323 (59.2%) | |
| | *Rarely* | 136 (24.9%) | |
| | *Never* | 18 (3.3%) | |

* Pearson Chi-Squared Tests; Significance level $P \leq 0.05$

The following paragraphs will provide details of each of the four ethical factors.

## Work Related Stress

Regarding the work-related stress questions, "how often do you find your work stressful, and COVID-19 put me in great stress at work" about 90% of the healthcare professionals agreed that COVID-19 had added stress where 65% were clinical and 35% were nonclinical employees. There was no significant association between clinical and nonclinical employees regarding the questions, "how often do you find your work stressful," with $\chi^2(4) = 5.772$, $p = 0.217$ and "COVID-19 put me in great stress at work," with $\chi^2(3) = 3.439$, $p = 0.329$. The Pearson's *r* value had no significant strength of association among the employment status for clinical and nonclinical employees.

## Psychological Wellbeing

In the quantitative correlational study, employees were asked, during the pandemic, how many days their poor physical or mental health keeps them away from doing usual activities. Workers complained of having more COVID-19 patients that had created additional work for many days a month and a workload that had an unsettling psychological effect. About 77% of employees responded that COVID-19 disrupted their regular recreational activities and self-care for weeks to months. Ten respondents commented that they were physically and emotionally depressed and very sad about their regular activities. Employees were concerned about patient suffering, quality of end-of-life support, high levels of death, and the disruption of communication between caregivers and families. All these issues shake up our ethical principles and lead to suffering for our healthcare professionals (Robert et al., 2020).

## Moral Distress

In this study, about 66% of employees (245 clinical and 121 non-clinical) were mandated by their employers to work extra hours, which was decreed by their employer. Mandating employees could unlikely impact workplace occupational health safety, moral distress, and a potential ethical dilemma for healthcare workers. In a meta-analysis study researchers reported that longest working hours adversely affect the employees' occupational health safely (Wong et al., 2019). Employees were mandated by their employer to wear surgical masks, gloves, and respirators, face shields, and other PPE for the longest period, and maintain social distancing regardless of level of transmission. Poor work-life balance could lower employee performance, lead to lack of attentiveness, fatigue, and tiredness. As a result, long working hours could lead to increased risk workers psychological, mental, and behavioral issues.

The survey finding revealed that 81% of employees (344 clinical and 198 nonclinical) do not have access to stress reduction management programs in their current workplace. There was a significant association between employment status and access to reduce stress management programs at the current workplace from hospital management with $\chi^2(1) = 10.439$, $p = 0.001$. The Pearson's $r$ value had a negative strong significance (Pearson's $r = -0.139$, $p=0.044$). Also, there was a significant association between employment status and mandatory overtime required by the employer, $\chi^2(1) = 4.214$, $p = 0.040$. The Pearson's $r$ value had a positive strong significance (Pearson's $r = 0.087$ $p=0.040$).

### Workplace Safety

About 97% of healthcare workers responded that during the pandemic they are having trouble going to sleep and/or of not getting enough sleep due to the fear and anxiety. There was a significant association between employment status and sleep disturbances within the past 12 months, $\chi^2(3) = 8.786$, $p = 0.032$. The Pearson's $r$ value had a positive no significance (Pearson's $r = 0.015$, $p=0.732$). Lack of sleep could increase burnout and lead to workplace safety issues towards a challenging ethical dilemma.

## Discussion

The novel coronavirus pandemic had a grip on the hospital functionality and career challenges among healthcare professionals. Every employee deserves to be safe in their workplace environments and federal law entitles them to a safe and healthy workplace environment. During the first wave of COVID-19 pandemic employees were assigned to work without adequate PPE, which put them at high risk of contracting and spreading diseases. The hospital administrator has the responsibility to keep the workplace free of known health and safety issues. In 1970, the United States Department of Labor enforced the Occupational Safety and Health Act (OSHA public law 91-596, as amended through January 2004), that each employee is free from recognized harm leading to death or serious physical harm. The healthcare providers have an ethical obligation for obtaining informed consent, telling the truth, valuing patient preferences, and avoiding harm. Healthcare professionals are being challenged by the lack of pandemic vigilance, allocation of clinical supplies, and application of ethical principles. Employers must comply and impose OSHA regulations to assure the greatest protection of the employees. Fear of the COVID-19 pandemic created unprecedented workloads and many frontline healthcare workers were even mandated by their employees to work harder than ever by extending their normal working hours. Employees have the right to speak up about their rights without fear of retaliation on issues such as insufficient PPE and exposure to grave danger from exposure to COVID-19 diseases.

Every healthcare organization has its own ethical standard to express their ethical norms and values. The ethical issues may be ingrained with workplace stress and empower healthcare professionals to respond positively to the distress of all complex ethical issues (Rushton, 2017). Work related stress is a particular form of suffering that reflects the torturing experience of failures, wrongdoing, and employee often feels that their integrity has been compromised. Also, healthcare workers' psychological wellbeing and safety at work is a vital part of an organization. Unfair labor practices of vulnerable workers may cause an occupational health and safety issue. During the pandemic, healthcare workers are disrupted and ill prepared to manage patient care while everyone demands equal and standard quality of care (Viens et al., 2020). Hospital administrators had to prioritize the treatment plan for the patients who are most likely to survive such as withhold or withdraw ventilators. This action violated equal rights for healthcare and raised questions on their Hippocratic Oath. The Hippocratic Oath refers to doing no harm to the patient which is the basic principle of healthcare ethics. Provider actions and practices are very important as long as they are in the interest of the patient care. In the midst of the pandemic, attention shifted towards treating patients who became seriously ill and sharing ventilators. This unethical practice could potentially cause stress among healthcare workers and weaken respect on their job. Employees' poor physical and mental health keeps them away from doing all usual activities such as self-care or recreational activities. Therefore, healthcare administrators should focus on reducing unethical activities and focus on increasing employees' productivity at work.

## Conclusion

The fear of COVID-19 pandemic had created an unprecedented workload and many frontline healthcare workers were even mandated by their employer to work harder than ever for extended hours. Employees were spending less time with their families and loved ones, which created unhappiness, poor job performance, and standard of patient care. The survey finding disclosed that 66% of employees (245 clinical and 121 nonclinical) were mandated by their employers to work extra hours, which was required for their employment. About 81% of the respondents felt that hospital management did not provide enough effort to reduce their stress which creates moral distress among frontline employees. The ethical factor, moral distress, could potentially increase employee turnover and intention to leave their positions, leading to an increase in the shortage of healthcare professionals. Work-life balance and safety approach is very important to all healthcare professionals. In response to workplace safety, 97% of employees believed that they had trouble going to sleep due to the fear of contracting COVID-19 diseases. Employees did not feel comfortable with their usual work ethics which led to major suffering among healthcare workers. About 90% of the healthcare professionals (493 out of 545) agreed that COVID-19 had added stress to healthcare professionals, where 319 of them were clinical, and 174 were from nonclinical areas. The COVID-19 pandemic continued to inflict damage on healthcare operations, finance, and workplace safety. In order to effectively manage future pandemics, epidemic outbreaks, or other unforeseeable healthcare crises, healthcare leaders need to focus on worker wellness, safety, and providing equitable support to those in need of care.

## References

Bowden, K., Burnham, E. L., Keniston, A., Levin, D., Limes, J., Persoff, J., Thurman, L., & Burden, M. (2020). Harnessing the power of hospitalists in operational disaster planning: COVID-19. *Journal of General Internal Medicine, 35*(9), 2732-2737. https://doi.org/10.1007/s11606-020-05952-6

Boyd, K. (2020). Ethics in a time of coronavirus. *Journal of Medical Ethics, 46*(5), 285-286. http://doi.org/10.1136/medethics-2020-106282

Ford, E. W. (2020). The next generational wave's experience viewed in 4-D. *Journal of Healthcare Management, 65*(4), 239-243. https://doi.org/10.1097/JHM-D-20-00147

Gebreheat, G., & Teame, H. (2021). Ethical challenges of nursing in COVID-19 pandemic: Integrative review. *Journal of Multidisciplinary Healthcare, 14,* 1029-1035. https://doi.org/10.2147/JMDH.S308758

Jia, Y., Chen, O., Xiao, Z., Xiao, J., Bian, J., Jia, H. (2021). Nurses' ethical challenges caring for people with COVID-19: A qualitative study. *Nursing Ethics, 28(*1), 33-45. https://doi.org/10.1177/0969733020944453

Labrague, L. J., & Santos, J. D. (2020). Fear of COVID-19, psychological distress, work satisfaction and turnover intention among front line nurses. *Research Square, 1*(1), 1-18. https://doi.org/10.21203/rs.3.rs-35366/v1

Lai, J., Ma, S., Wang, Y., Cai, Z., Hu, J., Wei, N., Wu, J., Du, H., Chen, T., Li, R., Tan, H., Kang, L., Yao, L., Huang, M., Wang, H., Wang, G., Liu, Z., & Hu, S. (2020). Factors associated with mental health outcomes among health care workers exposed to coronavirus disease 2019. *JAMA Network Open, 3*(3), e203976. https://doi.org/10.1001/jamanetworkopen.2020.3976

McGuire, A. L., Aulisio, M. P., Davis, F. D., Erwin, C., Harter, T. D., Jagsi, R., Klitzman, R., Macauley, R., Racine, E., Wolf, S. M., Wynia, M., & Wolpe, P. R. (2020). Ethical challenges arising in the COVID-19 pandemic: An overview from the association of bioethics program directors (ABPD) task force. *The American Journal of Bioethics, 20*(7), 15-27. https://doi.org/10.1080/15265161.2020.1764138

Patton, C. M. (September 2021). A phenomenological study of COVID-19's impact on U.S. nursing personnel. *Workplace Health & Safety*. https://doi.org/10.1177/21650799211030294

Robert, E., Kentish-Barnes, N., Boyer, A., Laurent, A., Azoulay, E., & Reignier, J. (2020). Ethical dilemmas due to the COVID-19 pandemic. *Annals of Intensive Care, 10*(84), 1-9. https://doi.org/10.1186/s13613-020-00702-7

Rushton, C. H. (2017). Cultivating moral resilience. *American Journal of Nursing, 117* (2), S11-S15. https://doi.org/10.1097/01.NAJ.0000512205. 93596.00

Turale, S., Meechamnan, C., Kunaviktikul, W. (2020). Challenging times: Ethics, nursing and the COVID-19 pandemic. *International Nursing Review, 67*(2), 164-167. https://doi.org/10.1111/inr.12598

Varkey, B. (2021). Principles of clinical ethics and their application to practice. *Medical Principles and Practice, 30*(1), 17-28. https://doi.org/10.1159/000509119

Viens, A. M., McGowan, C. R., & Vass, C. M. (2020). Moral distress among healthcare workers: Ethics support is a crucial part of the puzzle. *BMJ Blogs*. https://blogs.bjm.com/bmj/2020/06/23

Wong, K., Chan, A., & Ngan, S. C. (2019). The effect of long working hours and overtime on occupational health: A meta-analysis of evidence from 1998 to 2018. *International Journal of Environmental Research and Public Health, 16*(12), 2102. https://doi.org/10.3390/ijerph16122102

Zho, J., Stone, T., & Petrini, M. (2020). The ethics of refusing to care for patients during the coronavirus pandemic: A Chinese perspective. *Nursing Inquiry, 28*(1), e12380. https://doi.org/10.1111/nin.12380

# COVID-19 CONUNDRUMS: ETHICAL AND LEGAL ISSUES FACING THE MEDICAL COMMUNITY

**Sarah E. Nelson[1] and Emily J. Nelson[2]**

**Abstract:** Without a doubt, the COVID-19 pandemic has challenged the medical and legal communities in the ways they do business and their respective and often-intersecting responses to constantly changing and, sometimes, conflicting evidence and data. Particularly at the beginning of the pandemic, when little was known about the novel virus, what could be expected of healthcare workers who were tasked with taking care of patients with a contagious disease? How should healthcare providers triage resources (and also triage themselves) when faced with staffing and product shortages and still provide high-quality medical care? What are healthcare workers' and hospital visitors' obligations—ethically and legally--regarding masking and vaccination requirements? What ethical and legal considerations played into decisions to temporarily halt elective medical procedures at the start of the pandemic? This chapter will examine medical, legal, and ethical considerations on these critical issues and, in some cases, leave open questions that can perhaps inform future decision-making.

COVID-19, the disease caused by the novel coronavirus SARS-CoV-2, has created many challenges in daily life globally. As one example, the medical and legal communities have faced a number of ethical dilemmas throughout the pandemic, with intersecting responses to constantly changing and, sometimes, conflicting evidence and data. Such issues have included healthcare providers' responsibilities to care for patients with a potentially fatal disease (including with sometimes inadequate personal protective equipment), hospital visitor restrictions, and allocation of scarce resources (Nelson, 2020). How should these issues, including to whom to

---

[1] Assistant Professor, Icahn School of Medicine at Mount Sinai, New York, New York, USA

[2] Labor and Employment Attorney, GoodRx, Santa Monica, California, USA

allocate hospital beds and ventilators, be operationalized in the face of conflicting legal and ethical considerations?

While some healthcare providers may be legally obligated via contractual agreements or malpractice considerations to provide care, many healthcare workers likely feel a personal sense of obligation to care for patients beyond such legal documents. Indeed, such sentiment is reflected in the historical documents like the Hippocratic Oath—which doctors take upon graduation from medical school. In taking that Oath, providers commit to the following: "I will apply, for the benefit of the sick, all measures [that] are required" (Tyson, 2001). After the September 11, 2001 terrorist attacks, the American Medical Association reaffirmed that "it is a responsibility of health professionals to continue caring for patients even if doing so presents some danger to them" and "even in the face of greater than usual risks to physicians' own safety, health, or life" (Smith, 2020).

Yet coming into work for many healthcare workers has proved a daunting task since the beginning of the pandemic. At that time, very little was known about treatment for COVID-19 or the extent of measures that could be utilized to prevent its spread. Even scarier was the knowledge that several hospital systems lacked adequate personal protective equipment, especially in the early days of the pandemic. How could healthcare providers manage their moral and legal obligations while caring for patients in the face of these issues?

At the start of the pandemic in March 2020, reports about limited resources in European healthcare systems spurred startling concerns in the U.S. that vital critical care resources–including ventilators, dialysis machines, and critical care beds–would need to be triaged given limited supplies. Ventilators were, in fact, triaged in Italy (Rosenbaum, 2020). In the U.S., these concerns led to the development of hospital- and state-wide guidance on how to allocate resources to patients if supplies became limited. A group at Johns Hopkins had actually attempted prior to the onset of the pandemic to generate guidance on scarce resource allocation using community input (Biddison et al., 2018; Daugherty Biddison et al., 2019). A framework based on the two major ethical considerations identified (expected short- and long-term outcomes) was then developed (Daugherty Biddison et al., 2019).

During the pandemic, Johns Hopkins went a step further and convened a Scarce Resource Taskforce to flesh out available resources in Maryland and factors that might require initiating this allocation of scarce resources. Similar resource allocation discussions have been formalized in additional guidelines and recommendations (Feinstein et al., 2020; Fink, 2020; Truog et al., 2020).

Further, given the ramifications on patient care statewide, scarce resource allocation also reached the legal community, resulting in guidance provided by the governments of states including New York and Massachusetts (Commonwealth of Massachusetts, 2020; Klitzman, 2020). For instance, Massachusetts' guidance stipulates that saving lives as well as saving life-years are to be the priorities considered and that decisions may need to be made based on available critical care resources as well as severity of illness and comorbidities (Commonwealth of Massachusetts, 2020). New York State instituted legal immunity for physicians in the event that triage decisions for patients needed to be made (Klitzman, 2020). Given the need to decide who may "deserve" certain medical resources over others, many healthcare workers have been affected psychologically (Senior, 2020). Healthcare workers used to sparing no resource to cure and save their patients have been emotionally affected by the possibility of being unable to do so. New York City emergency room physician Dr. Lorna Breen's death by suicide amidst the stresses of the pandemic provides one tragic example, though one silver lining from her passing has been a renewed call to address healthcare providers' mental health (O'Connor, 2020).

As the pandemic has worn on longer than most of us anticipated, shortages of healthcare personnel have intensified for a variety of reasons, requiring further triaging of medical care. What are reasonable expectations for doctors, nurses, and other healthcare providers caring for patients, particularly those who have declined vaccination? Even before the pandemic, healthcare leaders predicted a future shortfall of nurses due to factors such as "baby boomer" nurses retiring, an increased aging population, and nurses moving away from direct patient care, among other reasons (Boyle, 2021). Unfortunately, the COVID-19 pandemic has only served to hasten this shortage amid nurses experiencing burnout and a feeling that subsequent COVID-19 surges could have been avoided by more voluntary compliance by individuals to don masks and undergo vaccination (Boyle, 2021)—which drives questions of personal and ethical responsibility. (Recent data suggest that vaccine mandates for medical professionals, discussed in more detail below, have not substantively contributed to the nursing shortage; Chidambaram et al., 2022). As a result, and given the vital role nurses play in patient care, the number of nurses available to care for patients has taken on added importance throughout the pandemic. Have any measures been suggested or put into place to mitigate healthcare provider shortages?

While Centers for Medicare and Medicaid Services (CMS) has mandated that hospitals ensure that there are sufficient numbers of nurses, licensed practical nurses, and other staff to provide adequate nursing care to patients, the government otherwise does not require specific nurse: patient ratios (Phillips et al., 2021). Several states have enacted legislation regarding nursing staffing, but only California (in 2004) has mandated specific ratios in different clinical settings (Phillips et al., 2021). For instance, while critically ill patients must be staffed at a nurse: patient ratio of 1:2 or fewer, general medical patients in the emergency room must be at 1:4 or fewer (*The Importance of the Optimal Nurse-to-Patient Ratio*, 2016). However, studies have shown that inadequate nursing staffing is associated with not only nurse burnout (Aiken et al., 2002) but also patient mortality (Griffiths et al., 2019; Needleman et al., 2011).

Perhaps most notable to the public eye, legal, ethical, and medical considerations have also converged on the subjects of mask-wearing and vaccines. The U.S. government cannot mandate that individuals receive the COVID-19 vaccine unless required to do so by a court. And while the U.S. Supreme Court blocked the U.S. Occupational Safety and Health Administration's (OSHA) mandate that workers of large (>100 employees) companies receive the vaccine or undergo regular testing, the Supreme Court did permit a CMS directive that requires healthcare workers at facilities utilizing federal funds to receive a COVID-19 vaccine, and states and cities may require that individuals receive the vaccine in certain cases (*Vaccine Mandates: What to Know*, 2022). For instance, California was the first state to mandate that all state and healthcare workers receive the vaccine or be tested at least once a week (*Vaccine Mandates: What to Know*, 2022). Hundreds of healthcare workers have been terminated from their jobs due to noncompliance with COVID-19 vaccine mandates (Gooch, 2022).

While hospitals have generally committed to treating patients regardless of vaccination status, states and institutions have taken different stances on whether visitors are permitted or whether they must be vaccinated or present proof of a negative COVID test. This situation, perhaps more than any other, is the most heartbreaking ethical crisis faced by decision-makers in the medical community. On the one hand, visitors are a source of comfort to patients, can help to alleviate patient anxiety, and can serve as advocates for the patient (Trogen, 2018). On the other hand, at least pre-vaccines, medical providers grappled with how to provide end-of-life patients a humane, comforting experience while hospital visitor restrictions were in place. In a decision that was likely far from easy, at the start of the pandemic, many hospitals banned visitors in an effort to curb the spread of COVID-19, leading to instances where patients oftentimes passed away without being surrounded by loved ones in a hospital in a tragic consequence of these policies (Wakam et al., 2020). Patients without COVID-19 also admitted to the hospital were similarly affected (Lamas, 2020).

While most visitor restrictions have eased, some hospitals continue to maintain visitor requirements intended to balance a patient's need for comfort and mental health support from visitors along with maintaining health and safety standards. For instance, California has required COVID-19 vaccination, testing, or proof of recent COVID-19 infection for hospital visitors (Aragon, 2022). Other hospitals may only require that potential visitors voluntarily report whether they are having symptoms that may be due to COVID-19 rather than objective evidence of vaccination or proof of recent testing; this of course relies on personal responsibility of these individuals to self-report, which anecdotally may not always be truthful and can thus cause great concern among healthcare workers and potentially also patients. Most recently, some states have enacted laws to better enable visitation, particularly in long-term care facilities, in light of evidence showing increased risk of death in long-term care patients as a result of neglect and social isolation due to COVID-19 visitation policies (Colombini, 2022).

Mandates for mask wearing in public have varied tremendously over the past 2 years since the pandemic began (with most states most recently dropping these mandates). Objections to mask and vaccine policies have included an infringement on the freedoms of individuals, religious exemptions, and others (Martin et al., 2021; Wheeler, 2021). However, there is strong evidence that mask mandates were indeed effective in reducing transmission and incidence of COVID-19 (Andrejko et al., 2022; Huang et al., 2022). Many hospitals and healthcare institutions required that healthcare workers and visitors wear masks. And while a Florida judge in April 2022 overturned a federal mandate that would have made masking mandatory on airplanes, trains, and other public transportation until May 3, 2022, many cities and states have instituted their own mandates - including continuing to require masks inside hospitals in New Jersey and Connecticut, for instance (Bove, 2022).

Yet another ethical and legal consequence to patients and healthcare included the fact that many medical procedures that were deemed "elective" or non-emergent were during the pandemic in an effort to free up resources for COVID-19 patients. Abortions were an example of such a procedure. For instance, Texas Governor Greg Abbott signed an executive order to halt elective surgeries including abortions early in the pandemic. Following a lawsuit by Planned Parenthood for Choice noting that adverse health risks were possible for the mother denied an abortion as well as a series of other legal steps, the order was later in essence abandoned (*Supreme Court of the United States: Search Results: Planned Parenthood Center for Choice, et al., Petitioners v. Greg Abbott, Governor of Texas, et al.*, 2021). Continued care including for cancer patients was also delayed by the pandemic that inevitably could lead to severe consequences for patients (Parmar et al., 2022; Riera et al., 2021). However, the perceived disruption in care may not have been true for other specialties, such as neurosurgery (Grassner et al., 2021; Schöni et al., 2022).

Medical and public health interventions instituted to help control the spread of COVID-19 have faced significant legal challenges and raise deep-seated ethical considerations, particularly in healthcare. Many of these decisions and policies will likely have long-lasting and often divisive effects on this country. Hopefully, the increased number of vaccinated individuals (vaccines still remain one of our greatest defenses against SARS-CoV-2, even if effectiveness may eventually wane after each dose; *COVID-19 Vaccines Work*, 2022) along with continued public education and being better cognizant of measures that can help mitigate disease overall (and not just COVID-19) such as social distancing and masking may lead us back to a somewhat more "normal" way of life and allow for the continued ability to safely care for patients.

## References

Aiken, L. H., Clarke, S. P., Sloane, D. M., Sochalski, J., & Silber, J. H. (2002). Hospital nurse staffing and patient mortality, nurse burnout, and job dissatisfaction. *JAMA, 288*(16), 1987–1993. https://doi.org/10.1001/jama.288.16.1987

Andrejko, K. L., Pry, J. M., Myers, J. F., Fukui, N., DeGuzman, J. L., Openshaw, J., Watt, J. P., Lewnard, J. A., Jain, S., & California COVID-19 Case-Control Study Team (2022). *Effectiveness of face mask or respirator use in indoor public settings for prevention of SARS-CoV-2 infection — California, February–December 2021*. CDC. https://www.cdc.gov/mmwr/volumes/71/wr/mm7106e1.htm?s_cid=mm7106e1_w

Aragon, T. (2022). *Requirements for visitors in acute health care and long-term care settings: State public health officer order: Amending the order of December 31, 2021*. California Department of Public Health. https://www.cdph.ca.gov/Programs/CID/DCDC/Pages/COVID-19/Order-of-the-State-Public-Health-Officer-Requirements-for-Visitors-in-Acute-Health-Care-and-Long-Term-Care-Settings.aspx?_cldee=Y2hlcnlsLmhhcmxlc3NAdGVuZXRoZWFsdGguY29t&recipientid=contact-41a5cda48

Biddison, E. L. D., Gwon, H. S., Schoch-Spana, M., Regenberg, A. C., Juliano, C., Faden, R. R., & Toner, E. S. (2018). Scarce resource allocation during disasters: A mixed-method community engagement study. *Chest, 153*(1), 187–195. https://doi.org/10.1016/j.chest.2017.08.001

Bove, T. (2022). Mask mandates are still in effect in a small number of places. Here's where. *Fortune*. https://fortune.com/2022/04/20/mask-mandates-where-are-they-stil-required/

Boyle, P. (2021). *Hospitals innovate amid dire nursing shortages*. AAMC. https://www.aamc.org/news-insights/hospitals-innovate-amid-dire-nursing-shortages

Chidambaram, P. & Musumeci, M. (2022). *Nursing facility staff vaccinations, boosters, and shortages after vaccination deadlines passed.* KFF. https://www.kff.org/coronavirus-covid-19/issue-brief/nursing-facility-staff-vaccinations-boosters-and-shortages-after-vaccination-deadlines-passed/

Colombini, S. (2022). New laws let visitors see loved ones in health care facilities, even in an outbreak. *NPR.* https://www.npr.org/sections/health-shots/2022/04/03/1086216581/visiting-patients-during-covid

COVID-19 Vaccines Work. (2022). *Centers for Disease Control and Prevention.* https://www.cdc.gov/coronavirus/2019-ncov/vaccines/effectiveness/work.html

Daugherty Biddison, E. L., Faden, R., Gwon, H. S., Mareiniss, D. P., Regenberg, A. C., Schoch-Spana, M., Schwartz, J., & Toner, E. S. (2019). Too many patients…A framework to guide statewide allocation of scarce mechanical ventilation during disasters. *Chest, 155*(4), 848–854. https://doi.org/10.1016/j.chest.2018. 09.025

Feinstein, M. M., Niforatos, J. D., Hyun, I., Cunningham, T. V, Reynolds, A., Brodie, D., & Levine, A. (2020). Considerations for ventilator triage during the COVID-19 pandemic. *The Lancet. Respiratory Medicine, 8*(6), e53. https://doi.org/10.1016/S2213-2600(20)30192-2

Fink, S. (2020). The hardest questions doctors may face: Who will be saved? Who won't? *The New York Times.* https://www.nytimes.com/2020/03/21/us/coronavirus-medical-rationing.html

Gooch, K. (2022). Vaccination-related employee departures at 55 hospitals, health systems. *Becker's Hospital Review.* https://www.beckers hospitalreview.com/workforce/vaccination-requirements-spur-employee-terminations-resignations-numbers-from-6-health-systems.html

Grassner, L., Petr, O., Warner, F. M., Dedeciusova, M., Mathis, A. M., Pinggera, D., Gsellmann, S., Meiners, L. C., Freigang, S., Mokry, M., Resch, A., Kretschmer, T., Rossmann, T., Navarro, F. R., Gruber, A., Spendel, M., Winkler, P. A., Marhold, F., Sherif, C., … Netuka, D. (2021). Trends and outcomes for non-elective neurosurgical procedures in Central Europe during the COVID-19 pandemic. *Scientific Reports, 11*(1), 6171. https://doi.org/10.1038/s41598-021-85526-6

Griffiths, P., Maruotti, A., Recio Saucedo, A., Redfern, O. C., Ball, J. E., Briggs, J., Dall'Ora, C., Schmidt, P. E., Smith, G. B., & Missed Care Study Group. (2019). Nurse staffing, nursing assistants and hospital mortality: retrospective longitudinal cohort study. *BMJ Quality & Safety, 28*(8), 609–617. https://doi.org/10.1136/bmjqs-2018-008043

Huang, J., Fisher, B. T., Tam, V., Wang, Z., Song, L., Shi, J., La Rochelle, C., Wang, X., Morris, J. S., Coffin, S. E., Rubin, D. M. (2022). The effectiveness of government masking mandates on COVID-19 county-level case incidence across the United States, 2020. *HealthAffairs*. https://www.healthaffairs.org/doi/10.1377/hlthaff.2021.01072

Klitzman, R. (2020). Doctors need room to make the wrenching decisions they face. *The New York Times*. https://www.nytimes.com/2020/04/04/opinion/coronavirus-doctors-lawsuits-prosecution.html

Lamas, D. J. (2020). I'm on the front lines. I have no plan for this. *The New York Times*. https://www.nytimes.com/2020/03/24/opinion/coronavirus-hospital-visits.html

Martin, S., & Vanderslott, S. (2021). "Any idea how fast 'It's just a mask!' can turn into 'It's just a vaccine!'": From mask mandates to vaccine mandates during the COVID-19 pandemic. *Vaccine*. https://doi.org/10.1016/j.vaccine.2021.10.031

Massachusetts, The Commonwealth of. (2020). *Crisis standards of care: Planning guidance for the COVID-19 pandemic*.

Needleman, J., Buerhaus, P., Pankratz, V. S., Leibson, C. L., Stevens, S. R., & Harris, M. (2011). Nurse staffing and inpatient hospital mortality. *The New England Journal of Medicine, 364*(11), 1037–1045. https://doi.org/10.1056/NEJMsa1001025

Nelson, S. E. (2020). COVID-19 and ethics in the ICU. *Critical Care, 24*(1), 10–12. https://doi.org/10.1186/s13054-020-03250-5

O'Connor, M. (2020). A doctor's emergency. *Vanity Fair*. https://www.vanityfair.com/style/2020/09/will-lorna-breens-death-change-doctors-mental-health

Parmar, A., Eskander, A., Sander, B., Naimark, D., Irish, J. C., & Chan, K. K. W. (2022). Impact of cancer surgery slowdowns on patient survival during the COVID-19 pandemic: A microsimulation modelling study. *CMAJ: Canadian Medical Association Journal = Journal de l'Association Medicale Canadienne, 194*(11), E408–E414. https://doi.org/10.1503/cmaj.202380

Phillips, J., Malliaris, A. P. & Bakerjian, D. (2021). Nursing and patient safety. *Agency for Healthcare Research and Quality: Patient Safety Network*. https://psnet.ahrq.gov/primer/nursing-and-patient-safety

Riera, R., Bagattini, Â. M., Pacheco, R. L., Pachito, D. V., Roitberg, F., & Ilbawi, A. (2021). Delays and disruptions in cancer health care due to COVID-19 pandemic: Systematic review. *JCO Global Oncology, 7,* 311–323. https://doi.org/10.1200/GO.20.00639

Rosenbaum, L. (2020). Facing Covid-19 in Italy - Ethics, logistics, and therapeutics on the epidemic's front line. *The New England Journal of Medicine,* 1–3. https://doi.org/10.1056/NEJMp2005492

Schöni, D., Halatsch, M.-E., & Alfieri, A. (2022). The impact of reduced operating room capacity on the time delay of urgent surgical care for neurosurgical patients during the COVID-19 pandemic. *Interdisciplinary Neurosurgery, 29,* 101544. https://doi.org/10.1016/j.inat.2022.101544

Senior, J. (2020). The psychological trauma that awaits our doctors and nurses. *The New York Times.* https://www.nytimes.com/2020/03/29/opinion/coronavirus-ventilators-rationing-triage.html

Smith, T. M. (2020). Doctors obliged to provide pandemic care. It wasn't always that way. *American Medical Association.* https://www.ama-assn.org/delivering-care/public-health/doctors-obliged-provide-pandemic-care-it-wasn-t-always-way?utm_source=twitter&utm_medium=social_ama&utm_term=3231454326&utm_campaign=Public+Health

*Supreme Court of the United States: Search Results: Planned Parenthood Center for Choice, et al., Petitioners v. Greg Abbott, Governor of Texas, et al.* (2021). https://www.supremecourt.gov/search.aspx?filename=/docket/docketfiles/html/public/20-305.html

*The importance of the optimal nurse-to-patient ratio.* (2016). Wolters Kluwer. https://www.wolterskluwer.com/en/expert-insights/the-importance-of-the-optimal-nursetopatient-ratio

Trogen, B. (2018). Do hospital visitors impact patient outcomes? *Clinical Correlations.* https://www.clinicalcorrelations.org/2018/08/03/do-hospital-visitors-impact-patient-outcomes/

Truog, R. D., Mitchell, C., & Daley, G. Q. (2020). The toughest triage - Allocating ventilators in a pandemic. *The New England Journal of Medicine, 382,* 1973-1975. https://doi.org/10.1056/NEJMp2005689

Tyson, P. (2001). The Hippocratic Oath today. *PBS.* https://www.pbs.org/wgbh/nova/article/hippocratic-oath-today/

*Vaccine mandates: What to know*. (2022). WebMD. https://www.webmd.com/vaccines/covid-19-vaccine/vaccine-mandates#1

Wakam, G. K., Montgomery, J. R., Biesterveld, B. E., & Brown, C. S. (2020). Not dying alone - Modern compassionate care in the Covid-19 pandemic. *The New England Journal of Medicine*. https://doi.org/10.1056/NEJMp2007781

Wheeler, L. (2021). Religious objections stand in path of mask, vaccine mandates. *Bloomberg Law*. https://news.bloomberglaw.com/health-law-and-business/religious-objections-stand-in-path-of-mask-vaccine-mandates

# U.S. HEALTHCARE WORKERS AND THE COVID-19 VACCINE: MANDATE TO VACCINATE OR NUDGE IF NO BUDGE?[1]

**Preeti John**[2]

**Abstract:** COVID-19 vaccines remain a key weapon in the fight against the deadliest modern-day global pandemic the world has experienced. Herd immunity for COVID-19 requires an estimated 55% to 82% vaccine uptake (Schaffer DeRoo et al., 2020), yet the willingness for vaccination is deeply influenced by several factors and vaccine hesitancy remains an important problem (Troiano & Nardi, 2021). The "duty to prevent" is not as undisputed as the "duty to treat", and there has been much debate about how measures to protect against COVID-19 infringe on individual liberties such as the right to autonomy and privacy. Decisions regarding whether to mandate a vaccine requires precise information about the safety and efficacy of the vaccine, transmission, severity and risks associated with the disease, and a comparative evaluation of alternatives to vaccination. A public health ethics framework is useful for analyzing ethical considerations regarding measures to promote public health, such as vaccine mandates. In this chapter, ethical considerations for COVID-19 vaccine mandates among healthcare workers (HCW) in the United States are summarized, with a brief overview of prior vaccination mandates for HCW.

## Overview of prior vaccination mandates for Health Care Workers (HCW)

### Federal and State Regulations in the United States

Since the advent of vaccines, mandates have been used to achieve herd immunity-levels of vaccination both in the general population and amongst HCW (Haviari et al., 2015; McClure et al., 2017).

---

[1] Modified with permission from the Society of Critical Care Medicine.

[2] Clinical Associate Professor, University of Maryland School of Medicine, and surgeon in the VA Maryland Healthcare System, Baltimore, MD, USA.

Current federal regulations do not include any mandatory vaccination programs; rather, vaccine mandates are generally within the purview of state and local governments. State vaccine requirements for HCW vary widely. In 1809, Massachusetts was the first state to pass a law requiring the general population to be vaccinated against smallpox (Salmon et al., 2006 ).

Some states have laws requiring HCW to be vaccinated against diseases such as measles, mumps, and rubella, with 'opt-out' provisions for when the vaccine is medically contraindicated or against the person's religious or philosophical beliefs (Megan et al., 2007). Mandatory requirements for influenza vaccination among HCW exist only in three states: Alabama, Colorado, and New Hampshire (CDC, 2014). Six states to date (Colorado, Maine, New York, Oregon, Rhode Island, Washington) have mandated COVID-19 vaccination for HCW with a "vaccinate or terminate" approach, only permitting healthcare workers to be unvaccinated if they have a valid religious or medical exemption as defined by the Equal Employment Opportunity Commission (EEOC; Pekruhn & Abbasi, 2019).

## Health Care Organizations

Many professional organizations endorse the proposition that HCW have a professional and ethical responsibility to help prevent the spread of infectious pathogens. The Society for Healthcare Epidemiology of America recommends that annual influenza vaccination is a condition of employment and professional privileges for HCW (Talbot et al., 2010). The American College of Physicians (2013) policy suggests that influenza vaccination is mandated for all HCW, unless there is a medical or religious objection.

In 2004, Virginia Mason Medical Center in Seattle, Washington, became the first health care system in the United States to make influenza vaccination a condition of employment. Within three years, the hospital reported 98% staff coverage. The remaining 2% of the staff who refused for medical or religious reasons were required to wear surgical masks when in the hospital during the flu season (Rakita et al., 2010). This influenza vaccine mandate is now followed by more than 400 healthcare organizations

(Dubov & Phung, 2015). With the COVID-19 vaccine, state and local laws are in flux; various state laws have imposed constraints on COVID vaccine mandates issued by employers (NASHP, 2022).

### Health care institutions: a unique environment

There is high risk for transmission of infections among vulnerable persons in health care settings: patients, HCW, as well as third parties with whom they come in contact.

The goal of a vaccine mandate would be 'community protection' or 'herd immunity'.

## Ethical Analysis

The root of the ethical dilemma behind a vaccine mandate is the conflict between public health ethics and the right to individual liberty and autonomy.

Utilitarian arguments for vaccine mandates claim that higher immunization rates result in a greater amount of good for all (lives saved, morbidity avoided). According to this view, mandating universal vaccination is 'morally right' because of the consequences: community protection and reduction in viral transmission resulting in reduction in infections, hospitalizations, and deaths. Critics of utilitarianism contend that it is limited to 'value monism' or the idea that there is only one fundamental 'super-value': utility - and that other values (e.g., individual liberty) do not have the same moral value (Navin & Attwell, 2019). Conversely, appealing to self-interest and individual liberty via lotteries and offering payment for vaccination (Groppe, 2021) - 'inducement' - could erode the sense of solidarity with public health and the willingness to take risks for the common good.

Mandating vaccines for HCW made on the basis of their "duty to care" draws on the utilitarian notion that this would allow maximum benefit to the public by keeping HCW healthy, thereby enabling them to provide care during the pandemic.

## Ethics Framework for Public Health

Public health aims to improve the health of populations rather than individuals. A six-step ethics framework was initially proposed in 2001 as an analytic tool to help public health practitioners assess ethical issues pertaining to proposed interventions, policies, and programs (Kass, 2001). The six questions posed in this framework are the following: what are the public health goals of the program? How effective is the program in achieving its stated goals? What are the known or potential burdens of the program? Can burdens be minimized and are there alternative approaches? Is the program implemented fairly? How can the benefits and burdens of the program be fairly balanced (Kass, 2001)?

The goal of HCW immunization programs is to influence group level transmission dynamics and reduce nosocomial transmission. Kass' ethics framework is well suited for developing and evaluating such programs. It allows for decision making within a morally pluralistic society and acknowledges that values underlying public health differ from values (such as beneficence, non-maleficence, and autonomy) that define clinical practice and research (Kass, 2001).

Childress et al. (2002) suggest that among the moral considerations most relevant to public health, the following three are critical to public health: producing benefits, preventing and removing harms, and utility (producing the maximal balance of benefits over harms and other costs). The ethical principles that are most likely to limit public health activities are justice, respect for autonomy and privacy.

## Advantages of a mandate - Beneficence, Non-maleficence

Healthcare institutions have a legal and ethical obligation to ensure a *safe* environment for patients, HCW, and visitors. Vaccination would reduce viral transmission and thereby promote health, enhance patient safety, and provide a sense of security.

HCW have an ethical/moral obligation to provide care for patients and to do no harm: vaccination would limit the spread of COVID infection to patients. The majority of burdens or harms with a vaccine mandate fall into three broad categories: risks to liberty and self-determination, risks to justice and risks to privacy and confidentiality, especially in data collection activities (Kass, 2001).

## Justice

Vaccines prevent hospitalizations and may reduce HCW shortages and protect health system capacity. This would enhance 'distributive justice' and enable healthcare organizations to fulfill their obligations to the sick and vulnerable.

'Distributive justice' requires the fair distribution of benefits and burdens. A single segment of the population cannot be subjected to disproportionate burdens, and therefore HCW cannot be the only 'frontline workers' subjected to vaccination mandates.

Considerations of 'procedural justice' are important: any mandates should be included in employment contracts; discussion of vaccine mandates during contract negotiations will provide an opportunity to employees or their representatives to express differing views (Omer, 2013). Staff/union representatives should be included in the creation of any proposed mandatory vaccination policies. Evaluation of exemption requests should be fair, consistent, and transparent. Policies regarding mandatory vaccination should be evidence based and should be responsive to changes in the relevant evidence base (Omer, 2013).

## Disadvantages of a mandate: disregarding autonomy

Administration of a vaccine requires verbal, informed consent. Mandates prioritize public health over individual autonomy, eliminate the right to informed consent or refusal of treatment. A mandate with no exemptions may infringe upon personal autonomy and privacy and leave people feeling disempowered. With regard to respecting personal autonomy, individuals should not be required to accept serious potential risks associated with the vaccine, (regardless of how rare they are), for the sake of public safety. A vaccine mandate may be counterproductive, negatively affecting morale and violating trust. The anti-vax movement sees vaccination programs as government interference in people's lives, with restriction of personal autonomy.

## Issues to Consider

### Availability of vaccines

A vaccine mandate requires unrestricted access to vaccines – therefore considerations for a mandate would apply only to areas where COVID vaccines are freely available, and supply is unlimited. Of note, the World Health Organization (WHO, 2022) does not presently support mandates for COVID-19 vaccination, instead favoring a focus on educational campaigns and universal availability of vaccines.

### "Dynamic justification"

The relative weightiness of reasons for mandating vaccines vary under different circumstances and epidemiological conditions - e.g., background vaccination rate, infectivity rate, and rate of hospitalizations (Navin & Attwell, 2019). Evidence for reduced viral transmission following COVID-19 vaccination is emerging. The incidence of new infections and hospitalizations in the United States has been steadily decreasing as more adults, adolescents and now children have been vaccinated (Moghadas et al., 2021).

## Availability of other options

If the use of personal protective equipment (PPE), physical distancing and physical barriers prevent the spread of COVID-19 and are available to HCW, mandating vaccinations may not be ethically warranted. Additionally, imposing a mandate may not be necessary for those HCW who do not interact physically with patients or can work from home. When other alternatives exist, coercion (Department of Health, 2014) - in the form of a mandate specifying threats or significant negative consequences for refusal - may not be justified.

Widespread education about the potential for vaccines to reduce transmission of a virus may even reduce the need for mandates. An "opt out" system (similar to that used for organ donation) would be an approach that would enable individual autonomy to be exercised (Blackmore, 2018).

Practical considerations should be taken into account when planning HCW immunization policies, such as efficient application of patient care based categories of HCW. Individual and union contracts can take into account differential patient contact while mandating vaccines to specific employees (Omer, 2013).

## Least Restrictive Alternative (LRA) Principle

This is a framework that provides protection for liberty in policy deliberations. When choosing between policies that are equal with respect to outcomes for public health, the policy option that least restricts liberty should be chosen (Navin & Attwell, 2019).

## 'Mandatory' vaccines and Exemptions

Contemporary forms of "mandatory" vaccination compel vaccination by direct or indirect threats of imposing restrictions in cases of non-compliance (Gravagna et al., 2020). Adverse action or termination of employment as a result of vaccine refusal could be considered 'coercion' (Department of Health, 2014), and the employer could be subject to legal action.

Per the U.S. EEOC and CDC guidance documents, vaccine mandates are subject to medical and religious-based exemptions (CDC, 2021; U.S. EEOC, n.d.). Providing exemptions for HCW would reduce their concerns and help them feel more empowered in their vaccination decision.

Facilities that opt for strict vaccine mandates should specify exemptions and offer alternatives to employment termination (i.e., teleworking when feasible, staying home without pay).

## Alternatives to Implementing a Mandate: Incentives, Nudges, Choice Architecture

Alternatives include education campaigns, 'inducement' in the form of incentives (financial or non-financial) and 'nudge strategies'. Some states have offered huge monetary incentives for people to get vaccinated (Groppe, 2021). There is no EEOC guidance specifying which vaccination incentives can be offered by employers. Thus these kinds of inducement may be legally problematic, given their potential for exploitation or 'undue inducement' and the differential effects they have on persons who may benefit more from monetary compensation (Emanuel, 2005). Nudges change behavior by means of 'choice architecture', a method of influencing choices by organizing the context in which healthcare professionals make their choices, without foreclosing other options. Using this strategy would likely increase vaccination rates in a less controversial manner than vaccine mandates (Dubov & Phung, 2015). Tax breaks or enhanced benefits packages and health insurance premiums for HCW who get vaccinated are nudge strategies that can be considered by healthcare systems (Dubov & Phung, 2015).

## Conclusions

Current EEOC guidance confirms that employers can mandate COVID-19 vaccination as long as they comply with the reasonable accommodation provisions of the Americans with Disabilities Act and title VII of the Civil Rights Act of 1964. The question faced by healthcare organizations is not so much whether vaccination can be mandated legally, rather whether it is always *ethically justifiable* to do so.

COVID-19 vaccine mandates should not be considered to be the 'magic bullet' that will ensure maximizing vaccine uptake amongst HCW. Reconciling the tension between optimizing public health, furthering social justice, and respecting personal autonomy requires that all ethical concerns regarding vaccine mandates should be taken into consideration. Engaging in an ethical analysis using a public health ethics framework is the most suitable approach to do this. Deliberations by institutional policy makers (including organizational ethics experts) and public health authorities should be transparent and should include navigation of social and cultural perspectives. 'Choice architecture' strategies including nudges, incentives and education should be utilized to enable a less paternalistic implementation of vaccine mandates.

## References


American College of Physicians (2013). Patient safety and health care provider immunization. https://www.acponline.org/acp_policy/policies/healthcare_provider_immunization_2013.pdf

Blackmore N. (2018). Flu vaccination: an opt-out system for healthcare workers. *BMJ (Clinical research ed.), 360,* k1143. https://doi.org/10.1136/bmj.k1143

CDC. (2014). *State immunization laws for healthcare workers and patients.* https://www2a.cdc.gov/vaccines/statevaccsApp/AdministrationbyVaccine.asp?Vaccinetmp=Influenza#221

CDC. (2021). *COVID-19 vaccine emergency use authorization fact sheets for recipients and caregivers.* https://www.cdc.gov/vaccines/covid-19/eua/index.html#:~:text= For%20each%20COVID%2D19%20vaccine,an%20informed%20decision%20about%20vaccination.

Childress, J. F., Faden, R. R., Gaare, R. D., Gostin, L. O., Kahn, J., Bonnie, R. J., Kass, N. E., Mastroianni, A. C., Moreno, J. D., & Nieburg, P. (2002). Public health ethics: Mapping the terrain. *The Journal of Law, Medicine & Ethics : A Journal of the American Society of Law, Medicine & Ethics, 30*(2), 170–178. https://doi.org/10.1111/j.1748-720x.2002.tb00384.x

Department of Health, Education, and Welfare, & National Commission for the Protection of Human Subjects of Biomedical and Behavioral Research (2014). The Belmont Report. Ethical principles and guidelines for the protection of human subjects of research. *The Journal of the American College of Dentists, 81*(3), 4–13.

Dubov, A., & Phung, C. (2015). Nudges or mandates? The ethics of mandatory flu vaccination. *Vaccine, 33*(22), 2530–2535.

Emanuel E. J. (2005). Undue inducement: Nonsense on stilts? *The American Journal of Bioethics, 5*(5), 9–W17. https://doi.org/10.1080/ 15265160500244959

Gravagna, K., Becker, A., Valeris-Chacin, R., Mohammed, I., Tambe, S., Awan, F. A., Toomey, T. L., & Basta, N. E. (2020). Global assessment of national mandatory vaccination policies and consequences of non-compliance. *Vaccine, 38*(49), 7865–7873. https://doi.org/10.1016/j.vaccine.2020.09.063

Groppe, M. (2021). Federal government gives OK for states to offer lotteries, cash incentives for vaccinations. *USA Today.* https://www.usatoday.com/ story/news/politics/2021/05/25/covid-vaccine-feds-ok-lotteries-cash-incentives-vaccinations/7436394002/

Haviari, S., Bénet, T., Saadatian-Elahi, M., André, P., Loulergue, P., & Vanhems, P. (2015). Vaccination of healthcare workers: A review. *Human Vaccines & Immunotherapeutics, 11*(11), 2522–2537. https://doi.org/10.1080/21645515.2015. 1082014

Lindley, M. C., Horlick, G. A., Shefer, A. M., Shaw, F. E., & Gorji, M. (2007). Assessing state immunization requirements for healthcare workers and patients. *American Journal of Preventive Medicine, 32*(6), 459–465. https://doi.org/ 10.1016/j.amepre.2007.02.009

McClure, C. C., Cataldi, J. R., & O'Leary, S. T. (2017). Vaccine hesitancy: Where we are and where we are going. *Clinical Therapeutics, 39*(8), 1550-1562. doi:10.1016/j.clinthera.2017.07.003

Moghadas, S. M., Vilches, T. N., Zhang, K., Wells, C. R., Shoukat, A., Singer, B. H., Meyers, L. A., Neuzil, K. M., Langley, J. M., Fitzpatrick, M. C., & Galvani, A. P. (2021). The impact of vaccination on coronavirus disease 2019 (COVID-19) Outbreaks in the United States. *Clinical Infectious Diseases: An Official Publication of the Infectious Diseases Society of America, 73*(12), 2257–2264. https://doi.org/ 10.1093/cid/ciab079

NASHP. (2022). *State efforts to ban or enforce COVID-19 vaccine mandates and passports.* National Academy for State Health Policy. https://www.nashp.org/state-lawmakers-submit-bills-to-ban-employer-vaccine-mandates/

Navin, M. C., Attwell, K. (2019). Vaccine mandates, value pluralism, and policy diversity. *Bioethics, 33,* 1042-1049. https://doi.org/10.1111/bioe.12645

Omer S. B. (2013). Applying Kass's public health ethics framework to mandatory health care worker immunization: the devil is in the details. *The American Journal of Bioethics, 13*(9), 55–57. https://doi.org/10.1080/15265161. 2013.825122

Pekruhn, D., & Abbasi, E. (2022, January 19). Vaccine mandates by state: Who is, who isn't, and how? https://leadingage.org/workforce/vaccine-mandates-state-who-who-isnt-and-how

Rakita, R. M., Hagar, B. A., Crome, P., & Lammert, J. K. (2010). Mandatory influenza vaccination of healthcare workers: A 5-year study. *Infection Control and Hospital Epidemiology, 31*(9), 881–888. https://doi.org/10.1086/656210

Salmon, D. A., Teret, S. P., MacIntyre, C. R., Salisbury, D., Burgess, M. A. & Halsey, N. A. (2006). Compulsory vaccination and conscientious or philosophical exemptions: Past, present, and future. *Lancet, 367*(9508), 436-442. doi: 10.1016/S0140-6736(06)68144-0

Schaffer DeRoo, S., Pudalov, N. J. & Fu, L. Y. (2020). Planning for a COVID-19 vaccination program. *JAMA, 323*(24), 2458–2459. doi:10.1001/jama.2020.8711

Talbot, T. R., Babcock, H., Caplan, A. L., Cotton, D., Maragakis, L. L., Poland, G. A., Septimus, E. J., Tapper, M. L., & Weber, D. J. (2010). Revised SHEA position paper: influenza vaccination of healthcare personnel. *Infection Control and Hospital Epidemiology, 31*(10), 987–995. https://doi.org/10.1086/656558

Troiano, G., & Nardi, A. (2021). Vaccine hesitancy in the era of COVID-19. *Public Health, 194,* 245-251. doi: 10.1016/j.puhe.2021.02.025

U.S. EEOC (n.d.). *Pandemic preparedness in the workplace and the Americans with Disabilities Act.* https://www.eeoc.gov/laws/guidance/pandemic-preparedness-workplace-and-americans-disabilities-act

WHO. (2022). COVID-19 and mandatory vaccination: Ethical considerations. https://www.who.int/publications/i/item/WHO-2019-nCoV-Policy-brief-Mandatory-vaccination-2022.1

# PART FIVE
# Healthcare management

# THE PUBLIC HEALTH PERILS OF FOLLOWING THE SCIENCE

**Molly Walker**[1]

**Abstract:** The U.S. Centers for Disease Control and Prevention (CDC) and the Food and Drug Administration (FDA) did not adhere to a single set of ethical principles and abandoned their ethical duty to the public with their ever-changing recommendations on masking and COVID-19 vaccine boosters in the U.S. These recommendations were neither based on deontological theory prioritizing individual autonomy nor utilitarian theory prioritizing benefit for the most people. Instead, they were based on limited scientific evidence and epidemiology. The agencies also ignored other public health principles, such as behavioral and social science. The result was less trust in public health agencies than ever, and unethical decisions such as assuming unvaccinated people would wear masks and denying boosters to healthy adults due to lack of evidence. Because CDC and FDA recommendations were solely based on "the science," which evolved with the pandemic, the public was left to deal with a patchwork of confusing, temporary and ever-changing decisions. Their lack of ethical principles during the pandemic opened other public health decisions, such as routine vaccination, to scrutiny, which raises questions about the future of public health and its function in society.

Public health ethics definitions are broad, and often conflicting because they must serve two sometimes conflicting principles: the public good and the right of people to maintain their autonomy. While Immanuel Kant's deontological theory prioritizes the rights of the individual over a broader public benefit, John Stuart Mill's utilitarian theory argues that an action is right if it benefits the most people (Coughlin, 2008).

The global COVID-19 pandemic saw those two principles clash repeatedly around the world. Nowhere was this more evident than in the United States. The U.S. federal government and its agencies began the pandemic following a more utilitarian philosophy, with lockdowns and mask

---

[1] Former deputy managing editor, MedPage Today, New York, New York, USA

mandates, which gradually eroded to lean more heavily on deontological theory when those mandates were lifted.

As the federal agency dedicated to public health in the United States, the Centers for Disease Control and Prevention (CDC) has its own definition of public health ethics, which it defines on its own website as "a systematic process to clarify, prioritize and justify possible courses of public health action based on ethical principles, values and beliefs of stakeholders, and scientific and other information" (CDC, 2017, para. 1).

The agency claims to take a "population-based approach" that targets "communities and populations" (para. 2). However, while the CDC discusses how their decisions serve "multiple stakeholders," they never elaborate on who those stakeholders are. Is the agency serving the community as a collective (which would fit Mill's theory) or the community as a group comprised of individuals (which would lean more towards Kant's)?

CDC goes on to contrast public health ethics with bioethics or medical ethics, claiming the latter two are "more patient or individual-centered" (para. 4). Yet the agency states that they use a variety of tools to guide their decisions, including "epidemiology, behavioral and social science, communication science, laboratory science," among others (para. 3). Most of these would lean towards a more utilitarian approach, but the CDC leaves wiggle room with the phrase "laboratory science," which focuses on data from the individual or patient, not the collective.

The agency refusing to define their "multiple stakeholders" nor take an entirely utilitarian or deontological approach to public health ethics led to confusing and often contradictory decisions during the pandemic. Instead of choosing personal autonomy or public good, CDC chose neither. They attempted to use both epidemiology and laboratory science (data based on the collective and data based on the individual, respectively). This created a morass of guidance that changed sometimes monthly. While deontological and utilitarian theories exist in a vacuum, the public does not. By choosing to focus purely on "science" without regard for how the public will act on and interpret that science, the agency sowed public distrust.

Both Kant and Mills have clear roles for the public in their definitions of ethics, but the CDC vacillated on what the role of the public was. Was it full of people with autonomy to be respected or a collective that needed to act as one to benefit society as a whole? One could argue that by refusing to pick a side, and instead focusing on the "science" as the driving principle, CDC abandoned its ethical duty to the public.

The CDC, as well as the U.S. Food and Drug Administration (FDA) are both guilty of confusing decisions that prioritized "science" without regard for how it might affect the public. By ceding recommendations to "science," they managed to violate both Kant's and Mills' ideologies, with decisions that alternately violated people's autonomy and were not in the best interest of the public.

In 2021, the CDC revised its recommendations for indoor mask usage twice in two months, first saying in May that certain people didn't have to wear masks indoors (American Hospital Association, 2021), and then taking that guidance back in July (Flaherty & Mitropolous, 2021).

In sticking completely with a data-driven decision on COVID-19 vaccine boosters for adults, both the CDC and FDA once again showed a dogmatic-like devotion to the data only, carving out specialized populations eligible for booster shots because they were the only groups where scientific evidence was available (FDA, 2021a). This resulted in a confusing patchwork decision where the FDA authorized boosters in a trickle-down fashion. Instead of giving the public simple, broad public health instructions with an eye towards behavioral and social science, they implemented a haphazard system based on age, perceived risk and in some cases, occupation, that relied on the public to determine for themselves whether they needed a booster shot.

In February 2022, the CDC once again "followed the science" on masking by changing metrics used to measure high COVID-19 case burdens and removing masking from any public health recommendation, shifting instead to an individual recommendation (Kalter & Ellis, 2021). Once again, instead of dictating a clear and effective policy to the public, the agency asked the public to make its own assessment of individual risk.

With this insistence on following laboratory science and epidemiology without regard for behavioral science or the community itself, CDC and FDA abdicated their responsibility to the public, and to tenets of public health ethics.

## A Prior History of Public Health Recommendations

While public health agencies have battled their fair share of skepticism through the years, the public has generally gone along with their recommendations, which have ranged from more utilitarian to more deontological theories. For example, when the inactivated polio vaccine was introduced in 1955, a year after clinical trials were conducted in 1.3 million children, uptake was immediate and widespread (historyofvaccines.org, 2022). Incidence of paralytic polio fell from 21,000 cases in 1952 to just 2,525 cases in 1960, a mere eight years later (Estivariz et al., 2021). In this case, the public saw polio vaccination in the utilitarian context. Polio was a public health threat, and a vaccine was developed to stop it.

In 2014, when cases of Ebola Virus were detected in the United States, states such as New York, New Jersey, and Illinois pushed for stronger quarantine recommendations than the voluntary quarantine recommended by the CDC (Yan & Botello, 2014). Famously, Dr. Nancy Synderman, former medical editor for the broadcast network NBC, violated a three-week quarantine upon returning from West Africa. She was widely ridiculed for putting those she encountered at potential risk of Ebola (Day, 2014). In this case, CDC took a deontological approach: not wanting to violate an individual's autonomy for the "greater good" of quarantine.

In both cases, the public was uninterested in the evidence behind them. Nobody insisted on a year or more of safety data before they would consider taking the polio vaccine. Nobody requested randomized clinical trials to prove that quarantine stops transmission of Ebola.

The COVID-19 pandemic changed all that, as the CDC and FDA were turned into political tools. Trump administration officials demanded rewrites, and in some cases completely suppressed data from CDC's house journal, the *Morbidity and Mortality Weekly Report,* that showed the coronavirus pandemic was getting worse, not better (Diamond, 2020). The administration interfered in the CDC's guidelines about opening schools (Mazzetti et al., 2020). Former President Trump famously refused to wear a mask himself until July 2020 after months of hedging on the necessity of masks in public spaces (Wise, 2020).

The FDA did not escape the heavy hand of the White House either, granting emergency use authorization (EUA) to anti-malarial, hydroxychloroquine, for COVID treatment in March 2020, which was later revoked when randomized controlled trials showed no benefit (FDA, 2020a, 2020b). Similarly, former FDA Commissioner, Dr. Stephen Hahn, was forced to walk back claims he made about the effectiveness of convalescent plasma to treat COVID patients, at a press conference where President Trump himself appeared to tout its benefits (Sagonowski, 2020). In 2021, FDA further limited the scope of convalescent plasma use after randomized trials again showed no benefit for most patients (Richards, 2021).

With CDC mostly sidelined or dealing with the heavy hand of government in its public health recommendations, and FDA bearing the weight of political pressure, public trust around both agencies dropped. A poll conducted from February 11 to March 15, 2021, found that 72% of those surveyed felt that public health agencies were important to the health of the nation. However, the percentage of people who gave the agencies "good or excellent" ratings declined from 59% in 2009 (the year of the swine flu pandemic) to 54% in 2021. Moreover, only half of those surveyed said they trusted the CDC, and only 37% said they trusted the FDA for public health information (Robert Wood Johnson Foundation, 2021).

The agencies had a reputation to restore. Unfortunately, in trying to burnish their own credentials, they swung the pendulum too far. And despite how well-meaning the latter approach might have been, one could argue that it, too, was unethical.

## "Follow the Science"

The incoming Biden administration made "follow the science" a big part of their plan to fight the COVID-19 pandemic (Pearce, 2021). This was embraced by newly minted CDC Director, Dr. Rochelle Walensky (Mandavilli, 2021). The idea was that the Trump administration had ignored the evidence and data from the medical community during the pandemic, choosing politics over science. Instead of sidelining the CDC, the Biden administration included the agency as part of their White House COVID-19 Response Team (White House, 2021a).

With this new administration came a new philosophy: no public health decision would be made without evidence to back it up. Data was divorced from policy and became the sole arbiter of public health decisions. By implementing evidence-based recommendations with no thought as to how they would be communicated to the public, these agencies failed to use all the tools they outlined for effective public health ethics.

Examined in a vacuum, CDC and FDA's recommendations are easily defensible when pointing to the data. But they take a haphazard approach to ethics, where it could be argued they are both violating personal autonomy and not doing the most good for the most people. This may be because there are no ethics built into science and data.

CDC's decisions on masking and COVID-19 vaccine boosters were driven almost solely by the "epidemiology" and "laboratory science" outlined by the CDC in its definition of public health ethics, but completely ignored behavioral and social science, and especially communication science. The agencies left the public with an unethical, unclear message about important public health interventions due to the CDC and FDA's overreliance on "follow the science."

## 2021-2022: Who Can Take Off Their Masks?

In May 2021, CDC issued new guidance that said vaccinated people in the United States could remove masks in indoor settings, but unvaccinated people had to continue to wear masks. This decision was indeed backed by science, as real-world evidence from Israel, as well as two smaller studies in the *Morbidity and Mortality Report*, that found vaccine effectiveness was 97% against symptomatic infection and 86% against asymptomatic infection in healthcare workers (Firth, 2021).

However, the decision appeared to exist in a vacuum that did not take personal decisions into account. CDC ignored the behavioral and social science part of such recommendations, not considering the massive resistance against masking, particularly among those who were resistant to getting vaccinated. Even a rudimentary understanding of behavioral and social science would indicate that since there was no way to determine who was vaccinated against COVID-19 or not, unvaccinated individuals would also take their masks off in public. The CDC's plan only worked if unvaccinated individuals kept their masks on. The effect was essentially lifting mask recommendations for the public during an active pandemic, a decision that "followed the science" but ignored the public health ethics of such a recommendation.

## July 2021: Masks Back On

In summer 2021, the American public had the blessing of the CDC to walk around maskless if you were vaccinated. Vaccines were effective against the original SARS-CoV-2 strain, but the same would not be true for later COVID-19 variants. Variants of concern, as defined by the World Health Organization (WHO), are when viruses "change and evolve" from the original strain (WHO, 2021).

The Delta variant (B.1.617), which originated in India, was 40%-60% more transmissible (Hagen, 2021). Data also showed infection with Delta linked to a higher rate of hospitalization and death than prior variants (Sheikh et al., 2021).

In July 2021, real-world evidence from 469 cases in Cape Cod, Massachusetts, found that three-quarters of COVID-19 cases were among the vaccinated, and that viral loads were similar in vaccinated and unvaccinated people who contracted the Delta variant (Brown et al., 2021). Based on those data, CDC adjusted their mask recommendations to say that people should mask indoors in areas of high transmission, regardless of vaccination status.

Technically, this recommendation was evidence and data driven. The understanding of the science changed, and CDC was "following the science." Yet, once again, the agency ignored behavioral and social science, as well as communication science.

The edicts were handed out with little explanation other than the science changed. There was no acknowledgment of how this might be confusing to the public, who were given leeway to remove their masks in indoor settings two months earlier. There was not even an admission that maybe, they were hasty in saying that masks could be removed in May 2021, which might have helped to assuage the public's concerns. Instead, it was the CDC once again failing to take anything beyond laboratory science and epidemiology into account.

## February 2022: Masks Back Off

As a public health agency, the CDC always used case numbers and infection rates to determine COVID-19 transmission, and those data guided their mask recommendations (Levensen & Firger, 2021). If people lived in a "substantial" or "high" transmission area, it meant they should be masking indoors, because there was a large amount of COVID-19 circulating in the community.

On February 25, 2022, the agency devised a new set of criteria to determine "risk," not transmission. "Risk" was now defined based on indicators of healthcare capacity: new hospital admissions, hospital bed utilization for COVID-19 patients and incidence of cases in a community (CDC, 2022b).

At a media briefing, Walensky couched the new guidelines in "following the science," claiming the agency had spoken to a variety of experts to determine the best criteria for evaluating severe disease (CDC, 2022c). However, she also mentioned that she wanted to "give people a break" from mask wearing.

The agency said that even in counties with enough COVID-19 transmission that they were classified as being at high risk of severe disease, masks were recommended for individuals, but not required. The nation's public health agency had finally picked a side: the deontological theory of respecting individual autonomy but refused to embrace it wholeheartedly. Instead, they hid behind "following the science" as a justification for their decisions.

## The Booster Blunder

The CDC was not alone in skirting public health ethics during the pandemic. FDA's Vaccines and Related Biological Products Advisory Committee (VRBPAC) voted down an application from vaccine manufacturer, Pfizer, for an additional dose of its COVID-19 vaccine in individuals ages 16 and up by a vote of 16-2 (Miller et al., 2021). This set off a cascade of events that would ultimately culminate in the FDA recommending boosters for all adults aged 18 and up two months later (FDA, 2021b).

In August 2021, President Biden announced at a White House media briefing that all Americans would have access to boosters by September 20, 2021 (White House, 2021b). Plagued by political interference from the last administration, the agency seemed determined to "follow the science," regardless of what the White House wanted. When FDA convened VRBPAC on September 17, 2021, the group had only real-world data available from Israel about the effect of boosters among adults ages 60 and up (Alroy-Preis & Milo, 2021).

Due to the lack of data, VRBPAC recommended limiting the scope of their authorization for boosters to a handful of groups, including older adults ages 65 and up and adults ages 18-64 with high-risk medical conditions that increased their risk for severe COVID-19. The committee expressed support for including healthcare workers and those with high occupational or institutional exposure to COVID-19, though it was not a part of their vote. FDA's resulting EUA for boosters included adults ages 18-64 with such occupational or institutional risks.

A few days later, the CDC's Advisory Committee on Immunization Practices (ACIP), a group of practicing clinicians throughout the country who act as an advisory board to the CDC on vaccines, disagreed with the FDA's decision (Branswell, 2021). ACIP claimed there was no "science" that adults with high exposure of COVID-19 contracted severe disease. They voted down a recommendation for boosters for high-risk occupational groups, such as teachers and healthcare workers. Like VRBPAC, ACIP claimed there was a "lack of data" to recommend boosters for this group.

The next day, Walensky overruled her own panel, arguing that it would be unethical to withhold boosters from people who wanted them, explaining at a media briefing: "We are tasked with analyzing complex, often imperfect data to make concrete recommendations that optimize health. In a pandemic, even with uncertainty, we must take actions that we anticipate will do the greatest good" (Walker, 2021a, para.6).

This was one of the first times where Walensky acknowledged that the agency was acting on "imperfect" data. On one hand, it could be argued that she followed the CDC's tenets of public health ethics by incorporating behavioral and social science. While there was no data that showed these professionals had higher risk of severe disease due to their occupation alone, a high risk of exposure could infer a high risk of infection and resulting serious complications. It was an ethical decision to protect those on the "front lines" of working with the public, such as healthcare professionals, teachers and those who worked at homeless shelters.

However, the die had been cast for confusion. By overruling her own panel, which cited "lack of data," Walensky did not "follow the science." This produced a patchwork of risk-based recommendations for boosters, leading to widespread public confusion (Flam, 2021).

Two months later, the FDA expanded its EUA for boosters to include "boosters for all" individuals ages 18 and up. This time, the ACIP had no qualms about endorsing this recommendation (CDC, 2021). Likewise, both CDC and ACIP endorsed boosters for individuals ages 12-17 (CDC, 2022a). In the agency's statement, Walensky said that "this booster dose will provide optimized protection" against the Omicron variant, but this begged the question of how the agency could only recommend boosters for limited populations two months earlier, but suddenly have enough data to recommend them now (CDC, 2022a).

As of early 2022, less than half of the fully vaccinated population, including individuals ages 12 and up and adults ages 18-64, had received a booster shot. This drove suspicion of the agency. Why were boosters not recommended two months ago, but suddenly recommended now? These evidence-driven recommendations muddied the messaging waters, even if they were technically supported by data.

## Upholding Ethical Standards: What Should've Been

At the ACIP meeting in September 2021 where the panel ultimately voted down a recommendation for a booster dose among adults ages 18-64 who were at high risk of occupational exposure, panel member Dr. Pablo Sanchez, of Nationwide Children's Hospital in Columbus, Ohio, voted no on the recommendation, with a prescient remark: "We might as well say just give it to everybody 18 and older" (Walker, 2021b, para. 8). He was suggesting something that was within the ACIP's power to do: a conditional recommendation. This type of recommendation meant that an individual could receive the vaccine based on their own assessment of benefits and risks, but it's not a full "recommendation" by the CDC (2019).

ACIP's conditional recommendations satisfy both ends of the ethical spectrum. They maintain an individual's autonomy, since it allows the individual to determine their own benefits and risks, but it also benefits the most people, since everyone who wants to protect themselves has that ability.

For two months, not making boosters available to adults who wanted them could be argued as an unethical decision by public health agencies. It both violated an individual's autonomy to choose to be protected and did not benefit the public good. The harms of COVID-19 vaccines are so rare, and in proportion to other approved vaccines such as influenza (Kim et al., 2022), that there is no ethical argument for saying that they aren't appropriate for a certain subset of the adult population. Pfizer's COVID-19 vaccine (Comirnaty) was originally authorized by the FDA for individuals ages 16 and up, and Moderna (Spikevax) was authorized for adults ages 18 and up. There was no scientific evidence that said an adult without a comorbid condition would be "harmed" by a booster shot. Yet, "follow the science" meant adults who did not fall into a particular category were left unprotected, because absence of data was interpreted as negative data.

While the White House should not have intervened in the decisions of public health agencies, FDA and CDC ultimately came to the same conclusion as the Biden administration. And the data that the agencies held out for was not iron-clad data from large phase III clinical trials, but piecemeal real-world evidence from other countries and immunogenicity data from boosters within subgroups of trial populations. They "followed the science," but it led them down an unethical path, and sowed more distrust among those across both sides of the ethical spectrum.

While one could argue that a medical intervention, like a vaccine, might violate an individual's autonomy, the same argument cannot be made for indoor mask use. This insistence on data to support recommendations that offered little to no harm was especially egregious. The CDC never should have said that vaccinated people could stop wearing masks since they knew unvaccinated people would stop wearing them, as well. Had they left the mask recommendation in place, they wouldn't have had to reinstate it two months later, when the real-world evidence changed. Letting unvaccinated people go without masks in the summer of 2021, as the Delta variant was increasing, was a violation of their own ethical principles.

In order to follow their own guidelines, CDC should've recommended wearing a mask indoors for at least while the U.S. government declared that COVID-19 was a public health emergency, which was still the case as of March 2022. To abruptly change metrics to fit their "follow the science" narrative seemed to be an excuse to lift mask recommendations while the country was still amidst a pandemic.

In trying to walk a tightrope between evidence-based recommendations and practical public health strategy, CDC and FDA have overcorrected for their shaky start at the beginning of the pandemic. The agencies erred on the side of "the science" without giving equal consideration to "the public," which was a violation of both deontological and utilitarian theories.

More worryingly for the public is the CDC moving a public health intervention like masking out of the realm of the collective good means they may have given tacit endorsement to this highly unethical slippery slope.

Public health recommendations – such as routine childhood vaccinations to enter school – were always considered in the public interest. Yet in March 2022, Florida's Surgeon General, Dr. Joseph Lapado, recommended against "healthy kids" receiving the COVID-19 vaccine, using the same "personal choice" narrative as the CDC used to lift mask mandates (Anderson et al., 2022). States like Texas have been trying to get required childhood vaccinations converted into "personal decisions" for years, using terms like "health freedom" (Hotez, 2021).

The CDC opened this can of ethical worms with their haphazard public health decisions based on weak ethical principles. With a mishmash of decisions that swung between individual autonomy and the collective good, based on the flimsy ethical notion of "following the science," they have truly lost the right to call themselves the nation's public health agency.

## References

Alroy-Preis, S., & Milo, R. (2021, September 17). *Booster protection against confirmed infection and severe disease: data from Israel*. Vaccines and Related Biological Products Advisory Committee, Food and Drug Administration, U.S. Department of Health and Human Services. https://www.fda.gov/media/152205/download

American Hospital Association (2021, May 13). *CDC ends indoor mask requirements for fully vaccinated people*. https://www.aha.org/news/headline/2021-05-13-cdc-ends-indoor-mask-requirements-fully-vaccinated-people

Anderson, Z., Rosica, J. L., Leake, L., Freeman, L., Bloch, E., & Fins, A. (2022, March 7). Florida to be the first state to recommend healthy kids not get COVID vaccine, contradicting CDC. *Sarasota Herald Tribune*. https://www.heraldtribune.com/story/news/politics/2022/03/07/florida-surgeon-general-joseph-ladapo-recommending-against-covid-vaccine-healthy-kids/9411801002/

Branswell, H. (2021, September 23). *Advisory committee recommends wide swath of Americans be offered Covid-19 vaccine boosters*. STAT News. https://www.statnews.com/2021/09/23/covid19-vaccine-boosters-cdc-acip/

Brown, C. M., Vostok, J., Johnson, H., Burns, M., Gharpure, R., Sami, S., Sabo, R., Hall, N., Foreman, A., Schubert, P. L., Gallagher, G. R., Fink, T., Madoff, L. C.,

Gabriel, S. B., MacInnis, B., Park, D. J., Siddle, K. J., Harik, V., Arvidson, D. & Laney, A. S. (2021). Outbreak of SARS-CoV-2 infections, including COVID-19 vaccine breakthrough infections, associated with large public gatherings – Barnstable County, Massachusetts, July 2021. *Morbidity and Mortality Weekly Report, 70*(31),1059-1062. http://dx.doi.org/10.15585/mmwr.mm7031e2

CDC: Office of Science. (2017, October). *Public health ethics*. U.S. Department of Health and Human Services, Centers for Disease Control and Prevention. https://www.cdc.gov/os/integrity/phethics/index.htm

CDC. (2019, October 8). *Update to the CDC and the HICPAC recommendation categorization scheme for infection control and prevention guideline recommendations*. Centers for Disease Control and Prevention, U.S. Department of Health and Human Services. https://www.cdc.gov/hicpac/workgroup/recommendation-scheme-update.html

CDC. (2021, November 19). *CDC expands eligibility for COVID-19 booster shots to all adults*. Centers for Disease Control and Prevention, U.S. Department of Health and Human Services. https://www.cdc.gov/media/releases/2021/s1119-booster-shots.html

CDC. (2022a, January 5). *CDC expands booster shot eligibility and strengthens recommendations for 12–17-year-olds*. Centers for Disease Control and Prevention, U.S. Department of Health and Human Services. https://www.cdc.gov/media/releases/2022/s0105-Booster-Shot.html

CDC. (2022b). *COVID-19 integrated county view*. U.S. Department of Health and Human Services, Centers for Disease Control and Prevention. Retrieved on March 31, 2022. https://covid.cdc.gov/covid-data-tracker/#county-view?list_select_state=all_states&list_select_county=all_counties&data-type=Community_Levels

CDC. (2022c, February 25). *Transcript for CDC media telebriefing: Update on COVID-19*. U.S. Department of Health and Human Services, Centers for Disease Control and Prevention. https://www.cdc.gov/media/releases/2022/t0225-covid-19-update.html

Coughlin S.C. (2008). How many principles for public health ethics? *Open Public Health Journal, 1*, 8-16. https://www.ncbi.nlm.nih.gov/pmc/articles/PMC2804997/

Day, P. K. (2014, October 14). Media react to NBC News' Dr. Nancy Snyderman violating Ebola quarantine. *Los Angeles Times*. https://www.latimes.com/

entertainment/tv/showtracker/la-et-st-media-reacts-nbc-news-nancy-snyderman-ebola-violation-20141014-story.html

Diamond, D. (2020, September 11). *Trump officials interfered with CDC reports on COVID-19*. Politico. https://www.politico.com/news/2020/09/11/exclusive-trump-officials-interfered-with-cdc-reports-on-covid-19-412809

Estivariz, C. F., Link-Gelles, R. & Shimabukuro, T. (2021, August 18). *Epidemiology and prevention of vaccine-preventable diseases: Poliomyelitis*. Centers for Disease Control and Prevention. https://www.cdc.gov/vaccines/pubs/pinkbook/polio.html#poliovirus

FDA Office of Media Affairs (2020, March 28). *Coronavirus (COVID-19) update: Daily roundup March 30, 2020*. U.S. Department of Health and Human Services, Food and Drug Administration. https://www.fda.gov/news-events/press-announcements/coronavirus-covid-19-update-daily-roundup-march-30-2020

FDA Office of Media Affairs (2020, June 15). *Coronavirus (COVID-19) update: FDA revokes emergency use authorization for chloroquine and hydroxychloroquine*. U.S. Department of Health and Human Services, Food and Drug Administration. https://www.fda.gov/news-events/press-announcements/coronavirus-covid-19-update-fda-revokes-emergency-use-authorization-chloroquine-and

FDA (2021a, September). *FDA authorizes booster dose of Pfizer-BioNTech COVID-19 vaccine for certain populations*. U.S. Department of Health and Human Services, Food and Drug Administration Office of Media Affairs. https://www.fda.gov/news-events/press-announcements/fda-authorizes-booster-dose-pfizer-biontech-covid-19-vaccine-certain-populations

FDA. (2021b, November 19). *Coronavirus (COVID-19) update: FDA expands eligibility for COVID-19 vaccine boosters*. Food and Drug Administration, U.S. Department of Health and Human Services. https://www.fda.gov/news-events/press-announcements/coronavirus-covid-19-update-fda-expands-eligibility-covid-19-vaccine-boosters

Firth, S (2021, May 13). *CDC drops most mask rules for the fully vaccinated*. MedPage Today. https://www.medpagetoday.com/infectiousdisease/ covid19 vaccine/92569

Flaherty, A, & Mitropoulos, A. (2021, July 29). *CDC mask decision followed stunning findings from Cape Cod beach outbreak*. ABC News. https://abcnews.go.com/Politics/cdc-mask-decision-stunning-findings-cape-cod-beach/story?id= 79148102

Flam, F. (2021, October 25). How to cut through the confusion on vaccine boosters. *Bloomberg/Washington Post.* https://www.washingtonpost.com/business/how-to-cut-through-the-confusion-on-vaccine-boosters/2021/10/25/350007b0-358b-11ec-9662-399cfa75efee_story.html

Hagen, A. (2021, July 30). *How dangerous is the Delta variant (B.1.617.2)?* American Society for Microbiology. https://asm.org/Articles/2021/July/How-Dangerous-is-the-Delta-Variant-B-1-617-2

Historyofvaccines.org (2022). *History of polio.* The College of Physicians of Philadelphia. https://www.historyofvaccines.org/timeline#EVT_100324

Hotez, P. J. (2021). America's deadly flirtation with anti-science and the medical freedom movement. *Journal of Clinical Investigation, 131*(7). e149072. https://doi.org/10.1172/JCI149072..

Kalter, L, & Ellis, R (2022, February 25). *CDC relaxes mask guidance for most of U.S. schools.* WebMD. https://www.webmd.com/lung/news/20220225/biden-administration-to-relax-face-mask-guidelines

Kim, M. S., Jung, S. Y., Ahn, J. G., Park, S. J., Shoenfeld, Y., Kronbichler, A., Koyanagi, A., Dragioti, E., Tizaoui, K., Hong, S. H., Jacob, L., Salem, J., Yon, D. K., Lee, S. W., Ogino, S., Kim, H., Kim, J. H., Excler, J., Marks, F. & Smith, L. (2022). Comparative safety of mRNA COVID-19 vaccines to influenza vaccines: A pharmacovigilance analysis using WHO international database. *Journal of Medical Virology, 94,* 1085-1095. https://doi.org/10.1002/jmv.27424

Levensen, E., & Firger, J. (2021, July 28). *What the CDC's 'substantial' and 'high' levels of Covid-19 transmission actually mean.* CNN. https://www.cnn.com/2021/07/28/health/substantial-or-high-covid-19-transmission-wellness/index.html

Mandavilli, A. (2021, June 10). The CDC's new leader follows the science. Is that enough? *New York Times.* https://www.nytimes.com/2021/06/10/health/walensky-cdc-covid.html

Mazzetti, M., Weiland, N. & LaFraniere, S. (2020, September 28). Behind the White House effort to pressure the C.D.C. on school openings. *New York Times.* https://www.nytimes.com/2020/09/28/us/politics/white-house-cdc-coronavirus-schools.html

Miller, S. G., Lewis, R., & Edwards, E. (2021, September 17). *FDA advisory group rejects Covid boosters for most, limits to high-risk groups.* NBC News.

https://www.nbcnews.com/health/health-news/fda-advisory-group-rejects-covid-boosters-limits-high-risk-groups-rcna2074

Pearce, K. (2021, January 15). *'Follow the science' and other principles of Biden's pandemic response plan.* Johns Hopkins University Hub. https://hub.jhu.edu/2021/01/15/biden-covid-response-hopkins-alums/

Richards, M. (2021, February 4). *FDA in brief: FDA updates emergency use authorization for COVID-19 convalescent plasma to reflect new data.* U.S. Department of Health and Human Services, Food and Drug Administration. https://www.fda.gov/news-events/fda-brief/fda-brief-fda-updates-emergency-use-authorization-covid-19-convalescent-plasma-reflect-new-data

Robert Wood Johnson Foundation. (2021, May). *The public's perspective on the United States public health system.* Harvard T.H. Chan School of Public Health. https://cdn1.sph.harvard.edu/wp-content/uploads/sites/94/2021/05/RWJF-Harvard-Report_FINAL-051321.pdf

Sagonowsky, E. (2020, August 25). *FDA chief walks back plasma claims, but his correction still missed the mark, experts say.* Fierce Pharma. https://www.fiercepharma.com/pharma/fda-chief-hahn-walks-back-plasma-claims-but-experts-say-correction-wasn-t-accurate

Sheikh, A., McMenamin, J., Taylor, B., & Robertson, C. (2021). SARS-CoV-2 Delta VOC in Scotland: demographics, risk of hospital admission, and vaccine effectiveness. *The Lancet, 397*(10293), 2461-2462. https://doi.org/10.1016/S0140-6736(21)01358-1

Walker, M. (2021a, September 24). *CDC overrules advisors on Pfizer booster for high-risk workers.* MedPage Today. https://www.medpagetoday.com/infectiousdisease/covid19vaccine/94692

Walker, M. (2021b, September 23). *CDC panel: Thumbs down on Pfizer booster for healthcare workers.* MedPage Today. https://www.medpagetoday.com/infectiousdisease/covid19vaccine/94681

White House (2021a). *Press briefing by White House COVID-19 response team and public health officials.* https://www.whitehouse.gov/briefing-room/press-briefings/2021/02/08/press-briefing-by-white-house-covid-19-response-team-and-public-health-officials/

White House (2021b). *Fact sheet: President Biden to announce new actions to protect Americans from COVID-19 and help state and local leaders fight the virus.* The White

House. https://www.whitehouse.gov/briefing-room/statements-releases/2021/08/18/fact-sheet-president-biden-to-announce-new-actions-to-protect-americans-from-covid-19-and-help-state-and-local-leaders-fight-the-virus/

Wise, A. (2020, July 11). *Trump wears mask in public for first time during Walter Reed visit*. NPR. https://www.npr.org/sections/coronavirus-live-updates/2020/07/11/889810926/trump-wears-mask-in-public-for-first-time-during-walter-reed-visit

WHO. (2021, December 4). *Coronavirus disease (COVID-19): Variants of SARS-CoV-2*. World Health Organization. https://www.who.int/emergencies/diseases/novel-coronavirus-2019/question-and-answers-hub/q-a-detail/coronavirus-disease-(covid-19)-variants-of-sars-cov-2

Yan, H., & Bothelo, G. (2014, October 27). *Ebola: some states announce mandatory quarantines. Now what?* CNN. https://www.cnn.com/2014/10/27/health/ebola-us-quarantine-controversy/index.html

# THE ETHICS OF COVID-19 VACCINES AND VACCINATION

**Michelle D. Fiscus**[1]

**Abstract:** The COVID-19 pandemic has been wrought with challenges, not the least of which have been the ethical considerations of COVID-19 vaccine development, distribution, incentivization, administration, and mandates. Guidance to states from the United States Centers for Disease Control and Prevention (CDC), especially as it pertained to the prioritization of populations and distribution of vaccines, was often incomplete or provided after states had determined how vaccines would be distributed. This resulted in approaches that differed considerably from state to state. Additionally, individual concerns around the ethics of accepting vaccination, along with the use of those arguments to justify opposition to vaccination, complicate messaging and create challenges to ensuring that all who are eligible for vaccination have access to vaccination and the scientifically based information needed to make an informed decision. This chapter will focus on the unique ethical considerations of COVID-19 vaccine development, distribution, incentivization, administration, mandates, and invoked exceptions to mandates in the United States through a review of existing publications and health policy, and detail the impact of these weighty issues upon the success of vaccination efforts in the United States.

## The Ethics of COVID-19 Vaccines and Vaccination

The ethics involving COVID-19 vaccinations are many—from the ethical manufacturing of the vaccines to the ethics of clinical trials, vaccine distribution, incentivization, administration, and mandates. Additionally, individual concerns around the ethics of accepting vaccination, along with the use of those arguments to justify opposition to vaccination, further complicate messaging and create challenges to

[1] Associate Clinical Professor, Children's Hospital at Vanderbilt University Medical Center, Nashville, Tennessee, USA

ensuring that all who are eligible for vaccination have access to vaccination and the scientifically based information needed to make an informed decision.

This chapter will focus on the unique ethical considerations of COVID-19 vaccine development, distribution, incentivization, administration, mandates, and invoked exceptions to mandates, in the United States through a review of existing publications and health policy, and detail the impact of these weighty issues upon the success of vaccination efforts in the United States.

## Ethics and COVID-19 Vaccine Development

Vaccine development is wrought with ethical dilemmas, especially when those vaccines are developed under the pressures of a pandemic caused by a novel virus like SARS-CoV-2. The ethics of an ongoing placebo arm in trials where the vaccine has been proven effective in preventing hospitalization and death, enrolling minors who are too young to provide informed consent, and enrolling participants from high-risk populations, such as those who are incarcerated, were all further complicated by the need to develop COVID-19 vaccines at warp speed (Wang et al., 2020). While much of this debate occurs within the scientific community, one ethical consideration has garnered significant public attention: the use of human fetal cell lines in vaccine manufacturing.

According to a Pew Research study of more than 10,000 U.S. adults surveyed in August 2021, White evangelical Protestants were less likely to have been vaccinated against COVID-19 than other religious groups (Funk & Gramlich, 2021). This may be due, at least in part, to the use of fetal cell lines in the development of some vaccines. Vaccines against varicella (chicken pox), rubella, hepatitis A, and rabies, and the COVID-19 vaccine developed by Johnson & Johnson are all produced by growing the targeted viruses in fetal cells which were obtained from fetuses that were electively aborted in the 1960s. Viruses that infect humans replicate best in human cell lines, and these fetal cell lines are essentially "immortal," with the same cell lines being used continuously since they were isolated decades ago. Once the virus is grown in the cells, the virus is purified, removing all traces of the fetal cells and their cellular DNA; therefore, while the viruses used to make the vaccines were produced using fetal cells, the vaccines themselves do not contain them (Children's Hospital of Philadelphia, 2021).

Many organized religions espouse tenets that oppose abortion, but support vaccination. Leaders of the Catholic church, the National Association of Evangelicals, the Orthodox (Jewish) Union, the American Society of Muslim Jurists, and the British Islamic Medical Association have issued statements in support of the Pfizer/BioNTech and Moderna vaccines, which are not manufactured using fetal cell lines (Stanford Medicine, 2021). In 2005, the Vatican released a statement, *Moral Reflections on Vaccines Prepared from Cells Derived from Aborted Human Fetuses*, in which Catholics were reassured they could receive vaccines developed using aborted fetal cell lines if there was no alternative available and if refusing to receive such a vaccine could result in serious harm (Sgreccia, 2005). In December 2020, the Vatican addressed concerns about COVID-19 vaccines specifically, saying:

> All vaccinations recognized as clinically safe and effective can be used in good conscience with the certain knowledge that the use of such vaccines does not constitute formal cooperation with the abortion from which the cells used in production of the vaccines derive. (Ladaria & Morandi, 2020, para. 6)

The document goes on to encourage pharmaceutical companies and governmental health agencies to "produce, approve, distribute and offer ethically acceptable vaccines that do not create problems of conscience for either health care providers or the people to be vaccinated" (para. 7). Since the first COVID-19 vaccines produced by Pfizer/BioNTech and Moderna were not manufactured using fetal cell lines, the ability to receive a vaccine that is without these ethical concerns already exists (Zimmerman, 2021).

When it comes to the use of religion as justification to refuse vaccination, three ethical issues arise: First, some use religious exemptions in lieu of philosophical or ideological objections to vaccination. In other words, when one is unable to legally exercise an objection based on conscience, some choose to falsely claim that the objection is based on their closely held religious beliefs. Second, there is the prioritization of one's claimed religious belief over the health and safety of that of the individuals they may go on to infect. Lastly, there is the prioritization of a parent or guardian's religious beliefs over the wellbeing of their child, who may have yet to make decisions about their own religious beliefs.

Where the line blurs is in the distinction between a sincerely held religious belief and an ideological one. Regardless of the support of COVID-19 vaccination by nearly all organized religions and the widespread availability of COVID-19 vaccines that do not utilize fetal cell lines in their manufacturing, COVID-19 vaccine mandates have driven large numbers of individuals who span different religions and backgrounds to request religious exemptions from vaccination. As COVID-19 and its vaccines have become politically polarizing in the United States, religious exemptions are commonly being used as a mechanism to exempt someone from a vaccine mandate based upon their political views (Fea et al., 2021).

While the Catholic Church does not support vaccine mandates, it does encourage vaccination, and Pope Francis has suggested that getting vaccinated against the coronavirus is a "moral obligation" (Winfield, 2022, para. 1). A leader within the Christian Science Church wrote, "...our practice isn't a dogmatic thing. Church members are free to make their own choices on all life-decisions, in obedience to the law, including whether or not to vaccinate. These aren't decisions imposed by their church" (Christian Science, 2022, para. 5). Despite support for vaccination from religious leaders, increasing numbers of individuals are claiming religious exemptions from vaccination for themselves or their children (Kaiser Health News, 2021).

When the New Mexico Department of Health surveyed parents who had filed for exemptions from school-required vaccinations, 54 percent of respondents said their objections arose from "philosophical" or "personal" beliefs. However, New Mexico allows only medical and religious exemptions to required vaccinations, not philosophical exemptions. The results of this survey suggest most respondents were untruthful when filing for a religious exemption to school-mandated vaccines (Reiss, 2014).

Merriam-Webster defines the verb *lie* as, "to make an untrue statement with intent to deceive; to create a false or misleading impression" (Merriam-Webster.com, n.d.). Representatives from four major religions, Judaism, Catholicism, Islam, and Protestantism, all agreed in interviews with the Religion News Service that lying is only acceptable when used to avoid evil (Winston, 2017). As vaccines that are recommended by the Advisory Committee on Immunization Practices (ACIP) are widely considered to be safe and effective, it is difficult to make the argument that falsely claiming religious exemption is ethical.

Most religions call for followers to "love thy neighbor" (Near Neighbours, 2018). Yet claiming religious exemption, whether sincere or not, prioritizes the beliefs of the individual over the wellbeing of neighbors and the community. In 1944, the U.S. Supreme Court concluded in *Prince v. Massachusetts* that, "The right to practice religion freely does not include liberty to expose the community or the child to communicable disease or the latter to ill health or death" (LawPipe, n.d., para. 6). Kriszta Sajber, Ph.D., assistant professor of philosophy at the University of Michigan, said in an interview with the *University of Michigan-Dearborn News*:

> When someone medically eligible with access to vaccinations does not accept a vaccine, they reserve to themselves the right to harm others. However, no one has the right to harm others.... Therefore, from an ethical perspective, no one has a 'right' to refuse a vaccine. (Tuxbury, 2021, para. 11)

Some health care organizations, however, may be relieved to have the option of approving religious exemptions, as doing so may help to keep hospitals from laying off critical staff during times when the medical system is under great stress (Levy & Messerly, 2022). In accepting ideological exemptions disguised as religious objections, those health care organizations may be creating their own ethical quandary: allowing unvaccinated health care workers to risk exposing patients to the virus versus laying off staff who will not comply with the mandate and risking not having staff to care for patients at all.

Parental refusal of recommended childhood vaccinations has increased in recent years, and the COVID-19 pandemic and politicization of its vaccines has only increased vaccine hesitancy. Historically, parents who have refused to provide their children with recommended childhood vaccinations have benefited from herd immunity, or the protection provided to unvaccinated individuals by a well-vaccinated community. In *Public Health and Personal Choice: The Ethics of Vaccine Mandates and Parental Refusal in the United States*, Rebecca Horan and Jonelle DePetro (2019) argue, "those who refuse vaccination yet benefit from herd immunity can be considered free-riders who are acting against the principle of fairness and, therefore, acting unethically" (p. 7). In their book, *Principles of Biomedical Ethics*, Thomas Beauchamp and James F. Childress (2019) outline four principles that are to be considered when faced with ethical dilemmas in medicine: autonomy (self-rule), nonmaleficence (the obligation to do no harm), beneficence (obligation to act for another's benefit), and justice (equitable treatment across population groups), all of which are to be considered with equal weight. As children are not considered to be autonomous, parents make decisions on their behalf. However, according to Douglas S. Diekema, MD, MPH and the American Academy of Pediatrics' Committee on Bioethics (2005), parents may make choices on behalf of their child unless those choices place their child at substantial risk of serious harm. When it comes to COVID-19, the risk to children who are infected with the SARS-CoV-2 virus is heavily debated. While serious illness and death among children with COVID-19 is rare compared to that of adults, the long-term effects of the disease are still unknown. As of May 2022, more than 13 million pediatric cases of COVID-19 had been reported in the United States, representing 19 percent of all cases (American Academy of Pediatrics, 2022). Based on these statistics and the unknown health impact of COVID-19 in children, there is an argument that withholding vaccination is not in the best interest of the child.

When considering only the principle of autonomy, the inability to refuse vaccination based upon one's personal or religious beliefs would appear to be unethical. However, when beneficence is considered, high vaccine uptake reduces cases and deaths and supports the exclusion of non-medical exemptions. Even when considering nonmaleficence and the risk of adverse reactions to COVID-19 vaccines, the risk is exceedingly small. So long as there is justice in access to COVID-19 vaccines, the balance when considering bioethical principles is shifted in favor of vaccination (Horan & DePetro, 2019).

## Ethics and U.S. COVID-19 Vaccine Distribution

A paper published in the *Journal of Medical Ethics* (Jecker, 2021a) outlined an ethical framework for the global distribution of COVID-19 vaccines—essentially stating that, while vaccines were limited in supply, they should first be provided to frontline and essential workers, those at greatest risk of infection, and those at greatest risk of severe disease or death. But in October 2020, nearly two months before the first Emergency Use Authorization (EUA) for a COVID-19 vaccine was given by the U.S. Food and Drug Administration (FDA), the 64 immunization programs across states, major cities, territories, and tribal nations were required by the Centers for Disease Control and Prevention (CDC) to submit their plans for the distribution of those vaccines across their jurisdictions. This meant developing a distribution plan before the details of vaccine storage, handling, and administration were understood and prior to the publication of ethical frameworks that could be used as guidance. As these jurisdictions developed their plans, they were tasked by the CDC to consider how these vaccines would be distributed to reach those populations most severely impacted by COVID-19, as well as those critical to the continued functioning of basic services. While the CDC provided an "interim playbook" to jurisdictions that outlined basic assumptions and hypothetical scenarios, it did not provide guidance as to how to go about prioritizing populations to receive a limited initial supply of vaccinations (CDC, 2020). According to an analysis of 47 of the 64 plans by the Kaiser Family Foundation (Kates et al., 2020), every plan prioritized health care workers, essential workers, and those at high risk for serious illness (older people and those with pre-disposing health risk factors), but jurisdictions varied in their ability to define and enumerate those categories. The KFF analysis found that only 53 percent of the reviewed plans mentioned incorporating racial and ethnic minority groups or disparities in health equity when identifying priority populations. Another review of 51 plans (all states and the District of Columbia) was conducted by researchers at the University of Chicago (Hardeman et al., 2021). Of the 51 reviewed plans, only 20 (39%) made mention of involving a health equity committee when creating their plans, and only four (20%) of those plans mentioned involving an ethicist. The study also found that 49 percent of states without health equity communities did not partner with organizations that served minority populations when developing their plans.

It wasn't until December 20, 2020, that the Advisory Committee on Immunization Practices (ACIP) published its *Interim Recommendations for Allocation of COVID-19 Vaccine*, which was well after jurisdictions had already made determinations about how they would prioritize "essential" populations and had communicated those decisions to the public (Dooling et al., 2021). While the prioritization of some frontline and essential workers, such as healthcare workers, was straightforward, the definition of "essential worker" varied by jurisdiction. Approximately half of the states with essential worker orders or directives deferred to the federal definition developed by the U.S. Cybersecurity and Infrastructure Security Agency (National Conference of State Legislatures, 2021). CISA states in its guidance that the "list of identified essential critical infrastructure workers is intended to be overly inclusive," placing the burden on jurisdictions to sub-prioritize within the list due to the limited availability of vaccines. Due to the exhaustive nature of the list, jurisdictions were often required to prioritize one type of "critical worker" over another, but may not have had data upon which to base those decisions. When ACIP's recommendations were released, jurisdictions were faced with the choice of proceeding with the priorities they had already established, despite the recommendations, or realigning their priorities to conform to the ACIP recommendations and, in some cases, informing previously prioritized populations that they were no longer at the front of the line.

Perhaps the most controversial group when it came to prioritizing populations for vaccination was that of incarcerated people. The *Framework for Equitable Allocation of COVID-19 Vaccine* (National Academies of Sciences, Engineering, and Medicine, 2020), published two months prior to the ACIP recommendations, prioritized those living and working in prisons, jails, and detention centers equally with teachers and other essential workers employed in settings that placed them at high risk for exposure to the virus. In mid-November 2020, the American Medical Association (2020) called for incarcerated populations to be prioritized in the initial phases of COVID-19 vaccine distribution. In the ACIP recommendations, however, corrections officers were classified as non-healthcare frontline workers and placed in Phase 1b of their prioritization plan, while incarcerated people were placed in Phase 2 with "all other persons aged ≥16 years not already recommended for vaccination in Phases 1a, 1b, or 1c" (Dooling et al., 2021, para. 10).

In a December 2020 white paper, *Recommendations for Prioritization and Distribution of COVID-19 Vaccine in Prisons and Jails*, published by Columbia University's Justice Lab and written by representatives of several academic centers, including Yale University, the University of North Carolina and Chapel Hill, and Columbia University, the authors argued that prioritizing the vaccination of those who live and work in correctional systems is critical to public health (Wang et al., 2020). The authors called for the prioritization of incarcerated people in the same phase as correctional officers, citing the disease burden and inability to implement mitigation measures in crowded and poorly ventilated settings. Black people, already disproportionately impacted by COVID-19 illness and death, are incarcerated at five times the rate of White Americans (Nellis, 2021). By December 2020, nearly 20 percent of the U.S. prison population had tested positive for the SARS-CoV-2 virus—an infection rate five times higher than that of the general population and with three times the age-adjusted mortality. According to the Prison Policy Initiative, a review of the available state prioritization plans in early December (prior to the release of ACIP recommendations) revealed that 11 states included incarcerated populations as part of Phase 1 of their vaccine rollout plans, 26 states included incarcerated populations in Phase 2, one state included the population as part of Phase 3, and eight states did not explicitly include incarcerated people in any part of their plans (Quandt, 2020).

While the argument to prioritize incarcerated people to receive COVID-19 vaccines was based on data demonstrating the population's risk of contracting the virus and suffering poor outcomes, politicians soon began weighing in on public health decisions. Colorado Governor Jared Polis stated during a joint news conference with National Institute of Allergy and Infectious Diseases Director Dr. Anthony Fauci on December 1, 2020, "There's no way that prisoners are going to get it before members of a vulnerable population" (Burness, 2020, para. 4). This statement ran counter to the plan published by the Colorado Department of Public

Health and Environment weeks earlier, which placed incarcerated people at the top of Phase 2, below "critical workforce" and "highest-risk individuals," but ahead of the general public and people deemed to be at high (but not "highest") risk (Burness, 2020, para. 2). As a result, Colorado deprioritized its incarcerated population and individuals were vaccinated according to their age bracket. In Wisconsin, Senate Bill 8 was introduced to direct the Department of Health Services not to prioritize an incarcerated person for vaccination and further directed the Department "not to prioritize incarcerated persons within an allocation phase" (WI SB8, 2021, p. 1). The bill was passed by the Senate but did not pass out of the House Committee on Health. In California and Ohio, officials allocated vaccines for individuals incarcerated in some prisons but not others. In February 2021, journalist Tamar Sarai Davis (2021) wrote:

> Such debates will likely continue to uplift ideas about deservedness, righteousness and mortality—arguments rooted in a punitive logic that fails to reckon with readily available data about the public health imperative of first vaccinating those most vulnerable within the facilities most liable for continuing the spread of COVID-19. (para. 18)

## Ethics and Incentivizing Vaccination

Early in the COVID-19 vaccine rollout, many states developed programs to incentivize individuals to receive a COVID-19 vaccination. Incentives such as $1 million giveaways, free college tuition, gift cards, and automobiles were offered to encourage individuals to prioritize getting vaccinated. In July 2021, the White House called on state and local governments to pay $100 to anyone willing to get their first vaccine dose (White House, 2021). Analysis of these programs has shown that most did not have the desired effect to increase vaccine uptake and have, instead, raised questions about the ethics of such programs.

Incentivizing vaccination is not unique to COVID-19 vaccinations efforts. Grocery stores and pharmacies often offer gift cards to those who receive an annual influenza vaccination, and families enrolled in the U.S. Department of Agriculture's Women, Infants, and Children (WIC) program receive education on vaccinations when they visit the clinic for monthly voucher pickup (Community Preventive Services Task Force, 2015). However, the degree to which state and local governments have been willing to incentivize COVID-19 vaccination far exceeds historical efforts to protect against other public health threats.

Much has been written on both sides of this debate, with ethicists and others weighing in heavily for and against incentivization of COVID-19 vaccination. Some argue that monetary incentives are exploitative and coercive, causing individuals enduring economic hardship to make the choice to receive a vaccine they may have declined were it not for the incentive (Jecker, 2021b, 2021c). This objection has been countered by those who argue that incentives encourage the individual to reduce their risk by choosing to become vaccinated rather than infected and, therefore, benefit the recipient more holistically. While some argue that modest cash awards do not unduly induce people to participate, others point out that providing cash incentives signals individual decisions can be manipulated and bought (Wertheimer & Miller, 2008).

Ohio's $5.6 million lottery has been estimated to have encouraged 80,000 individuals to get vaccinated. Brehm et al. (2022) estimated the lottery payout saved Ohio $66 million in intensive care unit costs and argued that incentives aren't meant to change beliefs, but to move people who were on the fence about getting vaccinated to take action. Brehm et al. went on to say that, since individuals who delay vaccination are comfortable with a degree of risk, incentivizing through a lottery may be appealing to them. Other researchers note, however, that financial incentives could set a bad precedent, setting public expectations that individuals are to take health precautions for selfish reasons rather than altruistic ones, and resulting in the expectation that participation in public health measures will be financially incentivized in the future (Campos-Mercade et al., 2021). A research letter published in January 2022 compared the daily first vaccination rate trends of 15 lottery and 31 non-lottery states and failed to demonstrate a significant increase in vaccination rates between the two groups (Law et al., 2022). This suggests the ethical debate around providing monetary incentives for vaccination may be moot, at least as it applies to the population at large.

Employers and health insurance plans have also provided incentives to employees and members over the course of the pandemic, but their efforts must comply with rules set out by the Affordable Care Act (ACA) and the Equal Employment Opportunity Commission (EEOC). Some ethicists argue that employer and health plan incentives have the potential to improve equity by encouraging historically more reluctant populations, such as Black Americans, to choose to get vaccinated. They also make the argument that financially incentivizing people to get vaccinated should be thought of no differently than incentivizing individuals to stop smoking or lose weight. Others argue that employer incentives have unequal impact upon different socioeconomic classes, with payments having limited impact upon those who receive high salaries but having potentially significant meaning to those who earn considerably less. They also point out that the employees and members may question the motives of employers and health plans who set the incentives, thereby increasing suspicion and mistrust (Jecker, 2021b, 2021c).

## Ethics and Vaccine Administration

In general, outside of a medical emergency, a parent or legal guardian provides informed consent prior to their child undergoing a significant medical intervention (Wilkinson & McBride, 2021). Most states allow minors who are emancipated, homeless or living apart from their parent or guardian, or who are married, to self-consent for medical treatment (Singer et al., 2021). Most states also have laws that explicitly allow minors to provide consent to receive diagnosis and treatment for sexually transmitted infections (CDC, 2021). Several states have policies in place that allow certain minors who do not meet those criteria to make healthcare decisions without the consent of a parent or legal guardian. Such "mature minor" doctrines allow health care providers to permit minors to self-consent to medical procedures if it is the opinion of the provider that the minor is mature enough to make that decision. As of October 2021, eight states, the District of Columbia, and the cities of Philadelphia and San Francisco, either allow certain minors to consent for COVID-19 vaccination without a parent or guardian or allow medical providers to waive parental consent (Kaiser Family Foundation, 2021).

Minor consent for health care decisions is grounded in both law and bioethics. From both perspectives, an adolescent must understand the risks and benefits of a medical procedure or treatment and have the capacity to give informed consent. While most minors involve their parents in their health care decisions, there are those who are separated from their parents, who disagree with their parents' views on a health topic, or whose parents are not available when health care decisions need to be made (English, 2021). An argument can be made that it is ethical for a minor to choose to protect themselves against a clear threat to their health, such as COVID-19. Ethicists also argue that it would be unethical for a parent to deny their child of such protection. As Kyle Brothers, MD, PhD FAAP, a member of the American Academy of Pediatrics' section on bioethics executive committee observed, "The fundamental idea is children don't have their $18^{th}$ birthday and suddenly change in terms of their ability to make decisions. The law has only imperfect solutions for respecting that continuous process of development" (Kusterbeck, 2021, para. 5).

While the rights of minors to make their own health care decisions vary by state, and sometimes by city, a position statement from the Society for Adolescent Health and Medicine states, "within ethical and legal guidelines, it will be important to develop strategies that maximize opportunities for minors to receive vaccinations when parents are not physically present, including opportunities for them to give their own consent" (English et al., 2013, p. 552). Regardless of the support of ethicists, the majority of states do not have provisions allowing for minor consent.

## Ethics and Vaccine Mandates

Perhaps the most contentious of topics concerning COVID-19 vaccines has been that of vaccine mandates. Vaccine mandates have been implemented (and challenged) since the early 1900s, but the political polarization of COVID-19 has created significant legal, political, and ethical debate.

In its 1905 ruling on *Jacobson v. Massachusetts*, the U.S. Supreme Court stated, "There are manifold restraints to which every person is necessarily subject for the common good. On any other basis, organized society could not exist with safety to its members" (Colgrove & Bayer, 2005, p. 572). In the 117 years since that decision, the courts have tended to protect individual freedoms, but consider limitations based on the risk of the disease versus the risk of restricting individual freedom, precedent, context (e.g., mandate of a vaccine under Emergency Use Authorization [EUA] versus full approval by the U.S. Food and Drug Administration [FDA], and sufficient access to a mandated vaccine; ACR Committee on Ethics & Conflict of Interest, 2022). Based on those four criteria, there may be legal justification for COVID-19 vaccine mandates, although mandates continue to be challenged at the level of the U.S. Supreme Court.

Arguably the most stringent mandate is that which applies to members of the U.S. military. On August 9, 2021, the Secretary of Defense issued a message indicating his intent to require COVID-19 vaccination for active and reserve servicemembers "no later than mid-September [2021] or immediately upon the U.S. Food and Drug Administration (FDA) licensure [of a COVID-19 vaccine], whichever comes first" (Austin, 2021, para. 2). By December 21, 2021, approximately 98 percent of active duty servicemembers had been vaccinated (Garamone, 2021). As of February 2022, the U.S. military had approved religious exemptions for 15 servicemembers out of approximately 16,000 applications—six from the Marine Corps and nine from the Air Force. The Army and Navy have approved zero of their nearly 6,500 requests for religious exemption (Liebermann & Kaufman, 2022).

In September 2021, the Biden Administration announced the requirement that federal workers and contractors be vaccinated. This was followed two months later by announcements that all eligible staff at health care facilities participating in Medicare and Medicaid programs be vaccinated (CMS, 2021), as well as all eligible employees of companies employing 100 or more individuals. The corporate mandate was eventually struck down by the U.S. Supreme Court; however, the Court upheld the mandate for health care workers (OSHA, 2022). The mandate for federal workers was blocked by the 5th U.S. Circuit Court of Appeals in January 2022 (Associated Press, 2022), and the mandate for employees of federal contractors was blocked in March 2022 by a U.S. District Court judge in Augusta, Georgia (Mulvihill & Lieb, 2022).

As the legal fights continue to play out through the courts, the ethical debates also wage on. In April 2021, the World Health Organization (WHO) published its policy brief on ethical considerations for COVID-19 vaccine mandates. The WHO argued that mandates may be necessary to achieve public health objectives if "less coercive or intrusive" public interventions have failed to achieve those goals (World Health Organization, 2021, p. 1-2). It also advised that mandates should be frequently re-evaluated to ensure they remain necessary and cautioned that the need for repeated vaccinations over time may make such mandates unrealistic. The WHO also commented on the importance of demonstrating vaccine safety and efficacy, especially for vaccines that are being used under FDA emergency use authorization and that may not yet have sufficient data to meet thresholds for safety. Finally, the WHO stressed the importance of ensuring sufficient supply of, and access to, vaccines for those affected by a mandate, as well as a transparent process for decision making about mandatory vaccination so as not to erode public trust (World Health Organization, 2021).

In July 2021, the National Catholic Bioethics Center (2021) released a document that pushed back against mandated COVID-19 immunization, stating, "Individuals must discern whether to be vaccinated or not in conscience and without coercion. Practical reason makes evident that vaccination is not, as a rule, a moral obligation and that, therefore, it must be voluntary" (para. 3). However, the Association of Bioethics Program Directors (2021), an association of "the leadership of nearly 100 academic bioethics programs at medical centers and universities across North America," argues the opposite: "…there is common agreement among both secular and religious ethical worldviews and traditions that preventing risk to others justifies enforcing limits to personal decision-making" (para. 4) and clearly states, "The ABPD supports the use of vaccine mandates as an essential measure against COVID-19" (para. 6).

Considerable debate also continues over the ethics of mandating COVID-19 vaccinations in children, especially while the vaccines are still under FDA EUA and when children, while still impacted by COVID-19, are much less likely to suffer serious or fatal illness than are adults (Zimmerman & Curtis, 2021). On the other hand, while children are themselves at low risk for serious disease, they can transmit the virus to adults who may not fare as well, and scientists do not yet understand the impact of SARS-CoV-2 infection, or repeated infection, upon the developing child (van Aardt, 2021). As of May 2022, only California and Washington, D.C. require children to receive the COVID-19 vaccine for K-12 school entry, although some counties and school districts have added the requirement for students who participate in some activities (NASHP, 2022).

While nearly 83 percent of the U.S. population has received at least one dose of a COVID-19 vaccine, the continued circulation of the virus has allowed for the development of many new variants, some of which have been significantly more infectious than the original SARS-CoV-2 virus (CDC, 2022). At the same time, the efficacy of COVID-19 vaccines against these variants has waned, prompting the CDC and ACIP to recommend additional vaccine doses to raise levels of immunity (CDC, 2022a). When it comes to mandating COVID-19 vaccines, the arguments on both sides are complex and the matter continues to be hotly debated.

## Discussion

The world has endured a pandemic unlike any other in modern history. Due to the ease of global transportation, the SARS-CoV-2 virus was able to spread from a cluster of cases of pneumonia in Hubei Province, China, to cause a declared pandemic in less than three months (World Health Organization, 2020). While the Trump Administration's *Operation Warp Speed* accelerated the development and distribution of COVID-19 vaccines in the United States within an unprecedented timeframe, vaccination rates in the United States are among the lowest in the western world (Holder, 2022).

In healthcare, the ethical principles of autonomy, beneficence, non-maleficence, and justice should be emphasized. As with vaccines introduced previously in the U.S., autonomy with respect to the decision to become vaccinated is well-preserved, except when it comes to children. There is no "forced vaccination" of adults in the U.S., although a decision to remain unvaccinated may impact one's employment or the ability to participate in some activities. However, for children, as with other vaccinations, the parent is typically the arbiter, weighing the risks and benefits of vaccination on behalf of the child. Vaccination against COVID-19 has been shown to reduce hospitalizations, deaths, and the incidence of multi-system inflammatory syndrome in children (MIS-C), while serious adverse events due to vaccination are extremely rare (Lewis, 2021). Safety data clearly show the benefits of vaccinating children, both to the individual, and to society with respect to decreased transmission of the virus.

When beneficence, or the expectation to act so as to benefit others, is considered, clarity can be brought to the discussions around the development of vaccines, as well as that of personal liberty versus societal obligation. Although some may espouse closely held personal beliefs around the use of fetal cell line technology in the development of some vaccines, the availability of vaccines that do not use this technology can remove this concern from consideration. The vaccines that are most widely available in the U.S. (mRNA vaccines) are not manufactured using fetal cell lines. The U.S. death toll from COVID-19, which exceeds 1 million, or 1 in 330 U.S. residents, makes the SARS-CoV-2 pandemic the deadliest in modern U.S. history (Lovelace, 2021). Given the demonstrated safety and efficacy of COVID-19 vaccines, limits upon individual liberty for the benefit of society are likely justified. Similarly, the principle of nonmaleficence, or "do no harm," can also be upheld so long as the risk of COVID-19 vaccination is significantly less than that of the disease. In the converse, it can be argued that there is individual responsibility to avoid maleficence. The WHO endorses that vaccines are "one of the most effective tools for protecting people against COVID-19" (2022). When an individual's choice to forgo receiving a safe and effective vaccination, regardless of their deeply held personal beliefs or fears, directly impacts the health and wellbeing of another, the principle of nonmaleficence is not upheld. Vaccine mandates are the government's way of attempting to limit maleficence resulting from individual decisions when a safe and effective vaccine is readily available and can be used to limit the spread of communicable disease.

Within the fourth principle, justice, is where much of the ethical debate resides– while COVID-19 vaccines are now abundantly available to the U.S. general population, there remain pockets of individuals who do not have equal access. Individuals who are incarcerated, and those who do not live or work near a vaccination site or who do not have access to transportation, who are unable to seek vaccination during the operating hours of most clinics, or who are experiencing homelessness are among these populations. Additionally, the control of the ability of some populations to access vaccination, whether through purposeful restriction to access or the denial of a minor's right to choose vaccination for themselves, violates the principle of justice (and nonmaleficence). Lastly, incentivization of vaccination should be designed in such a way that its impact is equitable and noncoercive to ensure justice is upheld.

## Conclusion

The COVID-19 pandemic has been wrought with challenges, not the least of which have been the ethical considerations of COVID-19 vaccine development, distribution, incentives, administration, mandates, and exemptions to mandates. As the pandemic forges on, the enduring ethical debate will be that of personal responsibility versus personal liberty as it relates to COVID-19 vaccination. This issue is sure to be the subject of considerable research and discussion for the foreseeable future.

## References

ACR Committee on Ethics & Conflict of Interest. (2022). Ethics forum: Vaccine mandates. *The Rheumatologist*. https://www.the-rheumatologist.org/article/the-ethics-of-vaccine-mandates/

American Academy of Pediatrics. (2022). *Children and COVID-19: State-level data report*. American Academy of Pediatrics. https://www.aap.org/en/pages/2019-novel-coronavirus-covid-19-infections/children-and-covid-19-state-level-data-report/

American Medical Association. (2020, November 17). *AMA policy calls for more COVID-19 prevention for congregate settings*. AMA. https://www.ama-assn.org/press-center/press-releases/ama-policy-calls-more-covid-19-prevention-congregate-settings

Associated Press. (2022, February 10). Vaccine mandate for federal workers blocked by 2nd court. *U.S. News & World Report*. https://www.usnews.com/news/health-news/articles/2022-02-10/vaccine-mandate-for-federal-workers-blocked-by-2nd-court

Association of Bioethics Program Directors. (2021, September 22). *ABPD statement in support of COVID-19 vaccine mandates for all eligible Americans.* https://www.bioethicsdirectors.net/wp-content/uploads/2021/09/ABPD-Statement-in-Support-of-COVID-19-Vaccine-Mandates_ FINAL9.22.2021.pdf

Austin, L. (2021, August 9). *Memorandum for all Department of Defense employees.* Secretary of Defense. https://media.defense.gov/2021/Aug/09/2002826254/-1/-1/0/Message-to-the-Force-Memo-Vaccine-FINAL.PDF

Beauchamp, T. & Childress, J. F. (2019). *Principles of Biomedical Ethics* (8th ed.). Oxford University Press.

Brehm, M. E., Brehm, P. A., & Saavedra, M. (2022). The Ohio vaccine lottery and starting vaccination rates. *American Journal of Health Economics.* https://www.journals.uchicago.edu/doi/epdf/10.1086/718512

Burness, A. (2020, December 1). Gov. Polis says Colorado prisoners shouldn't get COVID-19 vaccine before free people. *The Denver Post.* https://www.denverpost.com/2020/12/01/polis-covid-vaccine-prison-jail-colorado/

Campos-Mercade, P. M., Meier, A. N., Schneider, F. H., Meier, S., Pope, D., & Wengstrom, E. (2021). Monetary Incentives Increase COVID-19 Vaccinations. *Science, 374*(6569), 879-882.

CDC. (2020, October 29). *CDC COVID-19 vaccination program interim playbook.* https://www.cdc.gov/vaccines/imz-managers/downloads/COVID-19-Vaccination- Program-Interim_Playbook.pdf

CDC. (2021, January 8). *State laws that enable a minor to provide informed consent to receive HIV and STD services.* https://www.cdc.gov/hiv/policies/law/states/ minors.html

CDC. (2022). Vaccinations in the US. CDC COVID Data Tracker, https://covid.cdc.gov/covid-data-tracker/#datatracker-home. Accessed 30 May 2022.

CDC. (2022a). "ACIP Update to the Evidence to Recommendations for a 2nd COVID-19 Booster Dose in Adults Ages 50 Years and Older and Immunocompromised Individuals." CDC. https://www.cdc.gov/vaccines/acip/recs/grade/covid-19-second-booster-dose-etr.html. Accessed 30 May 2022.

Children's Hospital of Philadelphia. (2021, October 21). *Vaccine ingredients--fetal cells.* https://www.chop.edu/centers-programs/vaccine-education-center/vaccine-ingredients/fetal-tissues

Christian Science. (2022). *A Christian Science Perspective on Vaccination and Public Health.* https://www.christianscience.com/press-room/a-christian-science-perspective-on-vaccination-and-public-health

CMS. (2021, November 5). Medicare and Medicaid Programs; Omnibus COVID-19 health care staff vaccination. *Federal Register.* https://www.federalregister.gov/documents/2021/11/05/2021-23831/medicare-and-medicaid-programs-omnibus-covid-19-health-care-staff-vaccination

Colgrove, J., & Bayer, R. (2005). Manifold restraints: Liberty, public health, and the legacy of *Jacobson v. Massachusetts. American Journal of Public Health, 95*(4), 571-576.

Community Preventive Services Task Force. (2015, March). Increasing appropriate vaccination: Vaccination programs in the special supplemental nutrition program for Women, Infants and Children (WIC) settings. The Community Guide. https://www.thecommunityguide.org/sites/default/files/assets/Vaccination-Programs-WIC-Settings.pdf

Davis, T. S. (2021, February 3). *How politics and punitive logic are warping the debate over COVID-19 vaccines in prisons.* Prismreports.org. https://prismreports.org/2021/02/03/how-politics-and-punitive-logic-are-warping-the-debate-over-covid-vaccines-in-prisons/

Diekema, D. (2005). Responding to parental refusals of immunization of children. *Pediatrics, 115*(5), 1428-1431. doi: 10.1542/peds.2005-0316.

Dooling, K. M., Marin, M., Wallace, M., McClung, N., Chamberland, M., Lee, G. M., Talbot, H. K., Romero, J. R., Bell, B. P., & Oliver, S. E. (2021, January 1). The Advisory Committee on Immunization Practices' updated interim recommendation for allocation of COVID-19 vaccines-- United States, December 2020. *Morbidity and Mortality Weekly Report, 69*(5152), 1657-1660. https://www.cdc.gov/mmwr/volumes/69/wr/mm695152e2.htm?s_cid=mm695152e2_w

English, A. (2021, July). Ethics talk: Should adolescents be able to consent for COVID-19 vaccinations? *AMA Journal of Ethics.* https://journalofethics.ama-assn.org/videocast/ethics-talk-should-adolescents-be-able-consent-covid-19-vaccinations

English, A. F., Ford, C. A., Khan, J. A., Kharbanda, E. O., & Middleman, A. B. (2013). Adolescent consent for vaccination: A position paper of the Society for Adolescent Health and Medicine. *Journal of Adolescent Health, 53*(2013) 550-553. https://www.adolescenthealth.org/getattachment/Advocacy/Position-Papers-Statements/Adolescent-Consent-for-Vaccination-%E2%80%93-October-2013.pdf.aspx?lang=en-US

Fea, J., Mello, M., & Faskianos, I. (2021, November 30). *COVID-19 vaccines and religious exemptions.* Council on Foreign Relations. https://www.cfr.org/event/covid-19-vaccines-and-religious-exemptions

Funk, C. &. Gramlich, J. (2021). *10 Facts about Americans and Coronavirus Vaccines.* Pew Research Center. https://www.pewresearch.org/fact-tank/2021/09/20/10-facts-about-americans-and-coronavirus-vaccines/

Garamone, J. (2021, December 21). *Service members must be vaccinated or face consequences, DOD official says.* U.S. Department of Defense. https://www.defense.gov/News/News-Stories/Article/Article/2881481/service-members-must-be-vaccinated-or-face-consequences-dod-official-says/

Hardeman A., Wong, T., Denson, J. L., Postelnicu, R., & Rojas, J. C. (2021). Evaluation of health equity in COVID-19 vaccine distribution plans in the United States. *JAMA Network Open,* 4(7), e2115653. https://jamanetwork.com/journals/jamanetworkopen/fullarticle/2781618

Holder, J. (2022, May 30). Tracking coronavirus vaccinations around the world. *New York Times.* https://www.nytimes.com/interactive/2021/world/covid-vaccinations- tracker.html

Horan, R., & DePetro, J. (2019). *Public health and personal choice: The ethics of vaccine mandates and parental refusal in the United States.* The Keep: Eastern Illinois University. https://thekeep.eiu.edu/cgi/viewcontent.cgi?article=1006&context=lib_awards_2019_docs

Jecker, N. S. (2021a). Vaccine ethics: An ethical framework for global distribution of COVID-19 vaccines. *Journal of Medical Ethics,* 308-317. doi: 10.1136/medethics-2020-107036

Jecker, N. S. (2021b). Cash incentives, ethics, and COVID-19 vaccination. *Science, 374*(6569), 819-820. doi:10.1126/science.abm6400

Jecker, N. S. (2021c, April 2). What money can't buy: An argument against paying people to get vaccinated. *Journal of Medical Ethics.* doi: 10.1136/medethics-2021-107235

Kaiser Family Foundation. (2021, October 11). *State parental consent laws for COVID-19 vaccination*. State Health Facts. https://www.kff.org/other/state-indicator/state-parental-consent-laws-for-covid-19-vaccination/?current Timeframe=0&sortModel=%7B%22colId%22:%22Location%22,%22sort%22:%22asc%22%7D

Kaiser Health News. (2021, September 13). *Religious exemption claims on the rise with increased vaccine mandates*. KHN Morning Briefing. https://khn.org/morning-breakout/religious-exemption-claims-on-the-rise-with-increased-vaccine-mandates/

Kates, J., Michaud, J., & Tolbert, J. (2020, December 14). *How are States Prioritizing Who Will Get the COVID-19 Vaccine First?* Kaiser Family Foundation. https://www.kff.org/policy-watch/how-are-states-prioritizing-who-will-get-the-covid-19-vaccine-first/

Kusterbeck, S. (2021, September 1). *Complicated ethics of children self-consenting for vaccines*. Relias Media. https://www.reliasmedia.com/articles/148447-complicated-ethics-of-children-self-consenting-for-vaccines

Ladaria, L., & Morandi, G. (2020, December 21). *Note on the morality of using some anti-COVID-19 vaccines.* Congregation for the Doctrine of the Faith. https://www.vatican.va/roman_curia/congregations/cfaith/documents/rc_con_cfaith_doc_20201221_nota-vaccini-anticovid_en.html

Law, A. P., Peterson, D., Walkey, A. J., & Bosch, N. A. (2022). Lottery-based incentives and COVID-19 vaccination rates in the US. *JAMA Internal Medicine, 182*(2), 235–237. doi:10.1001/jamainternmed.2021.7052

LawPipe. (n.d.). *Prince v. Massachusetts*. LawPipe Online Legal Research Tool. https://www.lawpipe.com/U.S.-Supreme-Court/Prince_v_ Massachusetts.html

Levy, R. & Messerly, M. (2022, February 28). *Health workers' vaccine mandate undone by religious exemptions*. Politico. https://www.politico.com/news/2022/02/28/covid-vaccine-exemption-hospital-00011951

Lewis, T. (2021, December 2). *Vaccination is likely to prevent many more COVID cases than it is to cause a rare and nonfatal heart side effect in five-to-11-year-olds.* Scientific American. https://www.scientificamerican.com/article/the-benefits-of-vaccinating-kids-against-covid-far-outweigh-the-risks-of-myocarditis1/

Liebermann, O. & Kaufman, E. (2022, February 17). U.S. military has approved religious exemptions to vaccine mandate for 15 service members out of 16,000 requests. *CNN.* https://www.cnn.com/2022/02/17/politics/us-military-religious-exemptions-covid-vaccine/index.html

Lovelace, Jr., B. (2021, September 20). *COVID is officially America's deadliest pandemic as U.S. fatalities surpass 1918 flu estimates.* CNBC. https://www.cnbc.com/2021/09/20/covid-is-americas-deadliest-pandemic-as-us-fatalities-near-1918-flu-estimates.html

Merriam-Webster. (n.d.). Lie. In *Merriam-Webster.com dictionary.* https://www.merriam-webster.com/dictionary/lie

Mulvihill, G., & Lieb, D. A. (2021). *Southern district judge blocks vaccine mandates for federal contractors.* Law.com. https://www.law.com/dailyreportonline/2021/12/08/augustas-middle-district-judge-blocks-vaccine-mandate-for-federal-contractors/?slreturn=20220404192241

National Academy for State Health Policy. (2022). *States sddress school vaccine mandates and mask mandates.* https://apps.who.int/iris/handle/10665/340841

National Academies of Sciences, Engineering, and Medicine. (2020). *Framework for equitable allocation of COVID-19 vaccine.* The National Academies Press.

National Catholic Bioethics Center. (2021, July 2). *NCBC Statement on COVID-19 Vaccine Mandates.* https://www.ncbcenter.org/ncbc-news/vaccine mandatestatement

National Conference of State Legislatures. (2021, January 11). *COVID-19: Essential workers in the States.* NCSL. https://www.ncsl.org/research/labor-and-employment/covid-19-essential-workers-in-the-states.aspx

Near Neighbours. (2018, January 19). *Love thy neighbour on World Religion Day.* https://www.near-neighbours.org.uk/blog/2018/2/8/love-thy-neighbour-on-this-world-religion-day

Nellis, A. (2021, October 13). *The color of justice: Racial and ethnic disparity in state prisons.* The Sentencing Project. https://www.sentencingproject.org/publications/color-of-justice-racial-and-ethnic-disparity-in-state-prisons/

OSHA. (2022, January 25). *COVID-19 vaccination and testing ETS.* U.S. Department of Labor Occupational Safety and Health Administration. https://www.osha.gov/coronavirus/ets2

Quandt, K. (2020, December 8). *COVID vaccination plans.* Prison Policy Initiative. https://www.prisonpolicy.org/blog/2020/12/08/covid-vaccination-plans/

Reiss, D. (2014). Thou shalt not take the name of the Lord thy God in vain: Use and abuse of religious exemptions from school immunization requirements. *Hastings Law Journal, 1551.* http://repository.uchastings.edu/faculty_scholarship/1169

Sgreccia, E. (2005, June 9). *Talking about vaccines.* Immunize.org. https://www.immunize.org/talking-about-vaccines/vaticandocument.htm

Singer, N. K., Kates, J., & Tolbert, J. (2021, May 26). *COVID-19 vaccination and parental consent.* Kaiser Family Foundation. https://www.kff.org/policy-watch/covid-19-vaccination-and-parental-consent/

Stanford Medicine. (2021, September). *Show me the facts: Religion and the COVID-19 vaccine.* American Academy of Pediatrics Orange County Chapter. https://www.aap-oc.org/wp-content/uploads/2021/09/Religion-the-COVID-19-Vaccine_Fact-Sheet_vF.pdf

Tuxbury, S. (2021, September 20). What research surrounding COVID vaccination ethics tells us. *University of Michigan-Dearborn News.* https://umdearborn.edu/news/what-research-surrounding-covid-vaccination-ethics-tells-us

van Aardt, W. (2021). The mandatory COVID-19 vaccination of school children: A bioethical and human rights assessment. *Journal of Vaccines & Vaccination, 12*(3), 1-6.

Wang, E., Brinkley-Rubentein, L., Puglisi, L., & Western, B. (2020, December). *Recommendations for prioritization and distribution of COVID-19 vaccine in prisons and jails* [White Paper]. https://justicelab.columbia.edu/sites/default/files/content/COVID_Vaccine_White_Paper.pdf

Wertheimer, A., & Miller, F. G. (2008). Payment for research participation: A coercive offer? *Journal of Medical Ethics, 34(5),* 389–392.

White House. (2021, July 29). *Fact sheet: President Biden to announce new actions to get more Americans vaccinated and slow the spread of the Delta variant.* https://www.whitehouse.gov/briefing-room/statements-releases/2021/07/29/fact-sheet-president-biden-to-announce-new-actions-to-get-more-americans-vaccinated-and-slow-the-spread-of-the-delta-variant/

Wertheimer, A., & Miller, F. G. (2008). Payment for research participation: A coercive offer? *Journal of Medical Ethics, 34*(5), 389–392. https://doi.org/10.1136/jme.2007.021857

The White House. (2021, July 29). *FACT SHEET: President Biden to announce new actions to get more Americans vaccinated and slow the spread of the Delta variant.* The White House Statements and Releases. https://www.whitehouse.gov /briefing-room/statements-releases/2021/07/29/fact-sheet-president-biden-to-announce-new-actions-to-get-more-americans-vaccinated-and-slow-the-spread-of-the-delta-variant/

WI SB8. 2021-2022 Reg. Sess. (Wis. 2021, January 15). *Distribution of COVID-19 vaccines.* https://legiscan.com/WI/text/SB8/id/2243721

Wilkinson, D. & McBride, A. K. S. (2021). Clinical ethics: Consent for vaccination in children. *Archives of Disease in Childhood, 107*(1), 3-4. doi: 10.1136/archdischild-2021-322981

Winfield, N. (2022, January 10). Pope on COVID vaccines says health care a 'moral obligation'. *AP News.* https://apnews.com/article/coronavirus-pandemic-pope-francis-health-religion-093068b2ca50eb1680f8c440cff1fd18

Winston, K. (2017, February 16). *Thou shalt not speak alternative facts: Religion and lying*. Religion News Service. https://religionnews.com/2017/02/16/thou-shalt-not-speak-alternative-facts-religion-and-lying/

World Health Organization. (2020, April 27). *WHO Timeline-- COVID-19.* https://www.who.int/news/item/27-04-2020-who-timeline---covid-19

World Health Organization. (2021, April 13). *COVID-19 and mandatory vaccination: Ethical considerations and caveats.* WHO Policy Brief. https://apps.who.int/iris/handle/10665/340841

Word Health Organization. (2022, May 30). *COVID-19 and mandatory vaccination: Ethical considerations.* WHO Policy Brief. https://apps.who.int/iris/bitstream/

handle/10665/354585/WHO-2019-nCoV-Policy-brief-Mandatory-vaccination-2022.1-eng.pdf?sequence=1&isAllowed=y

Zimmerman, P., & Curtis, N. (2021). Why Is COVID-19 less severe in children? A review of the proposed mechanisms underlying the age-related difference in severity of SARS-CoV-2 infections. *Archives of Disease in Children,* 429-439. doi: 10.1136/archdischild-2020-320338

Zimmerman, R. (2021). Helping patients with ethical concerns about COVID-19 vaccines in light of fetal cell lines used in some COVID-19 vaccine. *Vaccine, 39*(31), 4242-4244.

# COVID-19 IN THE LONG-TERM CARE SETTING: ETHICAL CHALLENGES THAT REQUIRE LONG-TERM SOLUTIONS

**Cathy L. Purvis Lively**[1]

**Abstract**: The consequences of the pandemic will have a far-reaching effect on older adults and society. The unstable foundations of long-term care could not withstand the impact of the pandemic and created ethical challenges exacerbated by COVID-19. We have an ethical and moral obligation to address the issues and find solutions. Until we address the root causes, we will not improve long-term care. I will begin by summarizing the concept of healthy aging and then ageism as it intersects with the pandemic. The pandemic highlighted the societal perception of older adults as a burden on society and illuminated ageist views that shape public policy. When considering COVID-19 in the long-term care setting, I will consider three factors: (1) the high death rates within long-term care; (2) the lack of planning; and (3) the secondary harm from the public health measures. With each factor, we must consider how society responded and how we can ameliorate the harm, promote healthy aging, and better prepare for future public health emergencies. COVID-19 was a public health emergency requiring the enactment and imposition of drastic public health measures. The circumstances that existed may ethically justify the restrictions for long-term care as an emergency response in the early weeks of the pandemic but as the risks of extended isolation increased, the harsh restrictions became less defensible and increasingly more ethically problematic. We must rebuild the cracked foundation of long-term care and use the lessons learned from COVID-19 to better prepare for future public health emergencies.

COVID-19 disrupted life for older adults in long-term care. SARS-CoV-2 presented the risk of infection, severe illness, and death in long-term care facilities. The consequences of the pandemic will have a far-reaching effect on older adults and society. Returning to normal is likely to be slow

---

[1] Attorney and Mediator, Palm Beach County, Florida, USA

and challenging for long-term care residents after being intimidated by a deadly virus and isolated from family, friends, and other residents (Ayalon et al., 2020). The utilitarian approach to public health normalized, perpetuated, and exacerbated ageism and marginalization of older adults.

The pandemic threatened healthcare systems. The immediate emphasis was on "flattening the curve" by slowing the spread of the virus and protecting the most vulnerable populations. Public health officials identified older adults as vulnerable populations, especially those in long-term care. The factors that placed older adults at high risk during the pandemic existed long before the emergence of SARS-CoV-2. The social determinants of health, ageism, and the non-prioritization of long-term care contribute to the vulnerability of older adults. Vulnerable populations experience health disparities because of the inequalities secondary to age, medical conditions, race, ethnicity, or socioeconomic status (Berlinger et al., 2022). Outbreaks in long-term care facilities threaten residents and healthcare systems (Gardner et al., 2020).

Early responses to the pandemic advocated harsh restrictions on long-term care. Across the globe, long-term care facilities closed their doors to visitors and non-essential workers and stopped communal meals, group activities, and physical activities. The restrictions isolated residents of long-term care. The impact and the ethical implications of the restrictions intended to prevent the spread of the virus, protect the residents, and prevent overwhelming healthcare system inextricably intertwine with the preexisting social factors that devalue older adults and long-term care.

The unstable foundations of long-term care could not withstand the impact of the pandemic and created ethical challenges exacerbated by COVID-19. As ethicists, healthcare providers, and members of society, we have an ethical and moral obligation to address these issues and find solutions.

## Long-Term Care Residents at Risk

The heightened risk for long-term care residents is a combination of biological and psychological risk factors, such as impaired physical and mental ability, chronic illness, latent social, cultural, and demographic factors, such as socioeconomic status, and the lack of social network support. The physiological effects of the virus and the mitigation measures intersect with the latent social factors increasing the likelihood of adverse outcomes.

The pandemic highlighted health disparities and how, as a society, we should address the structural inequities (Berlinger et al., 2022). Until we address the root causes, such as social determinants of health and ageism, we will not improve long-term care. In addressing the foundational disparities within long-term care, I will begin by summarizing the concept of healthy aging.

## Healthy Aging

Before the pandemic, the WHO (2020a) proposed the Decade of Healthy Aging "to ensure that older people can fulfill their potential dignity and equality" (para. 3) and outlined three interconnected priorities, (1) create "age-friendly" communities; (2) promote person-centered health care; and (3) provide long-term care (Lloyd-Sherlock et al., 2019; WHO, 2020a).

In 2018, the American Geriatrics Society (AGS) identified five domains of healthy aging focused on (1) promoting health, preventing injury, managing chronic conditions; (2) cognitive health; (3) physical health; (4) mental health; and (5) facilitating social engagement and resilience (AGS, 2018; Batsis et al., 2021; Friedman et al., 2018). The priorities listed by the WHO and the AGS Domains of Healthy Aging apply as we consider the foundations of long-term care and the impact of the pandemic.

### Person-Centered Care

The WHO (2020b) recognizes person-centered care as a priority for healthy aging. Person-centered care focuses on the person and considers the individual's wishes, needs, and social aspects of care. Most long-term care facilities practice professionally directed and task-oriented institutional-centered care models, focusing on the illness or disease rather than the person.

A consortium of researchers in long-term care from 21 countries formed WE-THRIVE [2] to advance and support person-centered care in long-term care settings. Participants prioritized five concepts relevant to person-centered care, (1) relationships among all who are part of long-term care; (2) knowing the resident as a person; (3) identifying and addressing what matters most to the resident, (4) supporting meaningful engagement; and (5) supporting a positive environment (Corazzini et al., 2019).

The fifth factor identified by WE-THRIVE is supporting a positive environment. The comparison of long-term care to prisons is not unique to COVID-19 restrictions. Erving Goffman coined the term 'total institution' (Gawande, 2014; Goffman, 1961). Although Goffman's analysis reflected the circumstances in 1960, aspects of the total institution still exist throughout long-term care. Goffman compared basic social arrangements in which people separate aspects of life: they work, play, and sleep in different places, with different people, under a different authority, and without an overall plan (Gawande, 2014; Goffman, 1961). Total institutions break down barriers to separate spheres of life. All aspects of life occur in the same place under a central authority. Residents of a total institution carry out almost all phases of their daily lives in the close company of others and must do the same things together. Daily activity occurs on a pre-set schedule, with one activity leading at a pre-arranged time to the next.

Older adults are ethnically, socially, and economically diverse. Addressing their needs requires a multicultural approach. Gerodiversity considers cultural identity, heritage, social environment, community, family systems, and significant relationships (D'cruz & Banerjee, 2020; Iwasaki et al., 2009). Long-term care often fails to consider gerodiversity.

We must also consider the fundamental aspects of providing good care, outlined by Lopez et al. Good care extends beyond physical needs and includes (1) personalization; (2) humanization; (3) no-infantilization; and (4) no-victimization (López et al., 2021). Lopez et al. describe

[2] We-Thrive is an acronym for **W**orldwide **E**lements **T**o **H**armonize **R**esearch **I**n long-term care li**V**ing **E**nvironments.

dehumanization as a subtle form of mistreatment that violates fundamental human rights. Humanization recognizes human attributes and treats residents with sensitivity. It is speaking "to" and "with" rather than "at" the resident. Non-infantilization increases independence and maintains a sense of dignity and self-worth by establishing adult-adult relationships between staff and residents instead of parent-child relationships (López et al., 2021). The assumptions about residents' vulnerability and need for care promote paternalism, eclipsing humanization and non-infantilization. Promoting the highest level of care requires balancing physical care and patient safety with these factors.

The factors set forth by the WHO, AGS, WE-THRIVE and Lopez, provide a framework for analyzing, evaluating, planning, and implementing policies for long-term care. These factors apply to the entire aging population but are most relevant in long-term care, where ageism influences care delivery. I will now consider how ageism perpetuates the ethical challenges arising from COVID-19 in long-term care.

## Ageism

Ageism is socially normalized discrimination. The WHO (n.d.) defines ageism as stereotypes, prejudice, and discrimination towards others or oneself based on age. Including "oneself" in the WHO definitions of ageism is significant. Villanueva and Barber (2021) describe "internalized oppression" as when an individual absorbs and internalizes the cultural attitudes and stereotypes, adopts the oppressors' mindset, and develops feelings of inferiority, inadequacy, and self-hatred, invalidation, fear, and powerlessness. Older adults subjected to ageism are at risk of internalized oppression.

Van der Horst et al. (2021) suggest separating ageism from ableism and defining ageism using the "social relational approach" by recognizing the social oppression resulting from the unequal social relationship between various age groups. This unequal social relationship manifests through exclusion and oppression at the interpersonal, organizational, cultural, and social structural levels (van der Horst et al., 2021).

Under van der Horst's definition ageism stems from social relations rather than a characteristic of the individual and is differential treatment based on age, while ableism is differential treatment based on actual or expected impairments (van der Horst et al., 2021). Indeed, some older adults have impairments or conditions beyond age that fall under ableism rather than ageism.

The pandemic highlighted the societal perception of older adults as a burden on society and illuminated ageist views that shape public policy. Public health officials identified older adults, especially those in long-term care, as posing a risk of overwhelming the healthcare system and depleting limited resources, which added to the perception of older adults as a burden. Ageism pushes long-term care into the shadows of the healthcare spectrum (Houtven et al., 2020). Ageist attitudes and beliefs explain why long-term care was not a priority in pandemic planning and undermines the continuity of care for long-term care residents (Faghanipour et al., 2020).

## Deficiencies Within the Long-Term Care Sector

COVID-19 reignited concerns about the quality of care within the long-term care sector (Inzitari et al., 2020). The deficiencies in long-term care have existed for many years. As O'Neill (2018) argues, the quality of long-term care is not congruent with the complexity of care or the advances in geriatric care. Even before the pandemic, the shifting foundations of long-term care were moving toward an eruption, but we looked away.

Society can no longer look away. When considering COVID-19 in the long-term care setting, I will consider three factors: (1) the high death rates within long-term care; (2) the lack of planning; and (3) the secondary harm from the public health measures. With each factor, we must consider how society responded and how we can ameliorate the harm, promote healthy aging, and better prepare for future public health emergencies.

## COVID-19 Death Rates in Long-Term Care

In many countries, as many as half of the deaths from COVID-19 were long-term care residents (Inzitari et al., 2020.) As of March 31, 2021, in the United States, 179,000 long-term care residents and staff in long-term care died from COVID-19, representing 33% of total U.S. COVID-19 deaths (Galea, 2022).

Sepulveda et al. (2020) used publicly reported data on COVID-19 deaths for 12-Organization for Economic Co-operation and Development (OECD) member countries[3] to calculate and compare population-specific mortality rates and ratios for long-term care residents and community-dwelling older adults. Within the 12 countries, long-term care home residents accounted for 47.3% of COVID-19 deaths as of July 24, 2020. The substantial variations among these 12-OECD countries reflect levels of community transmission, policy response related to infection prevention and control in long-term care, and broader community factors. Denmark and Germany acted early to prevent the introduction of COVID-19 into long-term care facilities and had lower mortality. Spain and the United Kingdom, with less robust long-term care-related policy responses and higher levels of community transmission, had higher long-term care mortality rates. Canada had a higher mortality rate for long-term care residents than for community-dwelling older adults; Canada's long-term care home resident deaths accounted for a high percentage of its overall deaths, 78.4%, compared to the OECD 12-country average of 47.3% (Sepulveda et al., 2020).

Rates of death in long-term care facilities vary widely, with the lowest estimates at zero percent reported in South Korean long-term care hospitals and far higher rates between 40.3% and 71.7% in facilities in the United States, UK, and France (Salcher-Konrad et al., 2020). Research conducted at the London School of Economics reviewed various studies on the death rate from COVID-19 in long-term care in 14 countries (Salcher-Konrad et al., 2020). COVID-19 severely affected long-term care in several European

---

[3] Belgium, Canada, Denmark, France, Germany, Ireland, Italy, Netherlands, Spain, Sweden, United Kingdom, and the United States.

Union and European Economic Area countries,[4] with deaths among residents accounting for 37% to 66% of all COVID-19 deaths (Danis et al., 2020).

According to reports issued by the Finnish Institute for Health and Welfare, as of June 1, 2020, almost 50% of COVID-19 deaths were from long-term care (Forma et al., 2020). In Sweden, 47% of the COVID-19 deaths were long-term care residents, but there were striking regional differences–In the Stockholm region, 7% of long-term care residents died because of COVID-19, while hardly any deaths in long-term care in other regions (Szebehely, 2020).

We see the influence of ageism in the societal acceptance of the high death rate within long-term care. Tedros Adhanom Ghebreyesus, director-general of WHO responding to the social acceptance of the high COVID-19 death rate of older adults, stated, "[W]hen the elderly are dying, it's not fine. It's a moral bankruptcy" (Reynolds, 2020). SARS-CoV-2 was a novel virus, but the threat posed by infectious disease within long-term care is well known.

## Infectious Disease Outbreaks in Long-Term Care

Long-term care residents are vulnerable to complications and morbidity from viral infections (Lai et al., 2020; Louie et al., 2007; Lum et al., 2014; Gardner et al., 2020; Yen et al., 2020). From prior outbreaks in long-term care, we see common causative factors that increase the risk of the spread of infection, including, (1) residents may have multiple chronic diseases and comorbidities that increase susceptibility to infection; (2) residents share the same air and sources of food, water, medical care, and; (3) visitors, practitioners, and residents can come and go introducing pathogens; and (4) limited staff responsible for several residents' care (Lai et al., 2020; Thompson et al., 2020).

---

[4] Belgium 51%; France 50%; Germany 38%; Ireland 60%; Norway 59%; the Netherlands 31%; Spain 66%; Stockholm County Sweden 45%; Sweden 49%; UK England/Wales 26%; and UK Scotland 46%

The physical environment contributes to the spread of pathogens within long-term care facilities. The physical layout purportedly encourages socialization by sharing communal spaces (Ayalon et al., 2020; Cowper et al., 2020). The proximity of congregate living increases the likelihood of transmission and makes containment difficult. The culmination of staffing, resource shortages, and prolonged close contact contribute to heightened risk (Ayalon et al., 2020; Lai et al., 2020; Thompson et al., 2020).

The second factor to consider is the lack of planning for a pandemic, even though the threat of infectious disease in this setting was well established.

## Long-Term Care Settings Were Unprepared

Despite the known threat of infectious disease, long-term care facilities were unprepared. More than half of U.S. long-term care facilities lacked a plan to address a pandemic (Lum et al., 2014). Pandemic planning that existed was fragmented (Lum et al., 2014). Failing to adequately plan reflects ageism and the low priority of long-term care.

Government and public health officials scrambled to develop and implement policies to manage the spread of SARS-CoV-2. While there were some variations in the approaches, the focus was on avoiding overwhelming hospitals, preventing depletion of limited resources, and shielding vulnerable populations. The officials urgently implemented drastic measures that isolated older adults in long-term care.

### Public Health Measures and Restrictions

In the United States, the Center for Medicare and Medicaid Services (CMS) issued directives applicable to long-term care facilities on March 13, 2020 (CMS, 2020). The CMS measures included (1) restricting all visitors and non-essential health care personnel, except for compassionate care situations, such as end-of-life care; (2) canceling communal dining and all group activities; (3) implementing active screening of residents and staff for fever and respiratory symptoms; (4) ensuring residents practiced social distancing and performed frequent hand hygiene; (5) identifying staff working at multiple facilities, and actively screening and restricting them (CMS, 2020).

Some long-term care facilities devised window visits in which the residents remained inside the facility while the visitor remained outside. The individuals were separated by a wall and a window while talking on the phone. Gradually, CMS and long-term care administrators scaled back the restrictions. Residents could leave their rooms for meals but remained physically separated, preventing social interaction. In-person visits resumed with strict guidelines and limitations. The visits were limited. The pre-scheduled thirty-minute visits took place outside. Staff observed the visits to ensure the resident and visitor wore masks and maintained a six-foot distance. Staffing dictated the number of visits per day for the entire facility and the number of visits per week for a resident.

The European Centre for Disease Prevention and Control (ECDC) establishes regulations in the European Union (Thompson et al., 2020). On May 19, 2020, the ECDC reported on COVID-19 in long-term care. The ECDC identified primary factors contributing to COVID-19, long-term care staff working while contagious, staff working in multiple facilities, inadequate staff training, shortage of personal protective equipment and testing supplies, and testing only when an individual was symptomatic. The ECDC recommended screening residents and staff with daily monitoring and periodic testing. Nonpharmaceutical interventions included masks, strict adherence to hygiene, and isolation of sick individuals (Thompson et al., 2020).

The Finnish government declared a state of emergency on March 16, 2020. The initial guidelines aimed at protecting the population and safeguarding the economy recommended minimizing physical contact and quarantine-like conditions for those 70 and older (Forma et al., 2020). The guidelines evolved as the situation progressed. The government moved to a hybrid strategy, moving from extensive restrictions to enhanced management, consisting of testing, tracing, isolating, and treating, and convened a science panel to advise exit strategy measures and ways to mitigate the impacts. The panel included a wide range of experts but lacked expertise in aging and gerontology. Some restrictions were relaxed on May 22, 2020. The relaxed restrictions did not apply to older adults and still prohibited visits to long-term care facilities. In-room dining was the norm, and communal dining allowed for only a few residents at a time. Eventually, long-term care residents could see family and friends outside–2 meters apart.

On March 20, 2020, the Dutch government implemented visitor bans in all long-term care settings (Van der Roest et al., 2020). Long-term care facilities stopped social programs. Telephone calls, videoconferences, and window visits replaced in-person visits.

Interventions in Denmark and Germany included restriction of non-essential visitors, universal masking policies, improving staffing levels, preventing staff from working in multiple sites, implementing enhanced infection control training, auditing procedures, and widespread testing and isolation protocols (Sepulveda et al., 2020). Although Canada imposed forceful measures to prevent community transmission, the long-term care-related responses were diverse and less robust (Sepulveda et al., 2020).

Sweden's overall strategy was to minimize mortality and morbidity in the entire population and reduce threats caused by mitigation measures. (Szebehely, 2020). The initial focus was on limiting the spread of SARS-CoV-2 in the community and ensuring access to acute health care, with no specific attention to long-term care residents. Management of the pandemic was a combination of recommendations and legally binding rules (Szebehely, 2020). Examples of legally binding rules included a ban on visits to long-term care facilities, which began on April 1, 2020. The Public Health Agency did not mention the use of facemasks in elder care services until May 7, 2020, when support for masks and shields was published (Szebehely, 2020). While Swedish authorities and politicians stressed the importance of protecting older people, long-term care facilities reported difficulties in restricting spread because of staff shortages, scarcity of testing equipment and PPE, not prioritized for testing, and the physical layout of the long-term care with limited possibilities to stop infected residents from moving around (Szebehely, 2020).

Studies showed substantial variation in how COVID-19 spread among residents and staff and how many residents died because of COVID outbreaks in long-term care facilities. Some facilities successfully contained outbreaks (Salcher-Konrad et al., 2020). Other facilities were less successful and had high mortality rates.

The third factor to consider is the effect of consequences of these public health measures in long-term care.

## Consequences Of the Public Health Measures in Long-Term Care

The prioritization on prevention overshadowed residents' autonomy and overall well-being. The mandates applicable to long-term care deprived the residents of their agency and autonomy. Public health officials, government leaders, and long-term care administrators made decisions for the residents. The older adults' relocation into long-term care created a line of separation from their friends and family. The pandemic widened this division and created additional lines of separation.

The measures created other health risks. Physical distancing and reallocating health resources interrupted non-essential health care services. When exercise facilities closed and group activities stopped, residents could not remain active. Without stimuli, memory disorders progressed faster, and the risk of developing mental health conditions–depression, delirium, and behavioral problems increased. (Forma et al., 2020; McArthur et al., 2020).

Banning visitors and non-essential healthcare providers, prohibiting residents from leaving the facility, and restricting interaction among residents disrupted social connection. The restrictions promoted health by preventing infection, but interfered with managing chronic conditions and facilitating social engagement and resilience.

The restrictions interfered with monitoring, maintenance, and other routine health care. Family members assist in hands-on care, emotional support, and social support (Batsis et al., 2021; Gardner et al., 2020; Yeh et al., 2020). Without the day-to-day support from residents' families, the already-stretched staff divided their limited time between more residents, detracting from the quality of care (Bethell et al., 2021). Mandatory overtime led to high levels of burnout (Ayalon et al., 2020). The long-term care sector lost staff because of illness, death, and burnout.

The pandemic and various protective measures disrupted most of society's ability to take part in meaningful engagement. For those living in long-term care, the disruption was profound. The imposition and enforcement of restrictions escalated the likelihood of paternalism, dehumanization, and infantilization. The residents' primary communication was with members of the staff. Communication with the resident became more about speaking at them rather than having a conversation. Physical distancing limited the interaction between residents. Dehumanization was a significant risk during the pandemic. The public health mandates provided directives that the staff interpreted and carried out. Following the mandates, staff dictated what residents could and could not do and constantly monitored the residents, which increased the risk of falling into an adult-child relationship.

The most devastating and far-reaching harm is the social isolation associated with the visitor bans and physical distancing within the facilities

## Social Isolation and Loneliness

Human beings are instinctively connected (Campbell, 2020). This connection provides a safety net during adversity (Escalante et al., 2020). The pandemic presented adversity, and the restrictions frayed the safety net leaving older adults in long-term care socially isolated.

Society does not encourage older adults to remain connected and integrated into the community and instead allows older adults to become detached, leading to isolation (Galea, 2022). Pushed from their community into long-term care, older adults must try to adapt to a new community. Long-term care facilities are communities of residents, staff, and possibly others. Two aspects of social integration apply to long-term care residents: (1) a sense of belonging to the community and (2) active involvement in community life (D'cruz & Banerjee, 2020). Residents develop connections and a sense of belonging through group activities and communal dining. Qualitative studies with older adults in long-term care found that maintaining contacts and engaging in purposeful activity promote health and prevent loneliness (Batsis et al., 2021).

There are serious public health risks associated with social isolation and loneliness. Social isolation is a risk factor for loneliness, the subjective lack of meaningful relationships. Social isolation is "objective deficits in the number of relationships with and frequency of contact with family, friends, and the community" and is linked to increased rates of loneliness and emotional and physical health effects (Escalante et al., 2020, p. 520).

A study by Van der Roest et al. found that six to ten weeks after implementing the visitor ban, an alarming 77% of residents reported loneliness[5] (Van der Roest et al., 2020). More than half of the staff reported increased severity of agitation, depression, anxiety, and irritability (Van der Roest et al., 2020). Only 27% of relatives reported no changes in residents' mood status. Long-term care residents faced adversity but were alone, isolated, and without the safety net of human connection.

Recognizing the harm of the public health measures within a fractured healthcare system, we must now ask whether we can ethically justify the restrictions. Despite the efficacy of public health measures in slowing the spread of COVID-19, the ethical lines blurred as the pandemic lingered and the harms of isolation increased (Purvis Lively, 2021).

## The Ethical Challenges

COVID-19 was a public health emergency requiring the enactment and imposition of drastic public health measures. Thus, the ethical analysis should begin by looking through a public health lens.

### Public Health

Public health focuses on community rather than individual health through societal actions (Kass, 2001). Achieving a balance between an individual's

---

[5] 50% as moderately lonely, 16% as strongly lonely, and 11% as very strongly lonely.

interest and the common good presents ethical challenges. Public health officials justify exercising paternalistic compulsory powers by asserting the common good and protecting the public's health, reflecting the utilitarianism undergirding public health. A basic public health ethics analysis considers four principles: (1) harm, (2) proportionality, (3) reciprocity, and (4) transparency.

COVID-19 presented a credible threat of harm to health systems and society. Older adults were more susceptible to becoming infected and suffering severe physical effects. Healthcare systems worldwide faced being overwhelmed and the depletion of limited resources. The overwhelming harm from the virus created the need for drastic emergency measures to protect the vulnerable population, slow the spread, and preserve resources.

Proportionality requires balancing the burdens and benefits and considering the least restrictive alternative. The concept of the least restrictive alternative applies to public health and law. In the United States, challenges to infringements on Constitutional rights often include analyzing whether the infringement is the least restrictive means of achieving the intended result.

The argument proffered by Savulescu and Cameron (2020) that the selective lockdown of older adults in the UK was a proportionate way to reduce morbidity and limit social disruption applies to the restriction on long-term care. The restrictions burdened, but also benefited older adults. The benefits were significant and thus outweighed a *temporary* loss of liberty.

When the WHO first declared the pandemic, given the circumstances in long-term care and the high risk, I suggest the restrictions were the least restrictive alternative. However, this analysis does not stop with the initial implementation. Proportionality requires ongoing assessment and reevaluation. As the pandemic lingered and the risk of harm from the restrictions increased, the restrictions imposed on long-term facilities were no longer the least restrictive alternative. However, this community received little attention because of the influences of ageism and a history of low prioritization. At this point, the ethical pendulum begins to swing (Purvis Lively, 2021).

Reciprocity seeks to offset the burdens imposed on individuals from which others benefit (Viens, 2008). The restrictions that compromised residents' liberties protected society from the indirect harm of depletion of scarce medical resources. Viens differentiates between a narrow and wide view of reciprocity. Under the narrow view, reciprocity applies only to those who voluntarily acted and accepted the burdens. Under the wide view, reciprocity applies regardless of whether the individual voluntarily acted. Not applying the wide view to long-term care residents is unfair and perpetuates ageism. Societal devaluation forced their migration from the community into long-term care facilities in which SARS-CoV-2 posed a threat. Residents did not have the option of acting voluntarily. Public health officials decided for them. At the very least, society owes this population policy changes that counter ageism and promote healthy aging.

Transparency was hard to find during the pandemic. Communications from governmental leaders, public health officials, and long-term care administrators were opaque and often conflicting, leaving unanswered questions, doubts, and speculation.

Nancy Kass (2001) developed an ethical framework for public health using a six-step analysis. The Kass framework is much like the framework proposed by Gostin in 1997 in Human Rights and Public Health in the Aids Epidemic and, more recently in 2022, in Risk Trade-Offs and Equitable Decision-Making in the Covid-19 Pandemic (Gostin & Wetter, 2022).

Step one identifies the goals of a public health initiative (Kass, 2001). The overarching goal was to reduce morbidity and mortality from COVID-19. A related question is who benefits from the initiative? As seen in many public health initiatives, the restrictions targeted a specific group to protect other citizens' health. The restrictions benefited residents but also society by preserving limited resources.

Step two of the Kass framework examines the effectiveness of the initiative and the data supporting the assumptions (Kass, 2001). Under the Kass framework, morbidity and mortality rates cannot remain unchanged. Gostin proffers that the benefit is only worth the burden if it is likely to achieve the goal of controlling the viral spread. Gostin focuses on spread rather than morbidity, but, much like Kass, asserts evidence-based action is essential. Although the quality and volume of existing data will vary, the initiative depends on data, not speculation (Kass, 2001). The amount and quality of data required to support the initiatives correlate with the severity of the infringement of liberty or the impact on vulnerable populations. COVID-19 presented an immediate serious threat, leaving no time to gather new data. Public health officials had to rely on data from past epidemics. The existing data suggested the restrictions would effectively reduce COVID-19 morbidity and mortality in long-term care. While we do not have all the data and evidence, countries that acted quickly and imposed restrictions and provided infection control early reported lower long-term care COVID-19 deaths than countries that took less robust action. While data showed the efficacy of prior infectious disease prevention, the analysis should have included data on the global public health issues of social isolation and loneliness.

The third step of the Kass framework identifies potential burdens or harms. This step is critical since the measures targeted older adults, a vulnerable population, and infringed on their liberty. Kass identifies three broad categories of risks: (1) The risk to privacy and confidentiality, (2) The risk to liberty and self-determination, and (3) The risk to justice (Kass, 2001).

There may be questions about potential privacy risks given the attention directed to long-term care and the reporting of testing status and case counts. However, the information provided did not include identifying information. The profound universal risk was the infringement on liberty and justice. The restrictions that forced residents into their rooms or apartments prevented them from leaving the facility and restricted their contact with visitors, significantly restraining their liberty.

Public health initiatives sometimes threaten justice by design or inadvertently if the regulation imposes undue burdens on a particular segment of society (Kass, 2001). Older adults in long-term care were at higher risk than the general population or community-dwelling older adults. The burdens on older adults living in long-term care settings were unequal, but they were at a greater risk secondary to age, comorbidities, and congregate living.

The goal was to flatten the curve to prevent overwhelming healthcare facilities and depleting scarce resources. Long-term care residents suffered the burden for the benefit of society. The restrictions contradicted the domains of healthy aging, the WHO priorities for health aging, and Lopez's aspects of good care, including, but not limited to, dehumanization and infantilization. The burdens of the restrictions were unavoidable because of the weak foundation of long-term care and the threat of the virus.

Step four considers how to minimize burdens and whether there are alternative approaches without reducing the efficacy (Kass, 2001). If more than one effective option exists, ethically, we must choose the approach that poses fewer risks (Gostin & Wetter, 2022). SARS-CoV-2 is a highly contagious pathogen, and the physical layout of long-term care settings makes viral spread more likely within a vulnerable population. Given the circumstances that existed, any alternative may have less efficacy. Thus the need for better planning.

Step five of the Kass framework corresponds with the ethical principle of distributive justice. Distributive justice requires a fair distribution of benefits and burdens (Kass, 2001). Ethically imposing the measures requires ameliorating the disproportionate burdens (Gostin & Wetter, 2022). Distributive justice does not require equal allocation. Instead, the allocation must be fair (Kass, 2001). A proportionately greater benefit may justify an unequal and discriminatory allocation to achieve the benefit (Savulescu & Cameron, 2020). When comparing the restrictions imposed on long-term care residents to other groups, it is debatable whether it is an issue of "like cases" since older adults in long-term care were at higher risk.

Public health officials cannot impose the differences arbitrarily or based on historical assumptions (Kass, 2001). The history of infectious disease in the long-term care sector provided data, and the interventions were not arbitrarily imposed or not based on historical assumptions.

Gostin suggests it is possible to ameliorate the inequities in benefits and burdens. The lockdowns on long-term care settings created harm to the least well-off. Older adults living in long-term care are 'least well-off' because of ageism. Thus, long-term care residents should receive other advantages to achieve equalization, even if this means receiving some unequal benefits.

Several theories of justice allow for and even require unequal allocation of benefits to correct burdens and inequities. John Rawls proffers that justice requires allocating resources unequally to help the least well off. Daniels (2014) advances the general principle of ensuring the protection of equality of opportunities. Society should compensate older adults who cannot pursue society's opportunities because of deep-rooted structural inequalities exacerbated by the pandemic. John Harris's (1987) double jeopardy argument supports giving long-term care residents an advantage. Older adults experienced harm because of structural inequities that disadvantaged them before and during the pandemic. As a result, they are worse off and without an advantage will suffer double jeopardy.

Some philosophers and ethicists distinguish between societal inequities resulting from the wrongful actions of an identifiable source and inequities resulting from an act of God or other circumstances (Kass, 2001). Only the former are entitled to corrective intervention. For example, under Parfit's view of deontic egalitarianism, justification for giving an advantage to the worse off depends on the reason for the inequity. If the unequal status results from circumstances such as a genetic condition or an accidental injury, deontic egalitarianism does not support giving an advantage to the worse-off. If the unequal position results from unjust actions, such as discriminatory treatment, deontic egalitarianism supports providing an advantage. The inequity based on comorbidities associated with aging does not support giving them an advantage. In contrast, inequity and marginalization are consequences of the unjust actions of others, and therefore older adults in long-term care should receive some advantages.

In the sixth step, the Kass analysis determines whether the expected benefits justify the identified burdens, which requires societal input and deliberation. Procedural justice requires a democratic process and deliberations that ensure consideration of minority views (Kass, 2001). For older adults living in long-term care, procedural justice fell flat. The restrictions excluded residents from civic participation. They did not have the same opportunity as the rest of society to address their leaders about the imposed mandates and restrictions. Older adults in long-term care may be less likely to advocate for themselves because of the lack of opportunity, physical limitations, being removed from their community, and internalized oppression.

Having considered the ethical justification of the restrictions from a public health perspective, I will now consider the bioethics principles.

## Bioethical Principles

In contrast to public health ethics, bioethics focuses on the individual. We immediately see the collision between the restrictions and autonomy. The protection from a deadly virus falls within the parameters of beneficence. Ethically justified medical interventions that are primarily beneficent can also inflict harm, for example, surgical amputation or chemotherapy. The restrictions were far more oppressive for long-term residents, but the risks were not the same.

## Justification

The ethical justification of the emergency response does not excuse the pervasive ageism or the lack of preparation. Given the totality of the circumstances that existed in long-term care and the threat of a deadly virus, the restrictions for long-term care were ethically justified as an emergency response in the early weeks of the pandemic. As the immediate risk of infection decreased and the risks of extended isolation increased, the harsh restrictions became less defensible and increasingly more ethically problematic.

Savulescu and Cameron (2020) are correct that there were no good options for mitigating the effect of COVID-19. We cannot rewind history or undo the mistakes made before and during the pandemic, but we can mitigate the harm from the restrictions and ageism and change public policies affecting older adults.

## Moving Forward to Long-Term Solutions

It is time to move long-term care from the shadows to the forefront. We need candid and open societal discourse to reframe long-term care. In the *Sum of Us,* Heather McGhee (2021) argues that when public policy creates an inequity, public policy should solve it. Public policy created and exacerbated ageism and the resulting inequities. As a result, public policy must take corrective action. We need significant investments in new long-term care models and policies focusing on person-centered care. Improving older adults' quality of life requires collaborative efforts and recognizing them as stakeholders. We must repair and rebuild the cracked foundation of long-term care and use the lessons learned from COVID-19 to better prepare for future public health emergencies.

## Conclusion

SARS-CoV-2, COVID-19, and the restrictions are not the primary source of the ethical challenges. The totality of the circumstances created harm for older adults living in long-term care. Policymakers, planners, and providers need to understand the social variations and the aging population's characteristics, behaviors, and needs (Darlington-Pollock et al., 2020).

Galea describes looking away from the foundations that caused the problems in healthcare, and Gawande contends that the treatment of older adults in long-term care is a "consequence of a society that faces the final phase of by human life cycle by trying not to think about it" (Galea, 2022; Gawande, 2014, p. 76-77). We can no longer avoid thinking about older adults living in long-term care facilities. We are ethically and morally obligated to ask how society can handle the next public health emergency and provide good care for long-term care residents. The ethical challenges in long-term care demand long-term solutions.

## References

AGS. (2018). *American Geriatrics Society White Paper on healthy aging.* GeriatricsCareOnline.org Complex Care. Access to Resources Simplified.

https://geriatricscareonline.org/ProductAbstract/american-geriatrics-society-white-paper-on-healthy-aging/CL025

Ayalon, L., Zisberg, A., Cohn-Schwartz, E., Cohen-Mansfield, J., Perel-Levin, S., & Bar-Asher Siegal, E. (2020). Long-Term Care settings in the times of COVID-19: Challenges and future directions. *International Psychogeriatrics, 32*(10), 1239–1243. https://doi.org/10.1017/s1041610220001416

Batsis, J. A., Daniel, K., Eckstrom, E., Goldlist, K., Kusz, H., Lane, D., Loewenthal, J., Coll, P. P., & Friedman, S. M. (2021). Promoting healthy aging during COVID-19. *Journal of the American Geriatrics Society, 69*(3), 572–580. https://doi.org/10.1111/jgs.17035

Berlinger, N., de Medeiros, K., & Girling, L. (2022). Bioethics and gerontology: The value of thinking together. *The Gerontologist*. https://doi.org/10.1093/geront/gnab186

Bethell, J., Aelick, K., Babineau, J., Bretzlaff, M., Edwards, C., Gibson, J.-L., Hewitt Colborne, D., Iaboni, A., Lender, D., Schon, D., & McGilton, K. S. (2020). Social connection in long-term care homes: A scoping review of published research on the mental health impacts and potential strategies during COVID-19. *Journal of the American Medical Directors Association, 22*(2). https://doi.org/10.1016/j.jamda.2020.11.025

Campbell, A. D. (2020). Practical implications of physical distancing, social isolation, and reduced physicality for older adults in response to COVID-19. *Journal of Gerontological Social Work, 63*(6-7), 181–183. https://doi.org/10.4324/9781003138280-40

CMS. (2020, March 13). *Guidance for infection control and prevention of coronavirus disease 2019 (COVID-19) in nursing homes (revised)*. CMS. Retrieved March 6, 2022, from https://www.cms.gov/medicareprovider-enrollment-and-certification surveycertificationgeninfopolicy-and/guidance-infection-control-and-prevention-coronavirus-disease-2019-covid-19-nursing-homes-revised

Corazzini, K. N., Anderson, R. A., Bowers, B. J., Chu, C. H., Edvardsson, D., Fagertun, A., Gordon, A. L., Leung, A. Y. M., McGilton, K. S., Meyer, J. E., Siegel, E. O., Thompson, R., Wang, J., Wei, S., Wu, B., & Lepore, M. J. (2019). Toward common data elements for international research in long-term care homes: Advancing person-centered care. *Journal of the American Medical Directors Association, 20*(5), 598–603. https://doi.org/10.1016/j.jamda.2019.01.123

Cowper, B., Jassat, W., Pretorius, P., Geffen, L., Legodu, C., Singh, S., & Blumberg, L. (2020). Covid-19 in long-term care facilities in South Africa: No time for complacency. *South African Medical Journal, 110*(10), 962. https://doi.org/10.7196/samj.2020.v110i10.15214

Daniels, N. (2014). Justice, health, and health care. In R. Rhodes, M. Battin, & A. Silvers (Eds.), *Medicine and social justice essays on the distribution of health care* (pp. 17–33), essay, Oxford University Press.

Danis, K., Fonteneau, L., Georges, S., Daniau, C., Bernard-Stoecklin, S., Domegan, L., O'Donnell, J., Hauge, S. H., Dequeker, S., Vandael, E., Van der Heyden, J., Renard, F., Sierra, N. B., Ricchizzi, E., Schweickert, B., Schmidt, N., Abu Sin, M., Eckmanns, T., Paiva, J.-A., & Schneider, E. (2020). High impact of COVID-19 in long-term care facilities, suggestion for monitoring in the EU/EEA, May 2020. *Eurosurveillance, 25*(22), 1–5. https://doi.org/10.2807/1560-7917.es.2020.25.22.2000956

Darlington-Pollock, F., Dolega, L., & Dunning, R. (2020). Ageism, overlapping vulnerabilities and equity in the COVID-19 pandemic. *Town Planning Review, 92*(2), 203–207. https://doi.org/10.3828/tpr.2020.40

D'cruz, M., & Banerjee, D. (2020). 'An invisible human rights crisis': The marginalization of older adults during the COVID-19 pandemic—an advocacy review. *Psychiatry Research, 292,* 113369. https://doi.org/10.1016/j.psychres.2020.113369

Escalante, E., Golden, R. L., & Mason, D. J. (2020). Social isolation and loneliness: Imperatives for health care in a Post-COVID World. *JAMA Health Forum, 1*(12), 520521–521. https://doi.org/10.1001/jamahealth forum.2020.1597

Faghanipour, S., Monteverde, S., & Peter, E. (2020). Covid-19-related deaths in long-term care: The moral failure to care and prepare. *Nursing Ethics, 27*(5), 1171–1173. https://doi.org/10.1177/0969733020939667

Forma, L., Aaltonen, M., & Pulkki, J. (2020, June 23). *Covid-19 and clients of long-term care in Finland: Impact and measures to control the virus*. University of Helsinki. https://researchportal.helsinki.fi/en/publications/covid-19-and-clients-of-long-term-care-in-finland-impact-and-meas

Friedman, S. M., Mulhausen, P., Cleveland, M. L., Coll, P. P., Daniel, K. M., Hayward, A. D., Shah, K., Skudlarska, B., & White, H. K. (2018). Healthy aging:

American Geriatrics Society white paper executive summary. *Journal of the American Geriatrics Society, 67*(1), 17–20. https://doi.org/10.1111/jgs.15644

Galea, S. (2022). *The contagion next time*. Oxford University Press.

Gardner, W., States, D., & Bagley, N. (2020). The coronavirus and the risks to the elderly in long-term care. *Journal of Aging & Social Policy, 32*(4-5), 310–315. https://doi.org/10.1080/08959420.2020.1750543

Gawande, A. (2014). *Being mortal: Medicine and what matters in the end*. Picador, Metropolitan Books, Henry Holt & Company.

Goffman, E. (1961). *Asylums*. Anchor.

Gostin, L. O., & Wetter, S. (2022). Risk trade-offs and Equitable decision-making in the Covid-19 pandemic. *Hastings Center Report, 52*(1), 15–20. https://doi.org/10.1002/hast.1328

Harris, J. (1987). QALYfying the value of life. *Journal of Medical Ethics, 13*(3), 117–123. https://doi.org/10.1136/jme.13.3.117

Houtven, C. H. V., Boucher, N. A., & Dawson, W. D. (2020, April 24). *Impact of the COVID-19 outbreak on long-term care in the United States*. PDXScholar. Retrieved January 7, 2022, from https://pdxscholar.library. pdx.edu/aging_pub/54/

Inzitari, M., Risco, E., Cesari, M., Buurman, B. M., Kuluski, K., Davey, V., Bennett, L., Varela, J., & Prvu Bettger, J. (2020). Nursing homes and long-term care after COVID-19: A new era? *The Journal of Nutrition, Health & Aging, 24*(10), 1042–1046. https://doi.org/10.1007/s12603-020-1447-8

Iwasaki, T. M., Kimmel, Y. N., Baker, D., & McCallum, T. J. (2009). *Gerodiversity and social justice: Voices of minority elders*. American Psychological Association. https://psycnet.apa.org/record/2009-11474-005

Kass, N. E. (2001). An ethics framework for public health. *American Journal of Public Health, 91*(11), 1776–1782. https://doi.org/10.2105/ajph.91.11. 1776

Lai, C.-C., Wang, J.-H., Ko, W.-C., Yen, M.-Y., Lu, M.-C., Lee, C.-M., & Hsueh, P.-R. (2020). Covid-19 in long-term care facilities: An upcoming threat that cannot be ignored. *Journal of Microbiology, Immunology and Infection, 53*(3), 444–446. https://doi.org/10.1016/j.jmii.2020.04.008

Lloyd-Sherlock, P., Kalache, A., Kirkwood, T., McKee, M., & Prince, M. (2019). Who's proposal for a decade of healthy ageing. *The Lancet, 394*(10215), 2152–2153. https://doi.org/10.1016/s0140-6736(19)32522-x

Louie, J. K., Schnurr, D. P., Pan, C. Y., Kiang, D., Carter, C., Tougaw, S., Ventura, J., Norman, A., Belmusto, V., Rosenberg, J., & Trochet, G. (2007). A summer outbreak of human metapneumovirus infection in a long-term-care facility. *The Journal of Infectious Diseases, 196*(5), 705–708. https://doi.org/10.1086/519846

Lum, H. D., Mody, L., Levy, C. R., & Ginde, A. A. (2014). Pandemic influenza plans in Residential Care Facilities. *Journal of the American Geriatrics Society, 62*(7), 1310–1316. https://doi.org/10.1111/jgs.12879

López, J., Pérez-Rojo, G., Noriega, C., & Velasco, C. (2021). Personal and work-related factors associated with good care for institutionalized older adults. *International Journal of Environmental Research and Public Health, 18*(2), 1–12. https://doi.org/10.3390/ijerph18020820

McArthur, C., Saari, M., Heckman, G. A., Wellens, N., Weir, J., Hebert, P., Turcotte, L., Jbilou, J., & Hirdes, J. P. (2020). Evaluating the effect of COVID-19 pandemic lockdown on long-term care residents' mental health: A data-driven approach in New Brunswick. *Journal of the American Medical Directors Association, 22*(1), 187–192. https://doi.org/10.1016/j.jamda.2020.10.028

McGhee, H. (2021). *Sum of us: What racism costs everyone and how we can prosper together*. Profile Books Ltd.

O'Neill, D. (2018). Reflecting on our perceptions of the worth, status and rewards of working in nursing homes. *Age and Ageing, 47*(4), 502–504. https://doi.org/10.1093/ageing/afy065

Parfit, D. (1997). Equality and priority. *Ratio, 10*(3), 202–221. https://doi.org/10.1111/1467-9329.00041

Purvis Lively, C. (2021). Social isolation of older adults in long term care as a result of covid-19 mitigation measures during the covid-19 pandemic. *Voices in Bioethics, 7*. https://doi.org/10.52214/vib.v7i.8526

Reynolds, E. (2020, September 4). *It's the worst disaster of the pandemic, but WHO chief says our lack of concern shows' moral bankruptcy'*. CNN. https://edition.cnn.com/2020/09/04/health/elderly-care-coronavirus-who-tedros-intl/index.html

Salcher-Konrad, M., Jhass, A., Naci, H., Tan, M., El-Tawil, Y., & Comas-Herrera, A. (2020). COVID-19 related mortality and spread of disease in long-term care: A living systematic review of emerging evidence. *London School of Economics*. https://doi.org/10.1101/2020.06.09.20125237

Savulescu, J., & Cameron, J. (2020). Why lockdown of the elderly is not ageist and why levelling down equality is wrong. *Journal of Medical Ethics, 46*(11), 717–721. https://doi.org/10.1136/medethics-2020-106336

Sepulveda, E. R., Stall, N. M., & Sinha, S. K. (2020). A comparison of COVID-19 mortality rates among long-term care residents in 12 OECD countries. *Journal of the American Medical Directors Association, 21*(11). https://doi.org/10.1016/j.jamda.2020.08.039

Szebehely, M. (2020, July 22). *The impact of COVID-19 on long-term care in Sweden*. ltccovid,org.

Thompson, D.-C., Barbu, M.-G., Beiu, C., Popa, L. G., Mihai, M. M., Berteanu, M., & Popescu, M. N. (2020). The impact of COVID-19 pandemic on long-term care facilities worldwide: An overview on international issues. *BioMed Research International, 2020*, 1–7. https://doi.org/10.1155/2020/8870249

van der Horst, M., & Vickerstaff, S. (2021). Is part of ageism actually ableism? *Ageing and Society*, 1–12. https://doi.org/10.1017/s0144686x 20001890

Van der Roest, H. G., Prins, M., van der Velden, C., Steinmetz, S., Stolte, E., van Tilburg, T. G., & de Vries, D. H. (2020). The impact of covid-19 measures on well-being of older long-term care facility residents in the Netherlands. *Journal of the American Medical Directors Association, 21*(11), 1569–1570. https://doi.org/10.1016/j.jamda.2020.09.007

Viens, A. M. (2008). Public health, ethical behavior and reciprocity. *The American Journal of Bioethics, 8*(5), 1–3. https://doi.org/10.1080/152651608 02180059

Villanueva, E., & Barber, W. J. (2021). *Decolonizing wealth: Indigenous wisdom to heal divides and restore balance*. Berrett-Koehler Publishers.

WHO. (2020a). *Decade of healthy ageing (2021-2030)*. World Health Organization. https://www.who.int/initiatives/decade-of-healthy-ageing

WHO. (2020b, October 26). *Healthy ageing and functional ability*. World Health Organization.

https://www.who.int/news-room/questions-and-answers/item/healthy-ageing-and-functional-ability

WHO. (n.d.). *Ageing: Ageism.* World Health Organization. Retrieved February 21, 2022, from https://www.who.int/news-room/questions-and-answers/item/ageing-ageism

Wu, B. (2020). Social isolation and loneliness among older adults in the context of COVID-19: A global challenge. *Global Health Research and Policy, 5*(1). https://doi.org/10.1186/s41256-020-00154-3

Yeh, T. C., Huang, H. C., Yeh, T. Y., Huang, W. T., Huang, H. C., Chang, Y. M., & Chen, W. (2020). Family members' concerns about relatives in long-term care facilities: Acceptance of visiting restriction policy amid the COVID-19 pandemic. *Geriatrics & Gerontology International, 20*(10), 938–942. https://doi.org/10.1111/ggi.14022

Yen, M.-Y., Schwartz, J., King, C.-C., Lee, C.-M., & Hsueh, P.-R. (2020). Recommendations for protecting against and mitigating the COVID-19 pandemic in long-term care facilities. *Journal of Microbiology, Immunology and Infection, 53*(3), 447–453. https://doi.org/10.1016/j.jmii.2020.04.003

# CONTRIBUTOR BIOGRAPHIES

**Christiaan Alting von Geusau** holds law degrees from the University of Leiden (Netherlands) and the University of Heidelberg (Germany) with part of his studies conducted at the University of Steubenville, Ohio and the University of Notre Dame, Indiana (United States). He obtained with distinction his doctorate in philosophy of law from the University of Vienna (Austria), writing his dissertation on "Human Dignity and the Law in post-War Europe", which was published internationally in 2013. After first practicing civil and European law in Amsterdam and Brussels until 2004, he is now President and Rector of ITI Catholic University in Austria where he also serves as Professor of Philosophy of Law and Education. He holds a honorary professorship at the Universidad San Ignacio de Loyola in Lima, Peru and is founding President of the International Catholic Legislators Network (ICLN). In this latter function he mentors political leaders from around the world and leads international educational programs for legislators. Christian publishes and lectures extensively on matters of law, education, public policy and freedom of conscience and religion.

**Barry Cartwright** holds a BA and MA in Sociology and a PhD in Criminology. He was a Senior Lecturer in the School of Criminology at Simon Fraser University for many years, and continues to serve as the Associate Director of the International CyberCrime Research Centre at SFU. He worked for a number of years for the Solicitor General of Canada, and although not a lawyer, was a managing partner of an immigration law firm for much of his career. He has taught numerous university courses on cybercrime, cyberlaw, and the sociology of law, and has published extensively in the areas of cybercrime, cyberlaw, cyberbullying and online disinformation.

**Michelle Fiscus**, M.D., F.A.A.P., is a board-certified pediatrician and public health advocate who practiced general pediatrics in Franklin, TN for 17 years before transitioning to a career in public health. She joined the Tennessee Department of Health in 2016 and served as Deputy Medical Director for chronic disease prevention, health promotion, injury prevention, and comprehensive cancer prevention programs until 2018.

She then served as Medical Director of the Tennessee Department of Health's Vaccine-Preventable Diseases and Immunization Program from 2019-2021, where she was a leader of the state's COVID-19 pandemic response and responsible for the roll-out of COVID-19 vaccines across Tennessee. Dr. Fiscus is a graduate of Indiana University and Indiana University School of Medicine and completed her residency in pediatrics at the James Whitcomb Riley Hospital for Children in Indianapolis. She is an associate clinical professor in the Department of Pediatrics at Monroe Carell Jr. Children's Hospital at Vanderbilt University Medical Center. She is a past-president of the Tennessee Chapter of the American Academy of Pediatrics and serves on the board of directors of the American Academy of Pediatrics as District IV Chair, representing Tennessee, Kentucky, Virginia, and the Carolinas. Dr. Fiscus and her family moved from Tennessee to northern Virginia in 2021, where she provides consultation to national non-governmental organizations on matters of immunizations and public health.

**Richard Frank** is an Associate Professor in the School of Criminology at Simon Fraser University (SFU), Canada, and the Director of the International CyberCrime Research Centre (ICCRC). Richard completed a Ph.D. in Computing Science (2010) and another PhD in Criminology (2013) at SFU. His main research interest is cybercrime. Specifically, he is interested in researching hackers and security issues, the dark web, online terrorism and warfare, e-laundering and cryptocurrencies, and online child exploitation. He is the creator of The Dark Crawler, a tool for collecting and analyzing data from the open Internet, dark web, and online discussion forums. Through this tool the ICCRC has collected ~150 million posts from various right-wing, left-wing, gender-based and religiously-motivated extremist communities, leading to a number of projects and publications. Dr. Frank has publications in top-level data mining outlets, such as in Knowledge Discovery in Databases, and in security conferences such as Intelligence and Security Informatics (ISI). His research can also be found in Criminology and Criminal Justice, the Journal of Research in Crime and Delinquency and the Canadian Journal of Criminology and Criminal Justice, to name a few.

**Edward Hadas** is a Research Fellow at Blackfriars Hall, Oxford University. He was born in New York and raised in St Louis in the United States. He was educated at Columbia University (BA), Oxford University (MA) and the State University of New York at Binghamton (MBA). He worked for two decades in finance, first in Buffalo and Boston in the U.S., and then in Paris and London, where he has lived since 1993. He became a financial journalist in 2004, working as a commentator and editor at Breakingviews.com, the Financial Times, and Reuters Breakingviews. His first book. Human goods, economic evils: A moral look at the dismal science, was published by ISI Books in 2007. Retiring from full-time journalism in 2017, he settled in Oxford, where he is a Research Fellow at Blackfriars Hall, part of the University of Oxford. His second book, Counsels of Imperfection: Thinking through Catholic Social Teaching was published by Catholic University of America Press in 2020. A third book, His Money, Finance, Reality, Morality will be published by Ethics International Press in 2022. Edward's next book is tentatively titled Prometheus, Pandora, Philoctetes (and the Cross): Narratives of modernity. He taught the course "The political economy of COVID-19" for the Oxford University Department for Continuing Education in 2021.

**Oliver Hirsch**, Ph.D., graduated from the Institute of Psychology at Philipps University of Marburg, Germany. He was a Research Fellow at the Clinic for Childhood and Adolescent Psychiatry and Psychotherapy at Philipps University Hospital Marburg and a Senior Research Fellow at the Institute of General Practice/Family Medicine at Philipps University of Marburg. He wrote his Doctoral thesis in the field of Clinical Neuropsychology on Visual Cognition in Parkinson´s disease. His habilitation in the field of Medical Psychology addressed decision making in General Practice/Family Medicine. He is also a certified Behavior Therapist and a certified Clinical Neuropsychologist with 15 years of clinical practice. Currently he is a Professor of Business Psychology with a focus on fundamentals and methods at FOM University of Applied Sciences, Siegen, Germany. Dr. Hirsch has published 67 peer reviewed publications mainly in Health Services Research and Public Health (e.g. PLoS ONE, Scientific Reports, Journal of Attention Disorders, Assessment, Journal of Affective Disorders, Frontiers in Psychiatry). In memoriam Walter Hirsch (1936-2022). The current situation reminded him of his childhood experiences under a totalitarian regime.

**Preeti John** M.D. is a surgeon who practices at the VA Maryland Healthcare System in Baltimore. Dr. John is an intensivist with the VHA's Tele-Critical Care program and is clinical associate professor at the University of Maryland Medical center. She is fellowship trained in Trauma and Critical Care and is triple board certified in General Surgery, Surgical Critical Care and Hospice and Palliative Medicine. She is a health care ethics consultant, certified by the American Society of Bioethics and Humanities. Dr. John serves as vice-chair of the Society of Critical Care Medicine's Ethics Committee and is chair of the ethics consultation service at the VA Maryland Healthcare system. She is the editor of a book titled 'Being a Woman Surgeon – 60 Women Share Their Stories' and is on the editorial board of the American Medical Women's Association's 'Literary AMWA' publication.

**Ashley Metz** is an Assistant Professor of Organization Studies at Tilburg University (The Netherlands) and a Research Fellow at Human Futures Institute (International). She studies change on the field or industry level, often related to macro shifts and jolts (primarily ecological and technological), and organizations within fields. She also studies how foresight and futures methods can help organizations navigate these evolving spaces. Her work has appeared in the Academy of Management Journal and Technological Forecasting and Social Change, and recently published the book, Organizing for Sustainable Development, with colleagues.

**Alim U. Monir**, Ph.D., is an Administrator of Clinical Pathology & Laboratory Services at the Bellevue Hospital with New York City Health & Hospitals. Prior to joining Bellevue, he served as Associate Technical Director of Clinical Laboratories at the SUNY Downstate Health Sciences University. Over fifteen years of clinical services, he was engaged in managing day-to-day laboratory operations and directing the policy and procedures of laboratory services. He is a certified Clinical Laboratory Technologist by the American Society of Clinical Pathology (ASCP) and New York State Department of Education (NYSDOE). He is an active member for the American College of Healthcare Executive (ACHE). He earned his Doctor of Philosophy in Business Administration with a specialization in healthcare administration at Northcentral University and

Master of Arts in Chemistry from the City University of New York at Brooklyn College. He also received a Master of Science and Bachelor of Science in Chemistry from the University of Dhaka, Bangladesh. In August 2021, Dr. Monir was awarded the Delta Mu Delta regional scholarship for outstanding leadership skills in business studies. He published several research articles on the topics of lead poisoning on children bone femur, quantitative analysis of neurotoxic cytoskeletal components, and x-ray powder diffraction patterns on hexagonal tungsten bronzes. Dr. Monir was born and raised in Bangladesh and currently resides in the City of New York. In his spare time, he enjoys fishing, traveling, and socializing.

**Emily J. Nelson**, J.D. is a labor and employment attorney at GoodRx. She received her undergraduate degree in Psychology from Harvard University and her law degree from Boston College Law School.

**Sarah E. Nelson**, M.D., M.P.H. is an Assistant Professor in Neurosurgery and Neurology at the Icahn School of Medicine at Mount Sinai and Adjunct Assistant Professor in Neurology and Anesthesiology/Critical Care Medicine at Johns Hopkins University. She received her undergraduate degree from the Massachusetts Institute of Technology and medical degree at Stanford University School of Medicine. She then completed her neurology residency at Tufts Medical Center followed by fellowship training in neurocritical care at Massachusetts General Hospital and Brigham and Women's Hospital. She also holds a Master of Public Health from the Johns Hopkins Bloomberg School of Public Health. She has diverse clinical research interests in neurocritical care, ethics, and telehealth.

**Sherina Okoye** is a lawyer, a writer, and an activist with a passion for writing, courtroom advocacy and human rights activism especially as it relates to women and children. She founded an NGO, African Kids and Women Rights Empowerment Initiative (AKAWI) with focus on protection of women and children from abuse, reduction and/or prevention of maternal mortality, empowerment, anti-trafficking, free healthcare services, free legal services for indigent widows, access to education, promotion of religious tolerance and gender parity awareness. Sherina has over the years, sponsored several groundbreaking and impactful socio-economic projects through her NGO with funds gotten largely from her writing.

**Karmvir Padda** is currently a Ph.D. student in the Sociology and Legal Studies department at the University of Waterloo. She is also a researcher at the International Cybercrime Research Centre (ICCRC) and completed her MA in Criminology at Simon Fraser University. Her research mainly focuses on combating online foreign interference (disinformation/ misinformation), extremists' use of the internet, right-wing extremism, hate crime, research methods and methodology, and computational social science. She has published several peer-reviewed papers in the areas of social media and disinformation warfare. Her research is generously supported by the Social Sciences and Humanities Research Council (SSHRC CGS-D).

**Cheryl M. Patton** earned her Ph.D. in Organizational Leadership, with a business concentration, from Eastern University, St. Davids, Pennsylvania, where she currently teaches qualitative methods and advises several doctoral candidates in the dissertation process. Dr. Patton also works as a senior core, part-time professor at Northcentral University, San Diego, California, where she teaches Ethics, Qualitative Research, and serves on dissertation committees. Her background is in healthcare; she obtained her Bachelor's in Health Arts and Master of Science in Health Services Administration from University of St. Francis, Joliet, Illinois after working in the medical imaging field at a tertiary care center for two decades. Her academic pursuits led to a second career in higher education instruction in 2007. From 2007 to the present, Dr. Patton has taught students at the associate, bachelor, master, and doctoral levels. Her research interests include healthcare leadership, workplace conflict, and workplace ethics. Dr. Patton's interest in studying the experiences of healthcare workers during the COVID-19 pandemic stemmed from her employment in the medical imaging field during the onset of the AIDS epidemic in 1981, where unprecedented challenges in hospitals and the lack of knowledge of the disease led to healthcare workers experiencing fear, confusion, and multiple changes in the healthcare workplace.

**Cathy L. Purvis Lively**, Esq. is an attorney and mediator in Palm Beach County, Florida. Before attending law school, Ms. Lively was a nurse in critical care, case management, and a program director. She is on faculty at the Alternative Dispute Resolution Academy in Orlando, Florida, and an

Associate in Professional Studies in the Bioethics Program at Columbia University. She graduated from Columbia University with a Masters in Bioethics and is currently a doctoral student in Bioethics at Loyola University with a focus on clinical ethics.

**Devin J. Rapp** is a Ph.D. candidate in Organizational Behavior (Management) at the University of Utah in the David Eccles School of Business. Devin conducts qualitative field research primarily through semi-structured interviews and observation and loves to study entrepreneurs and workers who find their work meaningful like farmers during harvest season or healthcare workers during the COVID-19 pandemic. Devin researches topics like burnout, mental health, boundaries, identity, entrepreneurship, job-related stigma, and more, emphasizing how and why work and personal life impact one another. In all of Devin's research and teaching, he seeks to integrate academic theory and practical application to empower workers and students through evidence-based knowledge and motivation for lifelong learning and self-improvement. Before pursuing a Ph.D. in Organizational Behavior, Devin graduated magna cum laude in health sciences from Brigham Young University in Provo, Utah, and worked for six years in healthcare as a licensed nursing home executive director and entrepreneur in Utah and California. Devin is originally from San Diego, California and now lives near Salt Lake City, Utah with his wife and two young boys.

**Jayme L. Renfro** is an Associate Professor of Political Science at the University of Northern Iowa. Dr. Renfro enjoys teaching public policy and administration to both undergraduate and graduate students and has earned university- and college wide teaching awards. She published State and Local Politics: Cases and Topics in 2021 and co-authored State and Local Government 2013–2014 with Kevin B. Smith. Dr. Renfro has also written, published, and publicly presented numerous academic works in the areas of policy, political behavior, and political participation.

**Claus Rinner,** Ph.D., is a Professor at Toronto Metropolitan (formerly Ryerson) University in Toronto, Ontario, Canada, where he teaches geospatial data analytics, cartographic visualization, and decision support systems. He holds degrees in applied mathematics, systems sciences, and geography from German and French universities. His externally funded, peer-reviewed, and widely cited research develops methods and techniques to improve effective collaboration and decision-making in fields such as public health, urban planning, and environmental management. During the Corona crisis, Dr. Rinner has substantially engaged in critical public scholarship.

**Agnese Roda** is a South Africa-based Italian anthropologist and translator. She is the co-founder of the project Boo_decolonize gender to fight the gender binary from an African perspective. Immigration practitioner, and mother of a little girl, she is interested in identity, gender, leadership, ethics, community work and corporate social responsibility. Agnese is active in her community and engages at different levels as a communication and relationship project manager for more inclusive and efficient leadership.

**Sarah-May Strange** holds a BA and MA in criminology from Simon Fraser University. She has conducted research, including with the International CyberCrime Research Centre at SFU, into topics of online disinformation, conspiracy theories and cybercrime, as well as marginalized identities, Islamophobia, homophobia, transphobia, the global far-right and foreign interference campaigns. Her work explores areas such as the socio-historical context of modern events, the radicalization and de-radicalization of right-wing extremists, prejudice, disability and accessibility, conservative Christianity as a political force, and the Canadian far-right. She applies a "critical" lens, making use of queer theory, feminist theory and post-colonialism, as well as methods such as content analysis, network analysis and Open Source Intelligence (OSINT).

**Vurain Tabvuma** Ph.D., is the Sobey Professor in Management and an Associate Professor in the Sobey School of Business at Saint Mary's University. He is also a Research Fellow at the Human Futures Institute (HFI).Vurain's research focuses on intrinsic motivation, onboarding, job satisfaction, organizational change, adaptation, student success, public service and pro-social motivation. His research has been published in refereed international journals such as Human Resource Management, Journal of Vocational Behavior, Economics Letters, Gender in Management: An International Journal, Evidenced-based HRM: a Global

Forum for Empirical Scholarship, Population Research and Policy Review, Public Administration Review, Journal of Public Administration: Research and Theory, and Kyklos. His recent research has investigated whether the patterns of reporting private information vary, depending on the victim of the dishonest reports. The results indicate greater dishonesty when the over-reporting harms fellow subjects. The data also suggest that the subjects attempt to hide their over-reporting. Another paper investigates how social policies and cultural context impact the association of marital status with parental work-life balance satisfaction. The paper finds significant work-life balance satisfaction advantages for married mothers across Canada, except in the province of Quebec. For fathers, no consistent marital status-related gap is found, regardless of the province. His research has been funded by the Social Sciences and Humanities Research Council (SSHRC), the British Academy, The Research Fund for International Young Scientists under the National Natural Science Foundation of China, the David Sobey Centre for Innovation in Retailing and Services and institutional funding from Saint Mary's University.

**Michael Tomlinson,** FGIA, FCG, Ph.D., is an independent Higher Education Governance and Quality Consultant. He was formerly a Director at Australia's Tertiary Education Quality and Standards Agency (TEQSA), where he led case teams to conduct assessments of all registered providers and was decision maker for all their course applications. Before TEQSA, he worked for twenty years in Australian universities, for the last fifteen of these in senior positions at Swinburne University of Technology. Dr. Tomlinson is a Fellow of the Governance Institute of Australia and of the (international) Chartered Governance Institute. He has been an expert panel member or chair for a number of offshore reviews for the national accreditation agency in Timor Leste; the Fiji Higher Education Commission (re the University of the South Pacific); and the Department of Higher Education, Research, Science and Technology of Papua New Guinea. Dr. Tomlinson is Chair of the Human Research Ethics Committee at Australia's National Institute of Integrative Medicine. He also holds a number of other positions at Australian institutes and universities: Chair of the Academic Board, Nan Tien Institute of Higher Education; Member of the Board at Australian College of the Arts Pty Ltd ('Collarts'); Member of the Academic Board at

Victorian Institute of Technology; and Honorary (Principal) Fellow, LH Martin Institute at The University of Melbourne.

**Ameline Vandenberghe** is a master's student at the University of Tübingen, Germany. After completing her bachelor's degree in Applied Communication at the Institute for Higher Social Communication Studies of Brussels (IHECS), she moved to Germany and enrolled in the Master's program "Literatur- und Kulturtheorie". In parallel with her studies, she worked as a PR assistant for the Franco-German Cultural Institute in Tübingen (ICFA) and the International Center for Ethics in Science and Humanities (IZEW). Her research interests are broad and include narratology, oral literature, dialogism, cultures of the Global South, climate justice, and gender studies.

**Molly Walker** worked as deputy managing editor at MedPage Today from 2014 to 2022, where she covered infectious diseases, pediatrics, and ob/gyn. She began covering infectious diseases in 2017, reporting on such public health stories as the U.S. Zika outbreak, the nationwide E. coli outbreak linked to lettuce, the 2018-2019 severe flu season, and the "London Patient," the second person to be cured of HIV. In 2019, she wrote an exclusive article about the 10-year anniversary of the first HIV vaccine trial, RV144, after being approached by the U.S. National Institutes of Health (NIH). She interviewed U.S. National Institute of Allergy and Infectious Diseases (NIAID) Director, Dr. Anthony Fauci seven times during her career, including an exclusive interview during the COVID pandemic. Molly was the lead reporter covering COVID for MedPage Today and wrote over three-hundred articles on COVID during the pandemic from January 2020 to June 2022. She received the 2020 J2 Leadership award from her company for her coverage. Molly left in 2022 to work as an editor at a healthcare advertising agency, as she holds a B.S. in Advertising from the University of Illinois at Urbana-Champaign. She lives with her English teacher husband, Erik, and two sons, Charlie and Louis, in Massachusetts, and writes YA novels in her spare time. Her additional publishing credits include letters to the editor at the Boston Globe and Fortune magazine.